Erxin Scales: Child Developmental Scale of China

"*Erxin Scales: Child Developmental Scale of China*, a developmental assessment tool with national norm, is grounded in Chinese child development data and deeply embedded within the socio-cultural fabric of China. Its publication will enhance international scholarly exchange and promote the advancement of child developmental assessment tools across a spectrum of culturally diverse settings."

—Mark Simms, *Former Chief Professor of Child Development Department at the Medical College of Wisconsin. Former Director of the Child Development Center at Children's Wisconsin*

"The release of the English version *Erxin Scales: Child Developmental Scale of China* exemplifies the collaborative ethos and unwavering dedication exhibited by Chinese experts in developmental and behavioral pediatrics and child psychology research. The scale is the only child developmental measure within mainland China that possesses national norm. Notably, its revision witnessed a pioneering integration of developmental evaluation with screening for autism spectrum disorder risk, thereby elevating the clinical utility of the scale and expanding the research scope of child developmental assessment."

— Xingming Jin, *Founder of the Developmental-Behavioral Pediatrics of Chinese Pediatric Society, Chief Physician, Professor of Department of Developmental-Behavioral Pediatrics at Shanghai Children's Medical Center, Shanghai Jiao Tong University School of Medicine*

"'*Erxin Scales*' is an important and valuable achievement of the two-decade collaborative research between the Capital Institute of Pediatrics and Institute of Psychology, and Chinese Academy of Sciences. This book will not only provide a good assessment tool for pediatricians, but also enlighten educators, caregivers and parents to understand children's physical and mental development."

—Su Li, Professor, *Institute of Psychology, Chinese Academy of Sciences*

Chunhua Jin · Zhenmin Gao · Wenwen Liu

Erxin Scales: Child Developmental Scale of China

palgrave
macmillan

Chunhua Jin
Capital Institute of Pediatrics
Beijing, China

Zhenmin Gao
Capital Institute of Pediatrics
Beijing, China

Wenwen Liu
Peking University School
and Hospital of Stomatology
Beijing, China

Translated by
Chen Zhao
China Center for the Economics
of Human Development
China Development Research
Foundation
Beijing, China

ISBN 978-981-99-9996-5   ISBN 978-981-99-9997-2 (eBook)
https://doi.org/10.1007/978-981-99-9997-2

© The Editor(s) (if applicable) and The Author(s), under exclusive license to Springer Nature Singapore Pte Ltd. 2024, corrected publication 2025

This work is subject to copyright. All rights are solely and exclusively licensed by the Publisher, whether the whole or part of the material is concerned, specifically the rights of translation, reprinting, reuse of illustrations, recitation, broadcasting, reproduction on microfilms or in any other physical way, and transmission or information storage and retrieval, electronic adaptation, computer software, or by similar or dissimilar methodology now known or hereafter developed.
The use of general descriptive names, registered names, trademarks, service marks, etc. in this publication does not imply, even in the absence of a specific statement, that such names are exempt from the relevant protective laws and regulations and therefore free for general use.
The publisher, the authors and the editors are safe to assume that the advice and information in this book are believed to be true and accurate at the date of publication. Neither the publisher nor the authors or the editors give a warranty, expressed or implied, with respect to the material contained herein or for any errors or omissions that may have been made. The publisher remains neutral with regard to jurisdictional claims in published maps and institutional affiliations.

This Palgrave Macmillan imprint is published by the registered company Springer Nature Singapore Pte Ltd.
The registered company address is: 152 Beach Road, #21-01/04 Gateway East, Singapore 189721, Singapore

If disposing of this product, please recycle the paper.

Foreword 1: Developing Amid Inheritance

It has been over a century since psychological testing and assessment emerged internationally. An array of professional scales, with the target population varying from infants to adults according to different purposes and functions, have played an irreplaceable role in psychological assessment and even in special talent selection. In the 1980s, Chinese scholars engaged in child psychology and pediatrics started to introduce authoritative scales from abroad, such as the Denver Developmental Screening Test, Gesell Development Schedules, Bayley Scales of Infant Development, and Wechsler Intelligence Scale for Children, to evaluate the development behavior, psychological development, and intelligence level of Children in China. However, most of the introduced scales were outdated, and for the Gesell, it has only a standardized Chinese version for children under 3 years old, and Bayley scales only regional Chinese versions were developed, lacking standardized psychometric national norms study across all age group. Moreover, multiple studies have shown that the developmental process and rate of Chinese children are significantly different from those of children in other countries. China is a developing country with the world's largest population, the largest number of children, and a significant imbalance in regional development. Small-scale, regionalized revised scales thus are incapable of reflecting the full picture of child development in China.

Due to such factors as culture, knowledge system, family beliefs, and children's development environment, the use of foreign scales in

China suffers from a striking cultural mismatch. Assessing children from different countries with non-standardized international scales reduces the comparability of the results. Apart from cultural differences, regular updates and elimination of the adopted foreign scales are also worthy of particular attention. Owing to limited human and financial resources as well as copyright restrictions, it is often difficult for the introduced and revised scales to be up-to-date. Furthermore, the rights to data storage, explanation, analysis, and final interpretation of scales all belong to their developers, indicating that the utilization of foreign scales might compromise the security of population information. Therefore, it is of vital necessity to develop a diagnostic assessment tool that is aligned with the characteristics of Chinese children's development, objectively reflects Chinese children's developmental level, and is compatible with China's cultural traditions. The Erxin Scales is hence born on demand. It is the only diagnostic assessment scale for child development in China that has indigenous intellectual property rights and is supported by two sets of national normative data. The development and revision of the scale took two decades (1980-1990 and 2005-2016), and its assessment covers multiple aspects of child's growth, meeting the integrated needs for evaluating children's neuropsychological development in China. It has provided substantial assistance to clinical practitioners of pediatric health and developmental behavior in understanding the milestones of child development, serving as an important guidance on clinical practice. In addition to its auxiliary role in assessing the developmental level of children and diagnosing their neurodevelopmental disorders, the scale's clinical application is further expanded to predicting the risk of autism spectrum disorder (ASD) through the addition of the Communication Warning Behavior Subscale. This subscale, developed as a response to the increasing prevalence of ASD, can contribute to the early diagnosis of and early intervention for improving the developmental outcome of ASD, which has more clinical application values.

Research on childhood neuropsychological development involves frequently assessing children's developmental level. In this regard, Chinese scholars often adopt, though resignedly, foreign assessment scales to facilitate their communication with international peers. This is because employing indigenous diagnostic tools not adequately understood by the international academia would affect their publication of high-quality SCI journal articles. Translating the Erxin Scales into English will provide foreign peers with the opportunity to understand child developmental scales of China. The introduction of this highly reliable and valid professional instrument with indigenous intellectual property rights also reflects our cultural confidence, the significance of which is enormous. I believe its publication will promote communication with foreign colleagues in the application and evaluation of child developmental scales, thereby benefiting global child health.

Tingyu Li
The Head of the Developmental
and Behavioral Pediatrics group
of the Chinese Medical
Association
Beijing, China

Foreword 2: The Emergence and Development of China's Children Neuropsychological and Behavior Scales

Childhood witnesses the fastest growth of human brain, and is a particularly sensitive and critical period for the development of intelligence, personality, and social behavior. Regular assessment of children's psychological and behavioral development with age and timely detection of developmental disorders and related diseases are of great value for children's health maintenance. In this process, assessment scales play an important role. A scale is a ruler, and its precision varies with its purpose. Trained professionals in developmental-behavioral pediatrics, child psychology, child psychiatry, and child healthcare can provide objective and reliable assessment of a child's psychological and behavioral development levels using validated, multidimensional child developmental scales or instruments.

In the last century, the commonly used scales for children's neuropsychological and behavioral development in China mostly originated from the West, as China lacked indigenous comprehensive measures to be used to exchange with international scholars. Its introduction of relevant scales from abroad could be dated back to as early as the 1940s. Due to differences in cultural backgrounds as well as children's growth environments between the East and the West, the scales introduced were not entirely suitable for assessing the psychological and behavioral development levels of children in China. However, China's indigenous development of children psychological and behavioral assessment scales with national norms had lagged behind because of the long research cycles, high professional requirements, and great interdisciplinary difficulties. It was not until the 1980s that a team of child health experts at the Capital Institute of Pediatrics (CIP) made a breakthrough in this endeavor. They set up a national collaborative multicenter research team based on longitudinal observation of the developmental patterns and behavioral characteristics of infants and young children in China, and established a nationally representative database of the pass rates for child neuropsychological evaluation items, with reliability and validity tests conducted. On this basis, China's first scale for assessing its children's psychological and behavioral development, known as the "Erxin Scales," was devised with standardized norms. This scale, as the first indigenous psychological and behavioral assessment tool suitable for Chinese children, fills the gap in the development of such instruments in China. With a clear instruction manual and readily comprehended evaluation standards, the scale has been widely applied to relevant clinical disciplines in China.

Over the more than thirty years of widespread use of the Erxin Scales, China's economy has developed rapidly, and the living environment for its children has undergone dramatic changes. This highlights the necessity of revising the scale in accordance with international conventions to add measurement indicators closely associated with the growth environment and social development. In 2009, CIP formed another national collaborative multicenter research team to revise the Erxin Scales. Referring to the data from the 6th national census, stratified cluster random sampling was adopted for standardization and norm construction on a nationally representative sample from seven provinces and cities. After ten years, a revised edition of the Erxin Scales capable of assessing the psychological development of 1-month-olds to 6-year-olds was finally formed. Specifically, 38 of the original 177 items were revised and 8 were deleted to remedy the deficiencies in the original version resulted from the passage of time. Furthermore, 125 items were added to extend the target population to 6-year-olds and to perform the function of screening the risk for ASD.

The revised and re-standardized Erxin Scales has been in use in China for five years and is reportedly employed by nearly 600 hospitals nationwide. Translating the Erxin Scales into English and introducing it to international colleagues will enable them to understand the development background, process, and current status of the psychological and behavioral assessment scale for Chinese children. I hope that the publication of the scale will enhance the exchange between Chinese and foreign professionals with similar interests. I also hope that the scale can be further revised and standardized in diverse cultural contexts, so as to provide a more valid instrument for assessing children's psychological and behavioral development in different countries and thus to promote healthy child development worldwide.

Jing Liu
The Party Secretary of Peking
University Sixth Hospital
Beijing, China

Foreword 3: "It Takes Ten Years to Forge a Perfect Sword"

Since my acceptance of Professor Jin's invitation to write a preface for her revised English version of Erxin Scales half a month ago, I have been thinking about what to write to show the importance of the scale and also my deep respect for Professor Jin.

For the past two weeks or so, the Chinese idiom "It takes ten years to forge a perfect sword" has frequently appeared in my thoughts. This is a very common, almost household, and yet quite special idiom, for it represents a type of sheer perseverance that is easy to say but difficult to practice.

This idiom lingers in my mind mostly because of the special connotation of "sword" in traditional Chinese culture. It is revered by people from all walks of life in ancient society not only as a potent weapon but also as a symbol of sacredness.

As the idiom means literally, ten years of forging will certainly generate an incredibly sharp sword. Therefore, people often use it as a metaphor to describe the certainty of achieving positive results from long-term hard work, and also to praise the noble quality of perseverance exhibited by those who diligently hone their skills.

Around 16 years ago when Professor Jin proposed revising the Erxin Scales, I wholeheartedly agreed and supported her idea, because it was a highly meaningful endeavor.

As early as the mid-1980s, when I had just arrived at the Institute of Psychology of the Chinese Academy of Sciences (IPCAS) for my studies, I heard that Yuyan Mao, a highly respected professor of child psychology, was working on the development of the Erxin Scale. Later on, I learned the origin of the name "Erxin" and that this work was a collaborative effort with colleagues from the Capital Institute of Pediatrics (CIP). Even the name of a seemingly ordinary child developmental scale reflects the wisdom and virtue of cooperation, which makes me deeply admire the spirit of the older generations of Chinese scientists. It was thus without surprise that after the mid-1990s, the Erxin Scale became a unique psychometric tool for children in mainland China, completely independent of foreign instruments and widely applied in clinical and research settings.

Experts from CIP and IPCAS spent over a decade developing the Erxin Scales, and another decade has elapsed since Professor Jin's team embarked on the revision of the scale in 2005. Therefore, using the idiom "It takes ten years to forge a perfect sword" as a metaphor for Professor Jin's devotion to the revision of the scale is perfectly appropriate.

In addition, "To do a good job, a craftsman must sharpen his tools first" is another sentence that has come to my mind. This expresses perfectly the importance of Professor Jin's contribution in revising the Erxin Scales.

Since the establishment of the People's Republic of China and especially after the implementation of its reform and opening-up policy in 1978, the country has undergone tremendous development and changes. The growth of various industries in China has been phenomenal, and child healthcare and research on child psychological development and education are no exceptions.

Children are the future of the world and also the future of China. Their healthy development will make the future full of hope. This is why massive emphasis has been placed on children's medical care and psychological development as well as education worldwide. However, all of this begins with an understanding of children's physical and mental development. This highlights the vital value of a child developmental scale with good reliability and validity.

Over its 5,000 years of evolution, China has formed not only a unique language system but also unique social and cultural forms, and the physical characteristics of Chinese people greatly differ from those of Westerners. Therefore, a set of child developmental scales based on the physical development characteristics of Chinese children and Chinese social culture is extremely important.

Professor Jin and her team have spent more than a decade comprehensively revising the original Erxin Scales, and the revised edition is an asset for both child healthcare and basic research in the field of child psychological development and education in China. Undoubtedly, the revised Erxin Scale, like the original one, is an immeasurable achievement.

Jiannong Shi
The Institute of Psychology
Chinese Academy of Sciences
Beijing, China

Acknowledgments

The development, application, and revision of the Erxin Scale have been a culmination of forty years of dedication and effort by several generations of professionals at CIP. It represents their unwavering commitment to research, revise, and improve the scale. I would like to express my utmost respect and gratitude to the experts and scholars who have contributed their wisdom to the revision of the scales.

Gratitude is expressed to appreciate and carry forward the efforts of our predecessors, and to let history remember them. Due to the extensive duration of the revision process, if there are any omissions in the acknowledgments, please accept my sincere apologies.

First and foremost, I would like to express my greatest appreciation to the professors and experts who warmly supported and participated in the discussions, debates, and guidance during the revision of the Erxin Scales, and provided constructive suggestions and recommendations. The following individuals deserve special recognition: Zonghan Zhu, former Director of Beijing Municipal Health Bureau and CIP; Xingming Jin from Shanghai Children's Medical Center; Jin Jing from Sun Yat-sen University; Xiu Xu from Children's Hospital of Fudan University; Yufeng Yang from Xi'an Jiaotong University; Huishan Wang from National Center for Women and Children's Health; Hongwei Ma from Shengjing Hospital of China Medical University; Xiaoyang Dai from Shenzhen University; Zhixiang Zhang and Weilan Liang from Peking University First Hospital; Huimei Wang from Children's Hospital of

Shanxi; Meixiang Jia from Peking University Sixth Hospital; and Feng Zhang from Beijing Children's Hospital.

I am extremely grateful to the leaders of the national collaborative multicenter normative research team: Xueling Gao, Weimin Zhang, Qiyun Du, Lan Zhang, Jingjing Liang, Aimin Liang, Yixun Zhang, Zhuang Wei, Hong Cui, Haiyan Jiang, Junshuang Ren, Ling Bao, Yanan Kong, Ning Zhang, and Lu Zhao. Their dedication and strong support during the revision of the scale are invaluable.

Heartfelt thanks go to Vice Director Bowen Chen for his full support as the leader of the projects funded by Capital Medical Development Research Fund and the National Science and Technology Pillar Program during the Twelfth Five-Year Plan Period, in the revision of the Erxin Scales. Special thanks also go to Ruili Li from the Department of Child Health Development Research for her assistance in data analysis.

Thanks are particularly due to the members of the research team at CIP, including Yue Zhang, Lili Zhang, Na Li, Ruihua Yang, Xiaoyan Wang, Jianhong Wang, Huimin Lu, Lei Du, Chunxia Wang, Yanping Sun, Haitao Gao, Wenhong Song, Mei Li, Heru Wang, and Qi Xu, who overcame difficulties, sacrificed personal rest, and worked together tirelessly during the ten-year revision process.

A heartfelt thank goes to Shen Liu for his valuable assistance in graphics and illustrations.

I would like to express my gratitude to Mr. Zhuhua Cha, a software engineer with extraordinary endurance, for his immense support and assistance in data storage, processing, and analysis over the past decades, all for the healthy development of children.

I am thankful to Maohuai Fan, Ping Lu, and Yi Luo, the leaders of CIP, for their utmost support during scale revision.

Special thanks go to Professor Tingyu Li, the head of the Developmental and Behavioral Pediatrics Group of the Chinese Medical Association, Professor Jing Liu, the Party Secretary of Peking University Sixth Hospital, and Professor Jiannong Shi from the Institute of Psychology, Chinese Academy of Sciences, for writing the foreword for this English edition.

I express my gratitude to Chen Zhao, the English translator, a researcher of Development Research Center of the State Council, worked in China Center for the Economics of Human Development, for her hard work and efforts in translating the manuscript over the past two years.

I also want to give special thanks to Professor Su Li from the CAS Key Laboratory of Behavioral Science, Institute of Psychology, and the Department of Psychology, University of Chinese Academy of Sciences. I am grateful for her guidance and assistance in the translation and proofreading of the manuscript, both in Chinese and English, providing expertise in the field of psychology.

Looking back on the revision work of the Erxin Scales, I am filled with mixed emotions. It has occupied much of the time that should have been spent with my family for more than a decade. However, I am fortunate to have the silent support of my husband, Song Yang. Not only did he help in creating the assessment tools for new items during the scale revision, but he also provided significant assistance in data proofreading, text refinement, and polishing of the Chinese manuscript before its English translation. As the manuscript is completed, I sincerely thank my family for their understanding, support, and help, especially my husband, Song Yang.

I wholeheartedly wish everyone health and happiness.

Contents

1	Introduction		1
2	Theoretical Basis of the Erxin Scales		7
	2.1	An Overview	7
	2.2	Development of Nervous System in Children	9
		2.2.1 Development of Cranial Nerves	9
		2.2.2 Brain Functions and Neurophysiological Activities	10
		2.2.3 Brain Plasticity	12
	2.3	Cognitive Development	13
		2.3.1 Cognition	13
		2.3.2 Basic Operational Processes of Cognition	13
	2.4	Piaget's Theory of Cognitive Development	16
		2.4.1 Concept of Cognitive Operation	16
		2.4.2 Maturation, Experience, and Equilibration	17
		2.4.3 Process of Children's Psychological Development	18
		2.4.4 Piaget's Stages of Cognitive Development	18
		2.4.5 Concrete Operational Stage (7–11 Years Old) and Formal Operational Stage (12–18 Years Old)	19
	2.5	Other Theories in Developmental Psychology	19
	2.6	Theoretical Foundations of Erxin Scales Items for Each Age Group	20

		2.6.1	Birth to 2 Years of Age	20
		2.6.2	1–4 Months of Age	21
		2.6.3	4–8 Months of Age	21
		2.6.4	8–12 Months of Age	22
		2.6.5	12–18 Months of Age	22
		2.6.6	18–24 Months of Age	22
		2.6.7	2 to 7 Years of Age	23
	2.7	Basic Theories and Techniques for Scale Development		26
	2.8	Commonly Used Child Developmental Scales and Their Applicability Analysis		28
		2.8.1	Commonly Used Child Developmental Scales	30
		2.8.2	Applicability Analysis of the Commonly Used Developmental Scales	35
	2.9	Influence of Culture and Environment on Cognitive Development		38
		2.9.1	Literature Review and Follow-Up Case Study	38
		2.9.2	Environmental Impact on Child Developmental Rate	41
	2.10	Representative Scales in Developing Countries		45
		2.10.1	Characteristics and Advantages of the Erxin Scales	45
		2.10.2	Learning from International Scales	49
		2.10.3	Feasibility of Applying the Erxin Scales in Non-Western Countries	51
	References			55
3	**Development and Revision of the Erxin Scales**			61
	3.1	Background of the Erxin Scales		61
	3.2	Necessity for Scales Revision		63
	3.3	Grants from the Government and Professional Organizations		63
	3.4	Formulation and Implementation of the Technical Roadmap for Scales Revision		64
		3.4.1	Formulation of the Technical Roadmap for Scales Revision	64
		3.4.2	Item Management and Quality Control	66
		3.4.3	Proposals for patent application	68
	3.5	Preliminary Preparation		68
		3.5.1	Determination of Scale Revision Principles	68

	3.5.2	Clarification of Scale Structure and Domain Attribution	70
	3.5.3	Principles for Determining Main Test Ages	71
	3.5.4	Principles for Determining Scale Dimensions and Item Weights	72
	3.5.5	Examination of the Original Scale Items	72
	3.5.6	Increase of Supplementary Items and Extension of Applicable Age Range up to 6 Years	74
3.6	Implementation of Item Testing		75
	3.6.1	Pass Rates for Modified Items During Clinical Testing	75
3.7	Determination of Main Test Ages for New Items		76
	3.7.1	Establishment of a Preliminary Pool for New Items	82
	3.7.2	Quality Control During Scale Revision	86
	3.7.3	Formation of the Original Revised Scales	88
3.8	Standardization of Measurement Tools		90
	3.8.1	Selection of Measurement Tools	90
	3.8.2	Collaborative Production of Testing Pictures	91
	3.8.3	Accessibility of play materials	91
	3.8.4	Novelty and operability of new measurement tools	91
	3.8.5	Replacement of Measurement Tools	92
3.9	Research Sample and Sampling Criteria		92
References			93

4 Psychometric Analysis of the Erxin Scales — 95

4.1	Difficulty Distribution of Items Across Domains	95
4.2	Item Discrimination	96
4.3	Correlation Between Test Items and Month Age	97
4.4	Reliability Tests	97
	4.4.1 Inter-Rater Reliability	97
	4.4.2 Homogeneity Reliability	97
	4.4.3 Split-Half Reliability	98
	4.4.4 Test–Retest Reliability	99
4.5	Correlation with Criterion Scales	102
4.6	Factor Analysis	102
4.7	Confirmatory Factor Analysis	104
References		114

5	**Application Value of the Erxin Scales**		117
	5.1 Developing Child Assessment Scales: an Essential Requirement for Progress		117
	5.2 High Content Validity		119
	5.3 High Discriminability of the Newly Revised Scale Items		120
	5.4 Close Correlation Between Scale Items and Month Age		121
	5.5 High Internal Consistency of the Scales		122
	5.6 Solid Scale Structure as Revealed by Factor Analysis		123
	5.7 Good Fit Between Conceptual Model and Actual Data		125
	5.8 Selection of Criterion Scales and the Criterion-Related Validity		126
	5.9 Design and Standardization of Testing Tools		126
	References		129
6	**Research on the Communication Warning Behavior Subscale**		131
	6.1 Research Background		131
	6.2 Feasibility Analysis		133
	6.3 Formation of the Subscales		134
	6.4 Validity Re-evaluation of the Communication Warning Behavior Subscale		136
		6.4.1 Expanding the Sample	137
		6.4.2 Plotting the ROC Curve	138
		6.4.3 Comparison of Overall DQs and Subscale Scores Among Groups	139
		6.4.4 Composition Ratio of Subscale Scores in Each Group	141
		6.4.5 Factor Analysis and Scree Plot	141
		6.4.6 Internal Consistency of the Subscale and Its Correlation with the Criterion Measure	142
	6.5 Highlight of the Scales Revision		145
	References		146
7	**Data Analysis of Normative Sample for the Erxin Scales**		149
	7.1 Basic Data on the Normative Sample		149
		7.1.1 Sampled Participants	149
		7.1.2 Distribution of Overall and Subscale DQs	149

		7.1.3	Frequency Distribution, Histogram, and Probability Density Curve of DQs	150

	7.1.3	Frequency Distribution, Histogram, and Probability Density Curve of DQs	150
	7.1.4	Analysis of Data Distribution Among Children Aged 0–4 Years and 4–6 Years	153
	7.1.5	Frequency Distribution, Histograms, and Probability Density Curves of DQs for the Five Subscales	156
	7.1.6	DQs Corresponding with the Quartiles for the Sample	160
	7.1.7	Means and Medians of DQs for Children at Different Main Test Ages	162
7.2	Number of Items and Age Range for the Erxin Scales		164
	7.2.1	Number of Items in the Revised Erxin Scales	164
	7.2.2	Age Range for the Scales	165
7.3	Classification Criteria for DQs of the Erxin Scales		166
	7.3.1	Classification Criteria of Well-known Developmental or Intelligence Scales	166
	7.3.2	DQ Classification and Evaluation of the Erxin Scales	167
7.4	Normative Reference Values for the Erxin Scales		173
	7.4.1	Formation of Normative Reference Values	173
	7.4.2	Classification and Evaluation of DQ Norm Levels	173
	7.4.3	Percentiles for DQs at Main Test Ages	175
7.5	Risk Index Classification of the Communication Warning Behavior Subscale		175
7.6	Stepwise Age Correction for Preterm Infants		175
References			178

8	**Application and Administration of the Scales**		179
	8.1	Management	179
		8.1.1 Management of Examiners and Assessors	179
		8.1.2 Specific Testing Requirements	181
		8.1.3 Requirements for the State of the Child Being Assessed	182
	8.2	Specific Requirements for the Assessor	182
		8.2.1 Kind Reminders	182
		8.2.2 Establishing a Friendly Relationship	182
		8.2.3 Following an Ascending Order of Difficulty	183

		8.2.4	Recording the Scores	183
		8.2.5	Data Input and Report Output	183
	8.3	Be Proficient in the Assessment Procedure of the Erxin Scales		184
		8.3.1	Familiarizing Yourself with the Instructions	184
		8.3.2	Memorizing the Specific Assessment Procedure	184
9	Instruction Manual for the Erxin Scales			185
	9.1	Operations and Passing/Scoring Criteria for Items of Erxin Scales		185
10	Appendices A, B, and C			295
	10.1	Appendix A: Reference Percentiles for Overall and Subscale DQs at Different Main Test Ages for the Representative Sample		295
	10.2	Appendix B: Inventory of Testing Tools Used in the Erxin Scales		302
		10.2.1	Inventory and Photographs of Testing Tools Used in the Erxin Scales	302
		10.2.2	Staircase for Testing	304
		10.2.3	Bed for Testing	306
	10.3	Appendix C: Pictures of Children Undergoing Assessment for Several Items		307

Correction to: Erxin Scales: Child Developmental Scale of China	C1
Index	331

List of Figures

Fig. 3.1	Technical roadmap for scales revision	65
Fig. 3.2	Percentage trends of pictures with names correctly stated by children at ages of 30, 36, and 42 months	82
Fig. 3.3	Percentage trends of damaged or missing parts correctly identified by children at ages of 42, 48, and 54 months	83
Fig. 3.4	Trends of the percentages of differences spotted by children aged 48 months to 84 months	84
Fig. 4.1	Model fit indices for the 1–3 months subset (excluding Items #3 and #4 at 1 month)	113
Fig. 4.2	Model fit indices for the 66–78 months subset (excluding Item #257 at 66 months)	114
Fig. 6.1	ROC curve plotted based on DSM-5 criteria for diagnosing ASD	137
Fig. 6.2	ROC curve plotted based on the DSM-5 criteria for diagnosing ASD	139
Fig. 6.3	Scatter plot depicting the link between eigenvalues and the number of components	145
Fig. 7.1	Histogram and probability density curve of overall DQs grouped with an interval of 6 for the sample of 8,914 children	152
Fig. 7.2	Histogram and probability density curve of overall DQs grouped with an interval of 6 for the 8,612 children aged 2–84 months	155

Fig. 7.3	Histogram and probability density curve of DQs grouped with an interval of 6 for the 7,658 children aged 1–60 months	157
Fig. 7.4	Histogram and probability density curve of overall DQs grouped with an interval of 6 for the 2,872 children aged 4–6 years (36–84 months)	158
Fig. 7.5	Histogram and probability density curve of gross motor DQs grouped with an interval of 6 for the 8,612 children aged 2–84 months	159
Fig. 7.6	Histogram and probability density curve of fine motor DQs grouped with an interval of 6 for the 8,612 children aged 2–84 months	161
Fig. 7.7	Histogram and probability density curve of adaptability DQs grouped with an interval of 6 for the 8,612 children aged 2–84 months	163
Fig. 7.8	Histogram and probability density curve of language DQs grouped with an interval of 6 for the 8,612 children aged 2–84 months	165
Fig. 7.9	Histogram and probability density curve of social behavior DQs grouped with an interval of 6 for the 8,612 children aged 2–84 months	167

List of Tables

Table 3.1	Number of participants and pass rates for the item "Understand adult facial expressions" (n%)	76
Table 3.2	Number of participants and pass rates for the item "Hold onto the railing to squat down and pick something up" (n%)	76
Table 3.3	Number of participants and pass rates for the item "Make protective action" (n%)	78
Table 3.4	Number of participants and pass rates for the item "Engage in joint attention" (n%)	79
Table 3.5	Number of participants and pass rates for the item "Describe the picture contents" (n%)	79
Table 3.6	Number of participants and pass rates for the item "Summarize the theme of pictures" (n%)	80
Table 3.7	Percentages (%) of pictures with names correctly stated by children at ages of 30, 36, and 42 months	81
Table 3.8	Percentages (%) of damaged or missing parts correctly identified by children at ages of 42, 48, and 54 months	82
Table 3.9	Percentage (%) of differences spotted by children aged 48 months to 84 months	83
Table 3.10	Percentages of deleted and retained new items in each domain	86
Table 3.11	Distribution of modified and newly added items across domains in the original revised scales	89

LIST OF TABLES

Table 4.1	Difficulty coefficients and composition ratio of test items in the five attributes for children ages 0 to 6 years old	96
Table 4.2	Composition ratio of correlation between test items and month age in each attribute	97
Table 4.3	Homogeneity reliability coefficients of the overall scale for each main test age	98
Table 4.4	Homogeneity reliability coefficients of the subscales for each main test age	99
Table 4.5	Split-half reliability coefficients of the overall scale for each main test age	100
Table 4.6	Split-half reliability coefficients of the subscales for each main test age	101
Table 4.7	Test–retest reliability coefficients for the 0–4 years age group (n = 101) ($\overline{X} \pm s$)	101
Table 4.8	Test–retest reliability coefficients for the 4–6 years age group (n = 30) ($\overline{X} \pm s$)	102
Table 4.9	Correlation of the revised Erxin Scales with GDS and WPPSI-R ($\overline{X} \pm s$)	103
Table 4.10	Factor loadings matrix after rotation and the match with scale domains for items assessing infants aged 1–3 months	105
Table 4.11	Specific parameters of model fit for each combined age group	111
Table 6.1	Sensitivity and 1-specificity (false positive rate) obtained from the segmented ROC curve	140
Table 6.2	Comparison of Erxin scales overall DQs, communication warning behavior subscale scores, and CABS scores among the three groups	140
Table 6.3	Composition ratio of scores stratified for the three groups	141
Table 6.4	Rotated component matrix for the communication warning behavior subscale	143
Table 7.1	Descriptive statistics of overall and subscale DQs ($N = 8,914$)	150
Table 7.2	Frequency distribution of overall DQs among the sample of 8,914 children	151
Table 7.3	Descriptive statistics of overall and subscale DQs for the 8,612 children aged 2–84 months	153
Table 7.4	Frequency distribution of overall DQs grouped with an interval of 6 among the 8,612 children aged 2–84 months	154

Table 7.5	Descriptive statistics of overall and subscale DQs for the 7,658 children aged 1–60 months	156
Table 7.6	Descriptive statistics of overall and subscale DQs for the 7,356 children aged 2–60 months	156
Table 7.7	Descriptive statistics of overall and subscale DQs for the 2,872 children aged 4–6 years (36–84 months)	158
Table 7.8	Frequency distribution of gross motor DQs grouped with an interval of 6 among the 8,612 children aged 2–84 months	160
Table 7.9	Frequency distribution of fine motor DQs grouped with an interval of 6 among the 8,612 children aged 2–84 months	162
Table 7.10	Frequency distribution of adaptability DQs grouped with an interval of 6 among the 8,612 children aged 2–84 months	164
Table 7.11	Frequency distribution of language DQs grouped with an interval of 6 among the 8,612 children aged 2–84 months	166
Table 7.12	Frequency distribution of social behavior DQs grouped with an interval of 6 among the 8,612 children aged 2–84 months	168
Table 7.13	Overall and subscale DQs at the quartiles and the 5th and 95th percentiles for the sample of 8,914 children	168
Table 7.14	Means, standard deviations, and medians of DQs for the 8,914 children at different main test ages	169
Table 7.15	Intelligence/ IQ/DQ classification by different scales	172
Table 7.16	Sample sizes and composition ratios of the overall and subscale DQs at different norm levels	174
Table 7.17	Classification and evaluation of DQ norm levels for the Erxin Scales	174
Table 7.18	Risk index classification and evaluation of the communication warning behavior subscale	176
Table 7.19	Illustrations of the stepwise age correction for preterm infants	178
Table 10.1	Overall DQs at the 3rd-97th percentiles across the main test ages from 1 to 84 months	296
Table 10.2	Gross motor DQs at the 3rd-97th percentiles across the main test ages from 1 to 84 months	297
Table 10.3	Fine motor DQs at the 3rd-97th percentiles across the main test ages from 1 to 84 months	298
Table 10.4	Adaptability DQs at the 3rd-97th percentiles across the main test ages from 1 to 84 months	299

Table 10.5	Language DQs at the 3rd-97th percentiles across the main test ages from 1 to 84 months	300
Table 10.6	Social behavior DQs at the 3rd-97th percentiles across the main test ages from 1 to 84 months	301

CHAPTER 1

Introduction

There has been a dearth of self-developed child developmental assessment scales that can be used for equal communication with international peers. As a national research institution for child development, the Capital Institute of Pediatrics (CIP) has dedicated itself to this realm for more than 40 years, with the Erxin Scales as its representative work. The development and revision of the scale took two decades (1980–1990 and 2005–2016) and was the joint effort of several generations. The English version of the Erxin Scales aims to accomplish the mission of introducing the child developmental scale of China with fully indigenous intellectual property rights to the international community.

The predecessor of CIP was the Institute of Pediatrics of the Chinese Academy of Medical Sciences. In 1980, Qinbing Xue, the director of the Institute at the time, invited Professor Yuyan Mao from the Institute of Psychology, Chinese Academy of Sciences (IPCAS) to guide the development of a scale suitable for the growth patterns of children in China according to the international requirements for scale development. With 60 healthy newborns from Beijing selected as research participants, experts leading by Hong Xue, Jiajian Zhang, and Zhenmin Gao took charge of tracking and observing the neuropsychological and behavioral characteristics of the infants and young children. Regular household visits, starting from once a month to once every 2–3 months after the age of 1 year, were conducted to collect relevant data. The work lasted for three and a half years and resulted in a valuable neuropsychological and behavioral dataset on infant and toddler development, holding significant academic value in China. On this basis, another 1275 infants and toddlers within the same-age range were included to conduct a cross-sectional validation of the neuropsychological and behavioral items, and a preliminary developmental scale for infants and toddlers aged 0–3 years was compiled. In 1985, scale standardization was initiated nationwide, and a collaborative multicenter research team was established in 12 cities, including Beijing, Tianjin, Shanghai, Wuhan, Kunming, Fuzhou, Changchun, Baotou, Kaifeng, Zhengzhou, Guiyang, and Lanzhou. A total of 13,868 children aged 0–3 years were included in the study, and a nationally representative database on neuropsychological development of infants and toddlers was established. Subsequently, a cross-sectional approach was used, and 1185 children aged 4–5 years were added to the research data for reliability and validity tests and establishing the national norms. The age range of the scale was then extended to 6 years old, ultimately forming China's first comprehensive assessment scale for neuropsychological and behavioral development in children aged 0–6 years. This filled the gap in our country's diagnostic scales for child development.

The final work was named "Erxin Scales" ("Erxin" for short), exhibiting distinctive characteristics of Chinese language. "Er" (meaning "child" in Chinese) in "Erxin" stands for CIP, and "Xin" (meaning "psychology" in Chinese) for IPCAS. The name of the scale takes the two Chinese characters that best reflect the nature and scope of the two cooperating institutes. The combination of the two characters also clearly reveals the purpose of the scale, conforming to Chinese logic and expression habits. After years of extensive application in child healthcare and pediatric clinical settings, "Erxin" has become an established technical term in the industry with a specific meaning, just like "Gesell" and "Bayley." Erxin Scale is currently the most favored and widely used developmental assessment scale for children in China.

In over two decades of Erxin Scales' wide application, significant societal and economic transformations had occurred in China, resulting in notable changes in the living and growth environments of children. Some items in the scale failed to accurately reflect the full picture of children's behavioral characteristics, and certain assessment tools became outdated, highlighting the necessity of revising the scale by international conventions. In view of this, Chunhua Jin from CIP, entrusted by Dr. Zhenmin

Gao and Dr. Jiajian Zhang, the original developers of the Erxin Scale, started to form a team in 2005 to prepare for the scale revision work. Under the guidance of Dr. Gao and Dr. Zhang, the team established a clear foundation based on the theory of cognitive development and proposed increasing items related to social communication to reflect the neuropsychological characteristics of children, innovatively integrating the domains associated with core symptoms and manifestations of autism spectrum disorder (ASD). In the meanwhile, item revision process and principles were established, the overall structure of the scale were determined, and all the measurement tools were standardized. A new domain was added in addition to the existing five domains. With the support of the Beijing Municipal Government and national scientific research funds, a preliminary pool for the new assessment items was established in the first few years. Through repeated clinical testing, 479 items were modified, 232 items were discarded, 247 items entered the item testing phase, and finally 120 items meeting the required pass rate were retained. Five new items were derived from the deleted ones and directly incorporated into the original revised scale. After the original version was formed, it underwent standardization on a nationally representative sample.

The representative sample for standardization was obtained by referring to the data from the 6th national census in 2010. Stratified cluster random sampling was employed, with an age ratio for 0–1 year, 1–4 years, and 5–9 years consistent with the census data, and a 1:1 gender ratio. The nationally representative provinces and cities included Beijing, Guangzhou (Guangdong Province), Taiyuan (Shanxi Province), Shenyang (Liaoning Province), Xi'an (Shaanxi Province), Chengdu (Sichuan Province), Changsha (Hunan Province), and Hefei (Anhui Province). Collaborative research centers for norm construction were established in the sampled regions. To ensure accurate measurement of children's developmental levels and consistency in assessment standards, the project team invited experts proficient in using the original Erxin Scale and Gesell Development Schedules, as well as assessors experienced in operating the scales to participate in the specific implementation and provide guidance. Professor Xiaoyang Dai, who had previously been responsible for revising the Hunan version of the Wechsler Preschool and Primary Scale of Intelligence (WPPSI), was also invited to give guidance on quality control and calibration scale selection and adoption in the revision of the Erxin Scale. Altogether 8952 children's data were collected for the analysis, standardization, and norm establishment of the original revised scale.

Employing a case-control research design, 67 of the newly proposed items related to communication warning behaviors were selected based on preliminary investigations into parents or caregivers of children diagnosed with ASD while simultaneously surveying healthy children. Specifically, data of 178 ASD children and 666 healthy children from the sampled areas were collected. Then, methods such as factor analysis were employed to screen the items and determine their number, ROC curve was plotted using clinical diagnosis of ASD as the criterion, and the value exhibiting high sensitivity and specificity was set as the screening threshold or normative risk index.

The finally revised Erxin Scales encompassed six domains and subscales including gross motor, fine motor, adaptability, language, social behavior, and communication warning behavior. It covered ages ranging from 1 to 84 months, divided into 28 age groups, with a total of 294 items. Among the newly included 125 items, 52 were added to the section for children aged 1 month to 4 years (the part of the original scale with national normative data), 40 were for the extended age range from 5 to 6 years, and 33 were for assessing communication warning behaviors. Regarding statistical data analysis, the examination of various psychometric properties of the scale were completed in early 2016, including item difficulty coefficient and discrimination index, the link between test items and age, the reliability, validity, criterion-related validity, factor analysis, and confirmatory factor analysis, as well as the reliability and validity of the newly added Communication Warning Behavior Subscale. On the basis of these work, the Chinese monograph *Children Neuropsychological and Behavior Scale-Revision 2016 (CNBS-R2016)*, or *Erxin Scales-Revision 2016*, was published, marking the completion of a ten-year-long scale revision process. Noteworthily, as one of the primary authors, I submitted the revision outline and related materials (excluding the not-yet-completed Communication Warning Behavior Subscale) during the scale revision period to the National Health and Family Planning Commission of China to apply for an industry standard, which was then issued by the Commission in 2017 (The Developmental Behavior Assessment Scale for Children Aged 0–6 Years, WS/T 580-2017).

The Chinese publication *Erxin Scales-Revision 2016* covers the national industry standard, but further refines the operational guidance and adds the subscale capable of screening ASD. The content of the book is comprehensive and the assessment results are presented in an easily understandable manner. It used mental age to indicate developmental degree, and developmental quotient (DQ) to indicate developmental level. Information related to DQs and mental ages are provided for both the overall scale and the subscales. In addition to assessing children's overall developmental levels, the scale also incorporates a screening function for ASD, effectively improving the identification of children with developmental deviations, delays, uneven development, and communication disorders. In the present English version, percentile distribution data for DQs at main test ages are added, providing further reference for longitudinal follow-up studies on children's developmental status and increasing the scope and effectiveness of the scale in assessing child development. Currently, the Erxin Scale is the most authoritative and comprehensive assessment scale for child development in China, and its revised edition has received full recognition and recommendation from experts in the field. Moreover, its national industry standard (WS/T 580-2017) content has been endorsed by the National Health Commission (NHC) with an official document (Maternal and Child Affairs of the NHC Office [2022] No. 12) for application at the grassroots level.

To establish brand awareness for Chinese scales, Dr. Zhenmin Gao and Dr. Jiajian Zhang have provided special instructions regarding the scale's name in the final revision stage: to maintain naming continuity and add the year or revision edition. The name of the Chinese monograph *Erxin Scales-Revision 2016* thus retained the year of its completion. In the publication of this English version, the scale's English name was also highly valued by Dr. Gao, who emphasized that the English name should reflect the term "Erxin Scales." Considering that "Erxin Scales" has become a fixed term with a specific meaning in China, and to minimize ambiguity in translation and particularly in the written expression between Chinese and English, it was decided to follow the naming conventions of internationally renowned developmental scales. Therefore, the revised scale in this English publication was entitled "Erxin Scales: Child Developmental Scale of China" ("Erxin Scales" for short), which has won the recognition and support from Dr. Gao, the expert of the original version of the Erxin Scales.

The Erxin Scales comprises a set of comprehensive child developmental assessment tools that are widely representative, highly reliable, valid, scientifically rigorous, and highly practical, fully suited to the national conditions of China. Undoubtedly, it is necessary for the scale to keep pace with the times and be continually updated. Undertaking the task of revising the Erxin Scale is not only a great honor for me but also an undeniable historical responsibility. In the process of promoting the Erxin Scales, we fortuitously came across Dr. Chen Zhao, Researcher of the Development Research Center of the State Council, and the deputy director of the China Center for the Economics of Human Development, CDRF. She got doctoral degree under the supervision of Professor Jiannong Shi from IPCAS who served as the project leader of the collaborating institute for normative study during the revision of the Erxin Scales. This pleasant encounter led to our translation of the Erxin Scales into English. We are very pleased to introduce the Erxin Scales, which has indigenous intellectual property rights and has been used for nearly half a century, to our foreign peers. Hopefully, this book will enhance equal exchanges with international colleagues, increase the scalability and universality of the scales, and help achieve the goal that the medical pioneers at CIP have been striving for. We greatly cherish the developmental assessment scale that embodies the collaborative endeavor of several generations, and that possesses indigenous intellectual property rights and is suitable for children in developing countries. Carrying forward the spirit passed down by our predecessors over the past century, we will forge ahead, not squandering the precious time, and contribute to its further promotion and establishment of a national brand.

Here I would like to express my special thanks to the invaluable guidance and assistance given by experts in psychology and psychometrics during the several rounds of proofreading for this manuscript. In particular, I would like to thank Professor Su Li from the CAS Key Laboratory of Behavioral Science, Institute of Psychology, and the Department of Psychology, University of Chinese Academy of Sciences. Professor Li has provided crucial assistance in the translation and proofreading of the manuscript, and has dedicated her enthusiasm and wisdom to ensuring the accuracy of psychology-specific terminology and the precision of the translation between Chinese and English. Her meticulous scholarly attitude has guaranteed the high level and quality of this English edition. Please allow us to express our heartfelt gratitude and deep respect to Professor Li!

CHAPTER 2

Theoretical Basis of the Erxin Scales

2.1 AN OVERVIEW

The neuropsychological development of children is manifested in various forms of neuropsychological activities, including motor abilities, language comprehension and expression, emotional responses to people and objects in the surroundings, as well as memory, imagination, and mathematical skills. It is a response to internal and external stimuli, resulting from the interaction of innate, genetic, and social environmental factors. The tests assessing abilities and characteristics of children, such as perception, motor skills, language, cognition, emotions, personality, and social adaptability, are collectively referred to as psychological assessments. Psychological and neurological development are difficult to be distinguished from each other due to their close relationship during infancy and early childhood, and the manifestation of cognitive activities may not be entirely consistent across different ages. Developmental scales formulated through long-term tracking and observation are typically used to evaluate neuropsychological development in infants and young children, with a focus on visual-motor skills and mainly reflecting biological processes. They are mostly employed to differentiate between children showing normal development and atypical development. Though most developmental scales are applicable for children aged 0–3 years, several renowned Western scales have a wider applicable age range. For example, the Bayley Scales of Infant Development (BSID) are applicable for children aged

1–42 months, while the age range of the Gesell Development Schedules (GDS) and Griffiths Mental Development Scales (GMDS) reaches 6 years or above. Among them, GDS was developed through tracking and observing infants from mainstream Caucasian society and families with a higher socioeconomic status [1], whereas the normative sample for BSID was derived from a representative population in the United States. Owing to the diversity of child development, human development in general exhibits both similarities and differences across different environments, races, and cultural backgrounds, despite the basic similarity of human neurophysiological development patterns. For this reason, revisions and standardization are necessary when applying Western scales to assessing children in non-Western, low-income countries so as to avoid biases.

China is a developing country with a large population, great geographical differences, and a relatively low investment in healthcare. The introduction of foreign scales requires continuous investment of human resources, materials, and finances, and challenges resulted from copyright issues and constant updating of scales are also inevitable. Developmental assessment, as a part of the clinical diagnostic process, involves detailed observation and measurement of children's development in general or in a specific domain, focusing on identifying abnormalities or the degree of abnormality in the progress of child growth. Therefore, clinically there is an urgent need to provide a comprehensive and unified developmental assessment tool for children at various stages. Through assessment, it is possible to objectively distinguish whether an individual child's development is advanced or delayed compared to that of others of the same age, and this is of particular importance for children with significant developmental delays. All of this demonstrates that developing suitable developmental scales for Chinese children is an essential endeavor.

As the saying goes, skillful work demands good tools. Investigation into intellectual development falls within the research realm of advanced psychological processes. Intelligence tests should be administered within the frameworks of psychological and cognitive theories, but researchers in psychological measurement often focus on improving testing techniques while neglecting the exploration of intelligence theories. With this in mind, we invited Professor Yuyan Mao, a theoretical expert from IPCAS, to provide guidance on cognitive theories at the beginning of the scale development project. At our invitation, Professor Mao not only guided the project theoretically but also personally participated in the early observation of the neuropsychological development and motor behaviors in Chinese children to explore their developmental milestones. She has made enormous contribution to developing the Erxin Scales by referring to the procedures for developing internationally renowned child assessment scales including BSID and GDS.

Prior to initiating this round of revision, we had studied cognition and cognitive development theories systematically, with a focus on Piaget's theory of cognitive development. Accordingly, a clear picture has been obtained of various psychological schools' theories on cognition and mind, as well as of the theoretical foundations of measurement purposes, techniques, and items. Piaget's theory of cognitive development guided throughout the revision of the scale, and its theoretical tenets were incorporated into the construction of the test items. In addition, to enhance the theoretical cultivation of the research team, Professor Jiannong Shi was specifically invited to participate in the project and provide theoretical guidance, thereby avoiding an excessive focus on improving testing techniques while neglecting the theoretical basis of scale development.

2.2 Development of Nervous System in Children

2.2.1 Development of Cranial Nerves

The brain and nervous system are the material basis for the psychological development of children and serve as the foundation for their cognitive activities from primary to advanced levels. The organ systems of infants continue to grow and develop, with the cranial nerves having priority. After birth, nerve cells or neurons in the brain continue to differentiate and increase in volume, leading to an increased brain weight. The brain weight of a newborn is approximately 370–390 grams, which grows to around 900 grams by the age of 1 [2] and triples to 900–1000 grams by the age of 2 [3, 4]. The brain has the adult form at birth, but the gyri and sulci are shallow. In school-age children, the physiological structure of the cerebral cortex becomes basically mature. Although brain development is most rapid during infancy and early childhood, myelination of nervous fibers continues after birth, with increased number and length of synapses. From 6 months' gestation to 1 postnatal year in age, brain cells actively proliferate and increase in number [5]; from 1 to 2 years of age, they continue to undergo a rise in both number and volume; after approximately 2 years of age, however, their increase only occurs in volume [6, 7]. Myelination of cranial nerves is roughly complete by the age of 1.5 years, with that of cerebral white matter complete by the age of 2 and that of spinal cord complete by the age of 4, and by the end of age 6 all cortical pathways have undergone myelination [8]. The construction of neural pathways in the brain leads to an increasing functional capacity, and billions of new connections are established among neurons within the first two years of postnatal life, resulting in an increasingly complex network [9]. Nevertheless, the interaction network between neurons becomes more refined and gradually ordered by virtue of a "pruning" mechanism. The physiological growth of the brain and nervous system further develops their functions, leading to faster neural excitatory conduction, enhanced competence in motor coordination, language, social adaptation and comprehensive analysis, greater emotional stability, developed personality traits, and gradually matured psychological and behavioral characteristics with age.

2.2.2 Brain Functions and Neurophysiological Activities

2.2.2.1 Reflexes

Infants are born with an array of innate reflexes such as sucking, swallowing, and grasping. Reflex actions are primarily controlled by lower-level areas of the nervous system and regulated by the cerebral cortex. On the basis of innate reflexes develop conditioned reflexes, and the first conditioned reflex infants develop are sucking when their mother picks them up and puts her nipple in their mouth. After 9–14 days, they establish the first natural conditioned reflex, namely starting to suck as soon as they are picked up. Other conditioned reflexes are subsequently developed using various sensory organs. By the age of 7–8 months, infants respond to complex stimuli including words. Around the age of 1, words begin to serve as simple signals in conditioned stimuli, and vocabulary must be associated with specific stimulus [4]. After the age of 2, conditioned reflexes can be formed by both the children's first signal system and second signal system, enabling them to adapt more quickly to their surroundings [2, 10].

2.2.2.2 Functions of the Cerebrum

The cerebrum is the central organ, and the cerebral cortex is responsible for essential functions of the brain and the coordination of different parts of the body. Specifically, the frontal lobe is involved in body movement, speech production, executive functions, and higher-order thinking; the temporal lobe is associated with hearing, language comprehension, speech formation, and memory; the occipital lobe is related to visual processing and the motor functions of the eyes and head; and the parietal lobe is associated with somatosensory processing, fine motor skills, language, and the ability to compute. The cerebral cortex and subcortical structures together constitute the limbic system. Subcortical structures include the hippocampus, dentate gyrus, cingulate gyrus, insula, and posterior orbitofrontal cortex, which are involved in controlling bodily functions, emotions, motivation, learning and memory, and sleep.

Neural activities in children are unstable, with low intensity and regularity. The subcortical centers, such as the thalamus and globus pallidus, are relatively well-developed in infants, and thus are featured by high excitability. And the excitatory or inhibitory processes in infants can easily spread because the immature cerebral cortex does not exert effective control over the subcortical centers. However, with the increase in age, the cerebral cortex gradually matures and exerts inhibitory effects on the subcortical centers.

2.2.2.3 *Functions of the Brainstem*

The brainstem includes the medulla oblongata, pons, midbrain, and diencephalon, and it connects the 3rd to 12th pairs of cranial nerves. The brainstem reticular formation enables selective attention, consciousness, vomiting, arousal and sleep, as well as the regulation of muscle tone, heart rate, blood pressure, and vasoconstriction. The medulla oblongata is the primary respiratory control center, the pons plays a crucial role in integrating bilateral body movements, the midbrain contains the centers for visual and auditory reflexes, and the hypothalamus in the diencephalon is involved in regulating emotional activities.

2.2.2.4 *Functions of the Cerebellum*

The cerebellum primarily regulates body movements and is closely associated with the vestibular nuclei and the brainstem reticular formation. Together, they regulate proprioception and reflex activities, and maintain body balance and coordination. The cerebellum develops to adult levels at around 6 years of age [2].

2.2.3 Brain Plasticity

The plasticity and compensatory capacity of the brain peak in the first few years of life. Brain plasticity refers to its capacity to be shaped or modified by the environment or experiences, and hence appropriate stimulation is needed during the critical or sensitive periods of children's brain development. Sensitive periods are specific stages in which certain knowledge or behavioral experiences are most easily acquired or formed, and during which an individual is more sensitive to environmental stimuli compared to other stages. Numerous studies have shown that enriching environmental stimuli can promote the development of brain functions in children. Brain plasticity is evident in children who have recovered from brain injuries after early intervention, as the functional areas of the damaged nervous system can be partially compensated, resulting in significant improvements in brain functions [2, 4].

The development of the nervous system is influenced by both the internal and external environments, and individuals in the process of growth exhibit plasticity [11, 12], which nevertheless varies depending on the age and the location and severity of the brain injury. Prenatal malnutrition, for example, will adversely affect fetuses' brain development if not corrected promptly. Pathological changes such as brain ischemia and hypoxia in the perinatal period, maternal and childhood illnesses, and environmental pollution can all negatively impact children's intellectual growth. Cognitive development in children emphasizes the role of environmental stimuli in early stages, and the absence of specific environmental stimuli during critical periods may result in permanent and irreversible damage to developing individuals [9]. This has been verified by a study showing that if kittens are deprived of the opportunity to see vertical lines, they will be unable to perceive these lines in adulthood, despite their accurate perception of horizontal lines [9]. Lack of visual stimulation can lead to maldevelopment of the visual cortex and cause permanent visual impairment. For instance, the treatment of deprivation amblyopia in infants with congenital cataracts after 6 months of age will not be effective; similarly, the absence of language input and learning in the environment during the sensitive period for language development may lead to language delays in children [2]. These examples illustrate that the absence of specific environmental stimuli can significantly impede individual growth [9]. Children's neuropsychological development is subject to constantly dynamic changes. Infants and toddlers are particularly vulnerable to internal and external stimuli, so monitoring and assessing their development levels in neurological, motor, language, and social behavior domains are crucial.

2.3 Cognitive Development

2.3.1 Cognition

Cognition refers to the process by which individuals perceive and acquire knowledge about the external world. It involves sensory organs' information processing in response to external stimuli, encompassing the psychological experiences of sensation, perception, memory, and thinking. While the brain's nervous system, muscular sense, and even diet and sleep influence behavior, external sensations (visual, auditory, olfactory, gustatory, and tactile sensations) and internal sensations (kinesthetic, vestibular, and organic sensations) promote the brain to produce experiences and overall reflection of individual properties of objective entities. Cognitive development is continuous and sequential, progressing from simplicity to complexity and from lower levels to higher levels. Children's cognition develops through active interactions with others.

2.3.2 Basic Operational Processes of Cognition

2.3.2.1 Perception

Perception is the overall reflection of objective entities that directly interact with the sensory organs of the human brain [4]. Acquiring knowledge requires not only sensation but also perception. Sensation is the response of the sensory organs to physical stimuli and represents the individual attributes of objective entities in the human brain. On the other hand, perception is a psychological process that involves categorizing, interpreting, and integrating stimuli from the sensory organs and the brain. Perceptual activities involve matching sensory information with established schemas, representations, or concepts to understand objects. Perception extracts distinct features of objects from the background and constructs new schemas, representations, or symbols. Infants have the ability to integrate information from multiple sensory channels, 2.5–3-year-old children are capable of shape abstraction, and 4–5-year-old children reach a peak in color abstraction. After the age of 6, children can abstract shape and color simultaneously [4], which signifies the development of thinking and marks the beginning of true abstraction. School-age children recognize the letters b, d, p, and q by extracting their distinguishing features. With accumulated cognitive experiences, perceptual activities become more selective and accurate, leading to the ability to identify objects based on partial information or features [13].

2.3.2.2 Memory
Memory constitutes an important psychological process that reflects past experiences in the mind and serves as the foundation of intelligence. Through memory, past experiences are stored in the mind and function as the basis for thinking and imaginative activities in the forms of recognition and recall. The results of thinking and imagination are then stored as new experiences in the mind, further deepening and abstracting human thinking activities and promoting intellectual development to a higher level. According to the information processing theory, memory is viewed as the process of encoding, storing, and retrieving information under certain conditions. It can be divided into three stores based on the time from information input to retrieval: sensory memory, short-term memory, and long-term memory. Short-term memory can be transferred to long-term memory through consolidation. In infants and toddlers, unconscious memory dominates, and the memory content is limited to everyday contact with concrete, vivid, familiar, and visually distinct objective entities. Novel and interesting objective entities with strong emotions are more easily remembered and retained for a long time. Infants at the age of 5–6 months can distinguish their mother's face from a complex background and then recognize their mother. Children over 1 year old can recognize events that occurred 10 days or even 1 month ago, while those around 3 years old can recognize events from several months ago, and their recall can last for weeks [6]. Memory is also influenced by interest, as information that is interesting and engaging is remembered more quickly and retained for a longer time, whereas uninteresting information is difficult to remember or quickly forgotten. Young children rarely use memory strategies during encoding and retrieval and are unable to use words to aid memory. The memory of preschoolers develops based on infant memory. Generally, older children have more effective recall compared to younger children, because they use established cognitive strategies during encoding and retrieval, such as categorizing based

on object meaning and utilizing systematic methods in searching. These cognitive abilities vary among children of different ages.

2.3.2.3 Thinking
Thinking is the advanced stage of human cognition that develops based on perception and memory. It is the cognitive process through which the human brain comprehends the essence of objects and the intrinsic connections between them. Thinking is the subject of cognitive processing and is characterized by its indirect and abstract nature. Indirectness refers to the process by which humans use other things as a medium and rely on their experiences to reflect a particular object. Abstractness refers to the reflection of common, essential features among things of the same category and the connections and regularities between them in the human brain, and it is achieved through the use of language (such as in describing a picture, which not only involves speech production but also demonstrates the ability to generalize, classify, and categorize). Thinking is the core component of intelligence. With the development of symbolic operations, children gradually engage in advanced cognitive activities such as hypothesis formation, evaluation, and reasoning during thinking. They establish rich and diverse schemas or symbols based on their experiences, which facilitate their participation in creative thinking activities. However, young children have low problem-solving abilities, incapable of fully remembering or understanding the questions presented to them, and they may even struggle to repeat the questions. Their short-term memory capacities are limited, and the stored schemas, representations, and concepts are insufficient [13]. Thinking activities are ultimately expressed through behavior [14]. Infants only have perception of objects and lack basic thinking abilities [4], which only start to develop after the age of 1 [9]. In toddlers aged 2–3 years, thinking is closely tied to direct perception and actions, and it occurs in actions. From ages 4 to 7 years, concrete and imagistic thinking develops, mental representations and associations based on concrete objects can be used for thinking [6], and intuitive images can be used for problem-solving.

2.4 Piaget's Theory of Cognitive Development

2.4.1 Concept of Cognitive Operation

Swiss psychologist Jean Piaget established the theory of cognitive development and introduced the concept of cognitive operation, making substantial contribution to understand children's cognitive processes and promoting the development of contemporary child psychology. Piaget believed that early intellectual growth arises primarily out of children's interactions with surrounding objects, and knowledge is a direct product of motor behavior [9]. Children are active participants in their life and acquire knowledge through engaging in activities. By comparison, infants, through sensorimotor actions at the sensory-perceptual level, understand objects and acquire initial intelligence via assimilation and accommodation. As mentioned above, perception originates from the psychological process of sensory and brain stimulation, while memory involves storing past experiences in the mind. Piaget referred to the experiences retained in the mind and stored in the form of mental activities and mental representations as schemas, which are the smallest units of psychological operation. When a stimulus appears, individuals assimilate it by perceiving and understanding it in accordance with their existing cognitive frameworks. Infants constantly incorporate new experiences into pre-existing schemas through assimilation, which allows their schemas to become more complex and refined. However, when a new object or experience fails to be assimilated into existing schemas, the pre-existing schemas are modified to adapt to reality, the process of which is known as accommodation. On the other hand, the process of using new methods to deal with problems failed to be solved by previous methods is referred to as adjustment [6, 13].

Children's language skills develop with age. When they begin to use words to process schemas, intellectual activities enter the realm of conceptual symbols, indicating the beginning of symbolization of schemas. Operations refer to mental procedures and the transformation of information processing, involving linking two entities according to specific rules. Addition and subtraction are examples of operations, where "sum" and "difference" represent the rules of "adding" and "subtracting" quantities. One important characteristic of operations is reversibility, namely the reversible relationship between two entities. Operations are the primary forms of concrete and abstract thinking, and children must possess the concept of conservation when engaging in operations. Conservation signifies the inherent property of objects remaining unchanged, serving as the basis for mental operations. Only on the basis of conservation can children engage in cognitive operations such as comparison, classification, categorization, and ordering. Schemas, representations, concepts, symbols, and operations are fundamental cognitive units of human cognition. Most cognitive activities in humans are purposeful and directed processes. For example, problem-solving involves monitoring and coordinating perception, memory and reasoning, integrating existing experiences, formulating hypotheses, and making decisions. Directed thinking emerges during early childhood, and evolves into advanced forms in adolescence.

2.4.2 Maturation, Experience, and Equilibration

The emergence of certain behavioral patterns in children is dependent on the maturity level of the nervous system, as neurological maturation is a necessary condition for psychological development [13]. According to Piaget, apart from the neurological maturation and formation of children's own experiences through activities, the social environment and the social experiences acquired by them are also requisite factors influencing their psychological development. The social environment plays a crucial role in facilitating children's socialization, and Piaget observed that the stages, trends, and outcomes of children's intellectual development are similar, regardless of the specific social environment in which they live. He also believed that the social environment is not a determinant of children's psychological development, but only affects its rate; instead, it is equilibration, namely the process of continuous automatic adjustment and constant pursuit of balance, that determines psychological growth [13]. Equilibration ensures the coordination of maturation, physical experiences, and social experiences, and gradually progresses toward reversibility. Reversibility is a system for perfection and compensation, ensuring that the process of automatic adjustment always remains in dynamic equilibrium which allows for psychological self-regulation. During children's psychological development, if a state of equilibrium is disrupted and is not automatically readjusted to reach a new equilibrium for an extended period, it can lead to psychological abnormalities.

2.4.3 Process of Children's Psychological Development

According to Piaget, children's psychological development is a continuous and stage-based process, and each stage has its specific psychological structures and exhibits certain age-related characteristics. The stages develop in a predetermined sequence and cannot be skipped or reversed. Each stage is the result of the preceding stage and lays the foundation for the subsequent stage. Entering a new stage does not imply the disappearance of the previous stage but rather represents a positive inclusion and integration. Therefore, a higher stage always has more complex structures and more comprehensive functions than the preceding stage [9, 13]. Actions are the bridge connecting the subject and the surrounding objects, and children can only acquire actual knowledge through their concrete and spontaneous activities. Piaget's views on activity have significant implications for child education and pediatric clinical diagnosis and treatment. Adequately organized, guided, and facilitated activities will provide children with the necessary conditions for psychological development and promote their intellectual growth.

2.4.4 Piaget's Stages of Cognitive Development

Piaget divided the intellectual development of children into four stages: the sensorimotor stage, the preoperational stage, the concrete operational stage, and the formal operational stage.

2.4.4.1 Sensorimotor Stage (0–2 Years Old)

This is the earliest stage of cognitive development, where infants and toddlers establish connections with the external world via their initial reflexive actions, and then use habitual and generalized actions (such as touching, pushing, and pulling) developed through repeated practice to solve real-world problems. Piaget viewed generalized actions as a form of sensorimotor thinking and an expression of intelligence. It is evident that actions are crucial in children's intellectual development.

2.4.4.2 Preoperational Stage (2–7 Years Old)

In this stage, children learn to use language and to think with representations, capable of engaging in symbolic plays such as doll play or drawing. Language and representations allow children to extend their thinking beyond the immediate activities and into a broader sense of time and space. Although their thinking becomes more flexible, they still cannot grasp the essence of objects and lack the concept of "conservation" regarding changes in object form. For example, when plasticine is rolled into a long strip, they would think its quantity or weight has changed. Constrained by concrete thinking, they lack the systematic and logical thinking adults have.

2.4.5 Concrete Operational Stage (7–11 Years Old) and Formal Operational Stage (12–18 Years Old)

During these stages, children's thinking becomes more advanced. They begin to free themselves from the constraints of concrete objects and engage in abstract thinking using language, word, or symbols. By this point, children understand that the quantity of an object does not change with changes in its form or appearance. After the age of 12, they can engage in deductive reasoning based on hypotheses or propositions, and their intellectual development tends toward maturity.

2.5 Other Theories in Developmental Psychology

Theories of child psychological development explain the trends, patterns, dynamics, and processes of children's psychological development, but different schools of thought in the field have different theoretical emphases. Piaget laid particular stress on children's actions, considering them as the starting point of intellectual activity. He believed that the essence of actions lies in the subject's adaptation to the object, and that subject's adaptation to the object through actions is the real cause of child psychological development. Neo-Piagetian theorists, however, suggest that the equilibration resulted from social regulations is the primary factor impacting individual cognitive development, and social cognitive conflicts are the main mechanism underlying cognitive development. Other psychological developmental theories, such as Freud's psychoanalytic theory, J. Watson's classical behaviorism, and B. Skinner's neo-behaviorism, have endowed us with a deeper understanding of children's psychological and intellectual development from different angles. For example, Skinner proposed that behavior is determined by the results of the activity, and infants' behavior can be controlled through reinforcement. If they receive the same response from adults for their smiles and vocalizations, their social communication behavior will increase (paying attention to the face of caregiver). Learning must be accomplished through operating actions. A. Bandura, the founder of social learning theory, believed that in social contexts, individuals imitate the behavior of others through observation. Research on cognitive information processing theory has found that preschoolers have a good understanding of numbers, and most 4-year-olds can perform simple additions and subtractions by counting and successfully compare different quantities [9, 15, 16].

2.6 Theoretical Foundations of Erxin Scales Items for Each Age Group

Piaget's theory of cognitive development guides both the development and revision of the Erxin Scales. Considering that the scale is for assessing and monitoring children aged 0–6 years, the cognitive development in the sensorimotor and preoperational stages will be the focus here to delineate the theoretical foundations and underlying framework of the scales' item design.

2.6.1 Birth to 2 Years of Age

According to Piaget, the sensorimotor stage begins at birth, and the earliest schemas infants possess are conditioned reflexes, such as sucking. During the early exploration of their environment, infants engage in processes of assimilation and accommodation to modify their early simple schemas. As they grow older and their motor skills improve, these schemas become increasingly complex. The development of motor skills is indicative of the potential for higher-level cognitive development. Maturation is one of the determinants of psychological development, and the significance of both natural and social environmental influences increases as children grow.

2.6.1.1 Newborns

Innate reflexes play a central role in newborns' cognitive development and determine the nature of their interaction with the world. The sucking reflex, as the earliest schema in newborns, leads them to suck on toys or objects in a similar manner, allowing them to assimilate the objects into their existing sucking schema. Subsequently, newborns respond to the environment through reflexive activities, such as sucking any item placed near their lips.

2.6.2   1–4 Months of Age

Infants' activities during this stage focus primarily on their own bodies, constituting what Piaget called primary schemas. Infants aged 1–4 months begin to coordinate individual actions into unified and integrated activities. For example, when an infant grasps a teething stick, he/she may also suck on it, combining the grasping and sucking actions. Infants adjust their original schemas to accommodate to the essence of the world based on their reflexive experiences. In the case of mixed feeding, for instance, if a baby receives both breastfeeding and bottle feeding (using artificial nipple) in one feeding session, he/she may adjust or change the sucking posture based on the sensory difference between the mother's nipple and the artificial nipple to facilitate the feeding process.

2.6.3   4–8 Months of Age

During this stage, infants begin to interact with the external world by shifting their cognitive focus beyond their own bodies. When in contact with the objective environment, infants develop their understanding through active engagement and personal experiences, and exert intentional influences on objects through simple motor actions. For example, 4-month-olds may show excitement and attempt to grasp when hearing someone playing a bell stick or a rattle drum. Based on this phenomenon, a new item is added to the Erxin Scale to assess 6-month-olds' ability to imitate and produce sound by clapping objects in response to social cues and interactions. Another typical example is the "Peek-A-Boo" test for infants aged 6 months or older. In this test, if the tester peeks and makes a sound from the same direction where an A4 paper is placed horizontally along the long side for two times, the infant will then wait in the direction where the tester previously peeked. This demonstrates that infants incorporate their experience into their active schemas and adjust themselves to adapt to reality. As infants begin to act on the external world, their cognitive development accelerates.

2.6.4   8–12 Months of Age

After reaching 8 months of age, infants start to exhibit goal-directed behaviors. During this stage, they can coordinate the purpose and method of their actions, overcome obstacles, and solve problems. They develop a concept of object permanence and can combine multiple schemas to generate a single behavior to solve a problem. For example, infants can find a toy that was just hidden under a pillow in front of them or partially covered in a certain location. When their maturity reaches a certain level, indirect actions will be used to achieve their goals. Once they start crawling, infants can maneuver around obstacles such as chairs to reach toys in distant places.

2.6.5   12–18 Months of Age

According to Piaget, intentional behavioral changes during this period lead to the formation of result-oriented schemas. Intentional behavioral changes bring about desired outcomes. Toddlers in this stage exhibit new exploratory behaviors and utilize tools. They not only engage in repeated enjoyable activities but also explore the causes of events through trial and error. For example, toddlers around the age of 1 often repetitively throw an empty feeding bottle or a bottle with leftover milk, using eye contact to communicate to the adult that it has fallen, resulting in the adult picking up the bottle with a smile. Moreover, they may enjoy repeatedly changing the position of toys or pouring building blocks from one container to another. Their next attempt or repetitive action will occur despite that not all blocks may fall inside the container or the container may not be able to hold them all. When pouring blocks, toddlers may perceive the different sounds produced by different containers or explore the varied states that arise from placing blocks in different containers (e.g., the container being too large to fill or the blocks overflowing when the container is too small). Toddlers in this stage engage in unplanned exploration and understanding of objects. Their curiosity about the surrounding world attracts them to anything novel or unexpected.

2.6.6   18–24 Months of Age

Symbolic thinking emerges at this stage, marking the beginning of thinking. Piaget suggests that only entering this stage can toddlers imagine where objects they cannot see might be. They will search for things that have been hidden from their direct sight and can imagine the possible trajectory of unseen objects. For example, when a toddler tries to reach a faucet on a countertop (to play with water) but fails, he/she will bring a small chair to stand on. Similarly, when pushing a large toy car into a bedroom (where the width of the car is close to the width of the door, and the length of the car is approximately twice its width), the toddler will adjust the direction multiple times (moving the car left and right, pushing it forward, and pulling it back) until the car is successfully pushed into the bedroom. The acquisition of mental representations or symbolic thinking abilities is the focus of this stage. Mental representations, namely internal images of past events or objects [9], enable the development of the ability to pretend, such as pretending to feed a doll or pretending to be a pilot or driver. Deferred imitation, defined by Piaget as a child's ability to imitate someone's past actions, provides clear evidence for the formation of internal representation in children [9]. Based on this concept, a new item is added to the Erxin Scales which assesses the capacity for role-playing, and the lack of imagination (such as being incapable of pretending) is considered a communication warning behavior for 21-month-olds.

2.6.7 2 to 7 Years of Age

Operations are organized, structured, and logical mental processes. Children in the preoperational stage (2–7 years old) are not yet capable of operations, but they can use symbols to represent people, objects, and locations in their surroundings, and also use words to represent objects and actions. Noteworthily, differences in physical development, language development, and thinking forms exist between children in the early phase of the preoperational stage and preschoolers in the later phase. For example, 4- to 24-month-olds mainly rely on the visual system to control gross motor skills and maintain balance, whereas 3- to 6-year-olds begin to use somatosensory information to control their balance abilities. The cognitive developmental characteristics of 2- to 3-year-old toddlers and 4- to 7-year-old preschoolers will be elaborated separately.

2.6.7.1 2–3 Years of Age
When in contact with the surface phenomena of external objects, 2-year-olds start to develop a lower form of thinking known as sensorimotor

thinking. Children of this age start using their own rules to perceive and think about the things around them. They also begin to use symbols to represent people, objects, and locations, reacting to new stimuli or events and modifying their existing thoughts, understanding, or behaviors to accommodate new information. For example, a toddler at 2.5 years of age calls a nearly spherical pumpkin "ball." In this case, the children assimilates the pumpkin into his/her existing schema of balls (because he/she already has a similar-sized green ball). However, if told that it is a round pumpkin and shown how it rolls when pushed, the children may then say "pumpkin ball" when seeing a round pumpkin again. This demonstrates his/her accommodation of new knowledge and modification of the related schema.

Children after the age of 2 can separate themselves from objects and learn to use pronouns like "I," "you," and "he/she." Schema processing begins to take the form of words. The sensory perception of 2- to 3-year-olds becomes more refined, allowing them to discern colors, grasp some vocabulary related to space and time, and distinguish concepts like up and down, front and back, near and far, and more and less. Additionally, they gradually develop an understanding of object size, shape, and even weight based on external physical experiences (e.g., they may describe heavier objects as "too heavy" or say they cannot lift them). During imagination or role-playing games, they may anthropomorphize most objects, treating them as if they have life. For example, if they have experienced getting hurt from a fall, they may ask if a stuffed koala toy feels pain when they accidentally press it under a toy car. Similarly, if a leaf is torn, they may ask, "Does the leaf feel pain?".

From ages 2 to 3 years, human thinking emerges and starts to develop. During this phase, children are capable of using words to classify and generalize certain external features of objects, such as size, color, and shape. However, they are unable to generalize based on the essential characteristics of objects. For example, a 2-year-and-9-month-old child may have only a superficial understanding of the concept of a "little brother." When seeing a boy who is smaller in size, the child's parents may refer to him as a "little brother" or a "little kid." However, when the child's grandfather introduces his own brother by saying, "This is my little brother," the child may respond by saying, "He is grandpa, not a little brother." This is because, in the child's previous experiences, a little brother is synonymous with a little kid. After reaching 2 and a half years of age, children not only acquire the ability to say "This is mine," but they also invert pronouns in conversations. For instance, when an adult asks, "Should I give this to you?" the child would respond, "You give it to me."

By the age of 3, children's utilization of concepts expands, including the comprehension and correct application of temporal concepts such as morning and evening. Subsequently, there is a qualitative change in their thinking abilities, with the emergence of mental reasoning and an increasing proficiency in language usage.

Egocentrism is a cognitive characteristic of the preoperational stage and constitutes the core of children's behavior during this phase. Egocentric thinking refers to a mindset that cannot consider the perspectives of others, adopt or choose others' suggestions, and lacks awareness of seeing things from different viewpoints. In the preoperational stage, the most prominent manifestation of egocentric thinking is observed in hide-and-seek games. Children around the age of 3 may hide their bodies behind a curtain while their feet, hands, or clothes remain visible. They believe that they have successfully concealed themselves, assuming that if they cannot see others, others cannot see them either. During this period, children often persist in their own activities and overlook situations where someone speaking to them requires a timely response, and may even ignore the presence of others due to immersion in their games. For example, a 2-year-and-10-month-old child, upon being picked up from daycare by the mother, becomes ecstatic and dances around without considering the people around or whether he/she is blocking anyone's path. The child may even lie on the ground, roll around, and ignore or disregard the mother's warnings (about the ground being dirty or the street being unsafe) until he/she is done playing. While playing with building blocks, children at this age often disrupt the constructions made by others, refuse to share their preferred items, and are unwilling to let other children play with toys they themselves are not interested in. These behaviors are not indicative of disobedience or selfishness in young children, nor do they imply a lack of consideration for others or eccentricity. Instead, they reflect the characteristics of egocentric thinking. The children's disregard for others, actions ignoring the presence of others, and the self-directed nature of their thoughts and behaviors all indicate that they are not aware that their actions can elicit reactions from others, nor do they realize that the person speaking to them requires a timely response. This is because the majority of language behaviors in young children or preschoolers are not driven by social motivations but are only meaningful to themselves [9].

2.6.7.2   4–7 Years of Age

Preschoolers are in the later phase of cognitive development in the preoperational stage. Their sensorimotor skills become more refined, and they transition from symbolic thinking to intuitive thinking of the conceptual thinking stage. The use of language enables children's thinking to be freed from the constraints of the present and the future, and the application of symbolic representations through behavior allows for faster thinking. According to Piaget, progress in thinking at the sensorimotor stage is necessary for the development of language. Language and thinking are closely related, as language development stems from cognitive progress, and continuous growth in cognitive abilities provides a foundation for the development of language skills [9]. Preschoolers tend to focus only on the visible, surface-level, and salient parts of stimuli, without considering the whole. This leads to inaccuracies in their judgments. For example, when an equal amount of juice was distributed into two different cups—one short and wide, and the other tall and narrow—most 4-year-olds would believe that the latter cup contains more juice. The reason for this erroneous judgment is that children at this age have not yet mastered the concept of conservation [9]. However, by the age of 5 and a half, the majority of children have learned the conservation of length. For instance, if presented with a rope and a slightly shorter ruler, with the ends of the rope pulled to those of the ruler, preschoolers would perceive the rope as longer, whereas younger children would say they have the same length [6].

2.7   Basic Theories and Techniques for Scale Development

Piaget's theory of cognitive development and the gradually increasing cognitive abilities provided the theoretical foundation for the initial development of the Erxin Scales. Piaget's theory emphasizes the crucial role played by the constantly and automatically coordinated equilibration of maturation, experience acquired from activities, and social environment in cognitive development, which also highlights the necessity for scale revision. Incorporating negative indicators of social communication through observation and interviews helps reveal the impact on developing individuals when the dynamic state of equilibration is disrupted. The theoretical basis of cognitive development for the development of the Erxin Scales has been discussed earlier. Ensuring the construct validity of the scale requires not only a solid foundation in cognitive development theory but also scale development expertise and psychometric techniques such as quality control. Psychometrics is the science of psychological measurement [17], and the preparation of psychological tests is both a scientific and artistic endeavor [18]. Psychological tests represent a disciplinary means of inferring and quantitatively analyzing psychological characteristics that permeate all human activities based on the observation of a limited number of representative behaviors [19]. Scale development should first comply with psychometric requirements, which is a prerequisite for subsequent scale application. Therefore, it is equally important to be equipped with psychometric expertise regarding specific scale development procedure, such as the methods for analyzing psychometric properties. Guided by the theory of cognitive development, the Erxin Scales specifies the test purpose, subjects, and applications, and determines the test item design. The planning and procedure for scale revision and item development, including details such as the time window, must follow the psychometric scale development process. Quality control should also be conducted according to the technical specifications of the scale standards.

The original version of the Erxin Scales was developed by combining longitudinal tracking and observations of healthy newborns from ordinary families in Beijing with cross-sectional validations. After that, a nationwide collaborative multicenter research team was established, and specialized training in operating methods was given by core personnel. A nationally representative sample was then selected to conduct normative research on the scale, including reliability and validity tests, to establish standardized norms for the whole country.

To ensure the quality and validity of the revised Erxin Scales meet the psychometric requirements, a revision roadmap was developed following the scale development procedure. While considering the overall design, measurement dimensions, and item weights, universal research materials were collected, including observation methods and descriptions of milestones from famous developmental scales. The test items were designed and modified based on the observation of developmental milestones in infants and young children, as well as their living skills and social communication abilities. A special clinical testing phase for main test ages or target ages was added, where test items needed to pass clinical screening before entering the item pool, ensuring quality control throughout the revision process. An item pool was finally established after clarifying the dimensions to be added, new test items to be included to each dimension, as well as the items to be modified or removed. Item testing was then conducted to select those qualified to be included in the original revised scale, where the operations and passing criteria were modified further. Subsequently, another nationwide collaborative multicenter research team (similar to the one organized during the scale development phase) was formed, and specialized training in operational methods was provided by core personnel. Finally, a nationwide sample was selected to complete the test according to the designated time frame, and after a series of complex technical operations, reliability and validity tests were conducted, and the national norms and DQ evaluation criteria were established (see Chapter 7 for details). During the ten-year revision of the scale, the strict adherence to the revision roadmap and a full-cycle standardized quality control system together ensured that the revised scale reached the psychometric standards. In addition, from the viewpoint of modern psychometric development which emphasizes the construction of theoretical models for developmental scales, this revision not only performed basic psychometric analyses regarding discrimination, reliability, and validity, but also used LISREL, a specialized software for confirmatory factor analysis, to examine the relationship between the factors and conceptual models. The results showed good model fit for the revised scale data. Further details related to the specific psychometric properties of the revised scale are discussed in Chapter 4.

2.8 Commonly Used Child Developmental Scales and Their Applicability Analysis

Scales used for assessing infants and young children are called developmental scales. Though many frequently employed developmental scales are applicable for children aged 0–3 years, some have a wider age range which reaches 6 years or older. During children's psychological growth, intellectual development exhibits a sequential pattern, with the manifestation of cognitive activities differing across various ages. In other words, psychological abilities of children in different age groups possess distinct characteristics [18]. The reason most scales for comprehensively assessing children under 6 years of age are referred to as developmental scales is related to the brain development and especially its high plasticity in this population. In the first years of life, many regions of the brain have not yet differentiated for specific tasks, and the brain exhibits the greatest plasticity in that if one region is impaired, other regions can assume its function [9]. Hence, infants with brain damage are less affected and can recover more completely than adults with similar injuries [9, 20–23]. Due to the susceptibility of infants' psychological development to environmental influences, the abilities developed during infancy differ from the nature of intellectual development in later stages [24]. The intellectual development can be accelerated through good early education, or it can be slowed down if a child fails to receive a supportive environment and appropriate education during critical periods. In the absence of any brain injuries or abnormalities, children's intellectual development depends primarily on the environment and education, which cannot be predicted through scale testing. Therefore, all developmental scales chiefly aim to measure the current developmental status of infants and young children, with the core purpose being the screening or diagnosis of children with developmental delays, rather than predicting future levels of ability. Research has shown that parental education level and occupation have a better predictive value for later intelligence quotient (IQ) compared to test scores during infancy [18], indicating that the brain's plasticity provides room for early education and repair of brain damage, which in turn contributes to the poor predictability of early developmental assessment results in terms of children's IQ levels.

From a cognitive perspective, the psychological and physiological development during infancy and early childhood are closely intertwined, and psychological development depends on the maturation and functional improvement of the nervous system. However, school-age children's physical growth tends to stabilize, and their psychological activities become relatively independent. After the age of 6, the psychological development of children gradually separates from their physical growth. Cognitive assessment scales for children aged 6 and above are generally referred to as intelligence tests, but some of these are for children aged 4 and above, such as the Wechsler Preschool and Primary Scale of Intelligence-Revised (WPPSI-R) which is used to evaluate children aged 4–6 years. Another type of scales reflects individuals' practical application of cognitive functions. Collectively referred to as adaptive behavior scales, they quantitatively assess independent living skills and social communication abilities needed in normal daily living, and are commonly used as supplementary tools for assessing developmental delays or the extent of intellectual disabilities.

2.8.1 Commonly Used Child Developmental Scales

In China, the development and introduction of developmental scales have lagged behind. Most of the internationally renowned Western scales that have been previously introduced and are currently in use are outdated versions. The commonly used developmental scales in China, such as Bayley Scales of Infant Development, Gesell Developmental Schedules, Griffiths Mental Development Scales, and Denver Developmental Screening Test, are briefly introduced as follows.

2.8.1.1 Bayley Scales of Infant Development

The Bayley Scales of Infant Development (BSID) is one of the most widely adopted developmental assessment tools for infants and toddlers. The original BSID was developed in 1933 and standardized in 1969 [19]. A stratified sample of 1262 infants and toddlers was collected for scale development, taking into account variables such as age, gender, race, urban and rural proportions, and parental education level, ensuring good representativeness [18]. The original BSID released by the American Psychological Association in 1969 is applicable for 2- to 30-month-olds.

It comprises three parts: the Mental Scale, the Motor Scale, and the Infant Behavior Record.

The Mental Scale includes 163 items that can be classified into five categories: (1) sensory acuity and accuracy, discrimination, responsiveness, and memory; (2) object permanence; (3) learning and response ability; (4) vocalization, vocabulary, and communication ability; (5) concept formation and classification.

The Motor Scale evaluates both gross motor and fine motor skills, consisting of 81 items, which can be classified as: (1) control of one's own body; (2) coordination of gross body movements; (3) fine motor skills of the hands and coordination of movements.

The Infant Behavior Record consists of 24 items and covers aspects such as emotional development, attention span, social behavior, interests, personal orientation, and cooperative behavior. Noteworthily, it provides information on children's mental development and adaptive abilities to the environment but is not involved in scoring. The items in the scales are arranged in order of difficulty and scored dichotomously (pass or fail). The results are indicated by the Mental Development Index (MDI) and the Psychomotor Development Index (PDI). In 1992, a revision of the original BSID was completed in Hunan Province, China [25], and since then it has been frequently applied to the clinical and research settings in the country.

The original BSID was revised subsequently by its team as BSID-II in 1993 and BSID-III in 2006 [26]. The revisions expanded the age range of the original BSID to 1–42 months. Additionally, the number of items in the Mental Scale increased from the original 163 to 178 in the first revision and to 188 in the second revision, while that in the Motor Scale increased from the original 81 to 111 and 138, respectively. The Infant Behavior Record was expanded to 30 items in BSID-II, on the basis of which items assessing social emotions and adaptive behaviors were added to BSID-III. This in turn resulted in the 35-item Social-Emotional Scale which serves as a substitute for the Greenspan Social-Emotional Growth Chart: A Screening Questionnaire for Infants and Young Children, and also the Adaptive Behavior Assessment System-Second Edition (ABAS-II) [26].

Moreover, BSID-III further expanded the original Mental Scale and refined it into a 91-item Cognitive Scale; the Language Scale consists of 97 items (49 for receptive communication and 48 for expressive communication); in the 138-item Motor Scale, 72 items are for gross motor skills and 66 for fine motor skills. As for the ABAS-II, it evaluates infants and young children across ten skill dimensions: Communication, Community Use, Functional Academics, Health and Safety, Home or School Living, Leisure, Self-Care, Self-Direction, Social, and Work. Each dimension has different sub-domains. Taking the Communication dimension as an example, its sub-domains include speaking, language, listening, and nonverbal communication skills, each with four different response options [26] that should be filled out by parents or primary caregivers. Currently, we have not yet introduced the new edition for revision.

2.8.1.2 Gesell Development Schedules
The Gesell Development Schedules (GDS) is devised by Dr. Arnold Gesell, a pediatrician at the Yale School of Medicine, in collaboration with several co-workers, to assist in distinguishing between typical and atypical

child development by comparing their behaviors. If a child deviates significantly from the norms for a specific age, his/her development would be considered atypical (either delayed or advanced). Based on years of observation of developmental behaviors in infants and young children, Gesell identified 4, 16, 28, 40, and 52 weeks, as well as 18, 24, and 36 months as key ages featured by critical milestones in development. These key ages represent transitional periods in development, where dramatic behavioral changes occur, indicating the arrival of new developmental stages. Consequently, they are the most appropriate stages for observing and assessing children's development. Based on the concept of key ages, Gesell proposed the developmental progress charts, prescribed the operational procedures, and devised a developmental scale that was officially published in 1940 and then revised subsequently in 1947 and 1974 [1, 9].

The scale consists of four schedules focusing respectively on motor behavior (gross motor and fine motor), adaptive behavior, language behavior, and personal-social behavior. It emphasizes the importance of developmental sequences and effectively reflects the maturation patterns of the nervous system. It is designed to evaluate children with developmental abnormalities, and the 1974 revised edition covers the age range from 4 weeks to 5 years [26]. Based on observations and parental reports, the assessor can explore the scoring of each schedule and reveal the link between the resulting scores and actual age to calculate the DQs for the schedules. Moreover, developmental delays are categorized into mild, moderate, and severe levels to provide guidance for clinical interventions. The classic GDS can be used as a supplementary tool in medical examinations for neurological disorders and organic behavioral abnormalities.

The Gesell Institute of Child Development finished a three-year study nationwide by 2010 [27], which included the assessment of data from 1,287 children aged 3 to 6 years. In the next year, the institute released the research data and standards for the Gesell Developmental Observation-Revised (GDO-R), which is used to assess children at 3–6 years of age. However, this assessment tool has not been introduced to China to date.

Nevertheless, regional revisions of GDS's 1974 edition had been conducted in Beijing and Shanghai. Specifically, the revision in Beijing experienced two stages, one in 1985 and the other in 1992 [24, 26, 28], extending the assessment tool's age range to 6 years. Although only with regional norms, GDS has enjoyed wide clinical application in China.

2.8.1.3 Griffiths Mental Development Scales

The Griffiths Mental Development Scales (GMDS) is a child assessment tool based on the observation of natural activities of children in Western societies, such as walking, talking, playing, and learning [29]. It is used for the age group starting from birth to 8 years. R. Griffiths believed that play is a universal experience in all cultures. The standardization of the 0–2 years part of GMDS was completed in 1996, whereas the 2–8 years part was standardized in 2006. To date, the GMDS-ER (Griffiths Mental Development Scales, Extended Revised) has been widely used by pediatricians and psychologists in many Caucasian countries [29]. From 2009 to 2013, the GDS-C (Griffiths Development Scales-Chinese) was adopted to evaluate the developmental status of 815 typically developing children aged 7 days to 8 years (424 boys and 391 girls) sampled from seven cities in China (including Hong Kong) [30]. The results showed that the Chinese data exhibited similar trends as the British data which were collected using GMDS-ER. However, both similarities and differences existed between the developmental curves of the Chinese children and British children [30].

The comparatively late introduction of GMDS to China makes its application here currently in the exploratory stage. In the future, it needs to be validated nationwide in China and standardized on a representative sample according to the standards in psychometrics related to scale revision procedures, processes, and quality control.

2.8.1.4 Denver Developmental Screening Test

The Denver Developmental Screening Test (DDST), developed by W. K. Frankenburg and J. Dodds, is one of the commonly used tools for screening developmental delays in infants and young children. It is designed for children aged 2 months to 6 years, and has 105 items arranged by difficulty [19] to assess four developmental areas: (1) personal-social development, including early social interaction and self-care behaviors, such as responding to adults' cues and searching objects; (2) fine motor/adaptive development, including hand manipulation and hand–eye coordination; (3) gross motor development, reflected by gross body movement control, including sitting, standing, walking, running, and jumping; and (4) language development, which includes both expressive and receptive languages. The test scores are classified into three screening levels: normal, suspicious, and abnormal, aiming to identify potential developmental delays or abnormalities at an early stage.

In China, the standardization of DDST (1967 edition) had been conducted in 1978 and 1979 by administering the test to representative samples across the country. Unfortunately, some data in the southern region were damaged due to natural disasters (floods), and only the data from six provinces and cities in the northern region were analyzed to establish the Chinese version of the DDST [26]. Thanks to its ease of administration, scoring, and interpretation, as well as short testing time (typically 10–30 minutes), DDST is widely used in clinical practice in China. However, if the child being tested is not cooperative for various reasons and takes more than 30 minutes to finish the test, a result of "suspicious" may be presented, which fails to adequately adapt to Chinese culture and current medical development. Nevertheless, the original developers of DDST revised and standardized the tool in 1990, and in China regional revisions of DDST were conducted in Chongqing, Nanjing, and Shanghai in 1997 and 2002, respectively [26].

2.8.1.5 Self-Developed Child Developmental Scales in China

In mainland China, many assessment scales used for child development are introduced or adapted from outdated foreign versions, with slight modifications made to fit the domestic context, followed by standardization. Only a few of its developmental scales are self-developed based on large samples and conform to psychometric procedures with the reliability and validity tested. Two such scales are as follows.

(a) **CDCC Developmental Scales for Children Aged 0–3 Years**: This was developed under the leadership of Cunren Fan at IPCAS from 1985 to 1987 based on a national sample of 1,600 children ranging from 2 months old to 3 years old, and CDCC stands for the Child Development Center of China [26, 31]. The scales include 121 items in the intellectual domain and 61 items in the motor domain. Similar to BSID, it utilizes MDI and PDI to indicate the test results, so some consider it a simplified version of BSID. However, this tool has not gained wide application despite its standardization.

(b) **Developmental Scales for Chinese Children Aged 3–6 years (Urban Version)**: This was devised by Houcan Zhang on the basis of a pilot study conducted in 1988 with a sample of 500 participants. In 1992, the normative study was completed with a sample of 2,368 participants. It consists of two parts: the Intellectual Development Subscale and the Motor Development Subscale [26]. Likewise, its application is limited.

2.8.2 Applicability Analysis of the Commonly Used Developmental Scales

BSID and GDS, providing a series of ordered, continuous, and standardized quantitative data that give insight into children's developmental levels, can objectively distinguish whether the children are ahead of or behind their peers by assessing their development, and are particularly useful in screening significant developmental delays [9, 32, 33]. These scales are mostly adopted or revised in Europe, America, Asia, and Africa. Technically, BSID-III is deemed the best assessment tool for infants and young children because of its expanded test content, enriched details, and comprehensive scoring system. In addition to diagnosing developmental delays, it provides developmental index scores and reference percentages, as well as percentile ranks and confidence intervals for each subscale within their respective age range, allowing for the determination of the degree of deviation from the normative developmental level. Although it may be challenging to apply BSID-III to clinical settings, it is internationally favored as an assessment tool in psychological experiments and scientific research. BSID has its origins in the research conducted on infant samples from the most developed countries in the world, with better living environments and higher levels of education compared to underdeveloped countries and regions. Due to the complexity of the tool's test content and scoring system, strict and long-term training is required for operators to master its administration. Interpreting the test results also demands a solid theoretical knowledge base. It requires not only high professional competence of the assessors, but also high qualified parents or caregiver, because the portions of the tool designed to be filled out by parents or caregivers involve multiple rating levels. This poses significant challenges for its clinical application in China and other underdeveloped countries or regions.

Furthermore, considering that China's child health care management covers the age range of 0–6 years, BSID's applicable population is not wide enough and thus its use is relatively limited. The cost-effectiveness regarding health economics caused by its revision and administration in China needs to be further explored.

In terms of GDS, its 1974 edition consists of eight test sheets for eight key ages, with a total of 63 operational methods. The same operational item has different requirements at different ages, and the standards for passing the items also vary. Such a sequential test design is equivalent to expanding the number of the scale items several times [6], which in effect requires a higher level of proficiency and professional knowledge from the assessors. Owing to the complexity of the operational, observational, and scoring criteria of the scale, it is also challenging to promote its nationwide use. Despite being a classic developmental tool, GDS's 1974 edition is nearly 50 years old, and social changes necessitate timely updates and introduction of new standardized versions in order to accurately assess today's children.

In a study conducted by Shanshan Xu and others in China, 457 normal infants and young children were assessed using BSID-III. The results revealed higher scores for the Cognitive, Language, and Motor Scales ($P < 0.001$) whereas lower scores for ABAS-II ($P < 0.001$) compared with the American reference norms; additionally, girls outperformed boys in the Cognitive, Language, and Social-Emotional Scales ($P < 0.05$). It was hence concluded that certain differences existed in child development between China and the United States [26, 34]. The research data also demonstrated that the correlation coefficient between the Motor Scale's composite scores and GDS's motor quotients was 0.367, that between the Cognitive Scale's composite scores and GDS's adaptability quotients was 0.164, and that between the Language Scale's composite scores and GDS's language quotients was 0.119. From the above correlation coefficients, it is clear that only a low correlation was discovered regarding motor quotients when evaluating Chinese children using developmental scales from the same developed Western country (one being BSID-III with no revision in China, and the other being the 1974 edition of GDS revised in China in 1985). This indicates that many issues need to be explored in the application of developmental scales from developed Western countries in China.

DDST has simple administration and scoring procedures, and standardized norms are available in China, resulting in a relatively high clinical utilization rate. However, its classification of the screening levels (especially the "suspicious" level) does not come with easily understandable, intuitive, and comparable references. This makes it less acceptable to

Chinese parents, and may even lead to their doubts about the competence of assessors and, in turn, foster a sense of distrust toward doctors. In Chinese culture, parents prefer to receive reference data that can be compared with their child's peers after an assessment, because this would enable them to better understand the child's developmental level and whether further actions are necessary.

Cross-cultural research based on GMDS has demonstrated differences in various domains of child development, including gross motor, fine motor, language, social communication, performance, and practical reasoning [30]. The discrepancy in developmental characteristics between Chinese and Caucasian children may be attributed to multiple factors, including cultural factors, parenting styles, and educational systems, all of which have a significant impact on child development [30].

In summary, the commonly used foreign scales that have been revised and are now widely used in China include the 1992 revision of the original BSID (1969 edition), Beijing's revision of GDS (1974 edition) in 1985 (for ages 0–3) and 1992 (for ages 3–6) with local norms established, Shanghai's revision of the same edition, and 1978–1979 revision of DDST (1967 edition) based on data from six provinces and cities in northern China. Most of these foreign scales are more than 50 years old, and 30 to 40 years have passed since the introduction and standardization of them in China, with only DDST's new edition revised in Chongqing and Shanghai. The challenge ahead is to address the issues of outdated scales, introducing new scales, and nationwide standardization.

It is crucial to devise developmental tools that are suitable for the local culture [30]. Most traditional intelligence tests from abroad were developed with English-speaking white middle-class participants, and children from different cultural backgrounds may perform poorly on these tests [9]. The issue of comparability warrants particular attention when using foreign scales with no or merely regional standardization in China to analyze the developmental levels of Chinese children [34–36].

Considering the impact of cultural factors, parenting styles, and educational systems on child development, as well as the parents' understanding and attitudes toward assessment results, it is highly necessary to devise developmental scales that are more culturally appropriate or have greater universality for children in developing countries. Additionally, when investigating the applicability of well-known scales from developed Western countries, it may be more meaningful to compare and analyze them with scales that have Chinese norms, such as the Erxin Scales.

Developmental scales for infants have greater predictive validity for atypical children, which can reach 0.60–0.70 for IQ scores below 80 [18]. As with other developmental scales, the predictive validity of GDS is proportional to the age of its participants [24]. It is vital to emphasize once again that all developmental scales primarily aim to measure the current developmental level of infants and toddlers, with the core purpose of screening or diagnosing developmental delays, rather than predicting future abilities.

2.9 INFLUENCE OF CULTURE AND ENVIRONMENT ON COGNITIVE DEVELOPMENT

2.9.1 Literature Review and Follow-Up Case Study

Many aspects of brain development occur automatically as genetically predetermined, but they are also malleable and can change as s function of the environment [9]. Let us take the case of Jianqiang to illustrate, a normally born healthy male infant who we had the opportunity to observe during his ongoing development. The infant demonstrated gross motor development: at 1 month of age, he could purposelessly lift both upper limbs and place them on the sides of his chest when lying supine; while lying prone, he responded to sounds, lifted his head off the bed surface, and occasionally raised his head upwards for a brief moment. He could raise his head to a 45° angle at 3 months of age, and to a 90° angle at 4 months (16 weeks). Moreover, he could roll over at almost 5 months (3 days shy), sit upright at 7 months, and crawl at 8 months. His motor development was consistent with the developmental norms of his same-age peers. However, Jianqiang only achieved the ability to stand with support at 10.5 months and began walking independently at 14 months, which were approximately 1.5 and 2 months later than his peers, respectively. At 2 years old, he was unable to jump off the ground with both feet, and even in the following months, he struggled to learn this skill. However, at 2 years and 7 months, he suddenly imitated others and could jump off the ground with both feet, achieving this skill 6 months later than the norm, almost approaching DDST's warning age. After approximately 3 weeks, he could jump down from a platform of about 3 cm in height without falling, and one month later (at 2 years and 9 months), he could continuously jump off the ground with both feet. At 2 years and 10 months, he could jump over a threshold approximately

3 cm high and 7–8 cm wide. This illustrates that the motor development in children is non-linear. Previous psychological studies show that color abstraction development predominates after the age of 3, and 3-year-old children can recognize 1–2 colors besides red. In the case of Jianqiang, he was observed at 2 years and 7 months to clearly and accurately identify four colors: red, black, yellow, and blue. He even distinguished orange from light yellow in various situations, consistently recognizing all four colors correctly. As regards language development, at 13 months old, he spontaneously extended his hand and said "nana" (meaning "take" in Mandarin) when seeing strawberries. At 14 months old, when asked how birds sound after he saw many sparrows chirping and flying in the trees during outdoor activities, he would respond with "jijizha" (imitating bird sounds). At 18 months old, he could understand daily instructions containing prepositional phrases, such as "put it in the box" or "grandfather is in the kitchen." At 2 years and 9 months old, he could construct simple compound sentences with hypotheses, such as "if the car is broken, let's ask grandfather to fix it," and he could also use object complements in Mandarin to express logical relationships, such as "Grandfather is too tall, so he cannot enter (a space that he can enter himself)." Clearly, the developmental rate in different domains varied for the same child. Jianqiang's gross motor development slowed down after he learned to crawl, while his language and color recognition developed significantly better than his gross motor skills. This may be related to excessive protection from the family to prevent falling and influenced by cultural and educational factors (the parents' emphasis on early education, starting to read picture books to the infant from 4 months of age during noon and evening every day).

Children are unique and although they develop at their own pace, the social and cultural background has a substantial influence on their growth, including the speed at which they reach different developmental milestones. As early as 1986, a longitudinal follow-up study conducted by Yuyan Mao [37] in China found that during the age range of 24–30 months, children were most susceptible to environmental influences, with a greater number of significant differences observed in language and adaptive behavior domains compared to fine motor skills. In the field of language skills, it was also found that there were gender differences in the expression of "don't want" among Chinese children, with girls exhibiting this ability earlier than boys, which differs from studies conducted in the United States at the time [37]. Chu-Sui Li, while revising the

Chinese version of the *Communication and Symbolic Behavior Scales*, pointed out that children developed in Chinese cultural backgrounds received significantly different scores on multiple subscales compared to the norms of American children, suggesting that infants and toddlers from different cultural backgrounds have differed levels of development in body movements, social communication, and other domains [38]. A study on Chinese language development in 2008 [39] indicated that among children aged 8–16 months, those from Beijing had a larger vocabulary repertoire than those from Hong Kong. From 16–30 months, children's vocabulary gradually expanded with age, but the total number of words produced by Hong Kong children was less than that by Beijing children. Additionally, during this stage, girls were 1–2 months ahead of boys in vocabulary and sentence development [39]. In terms of early speech production, a study on imitating parental words or phrases reported in the original English project showed that there were differences in the developmental levels between English-speaking children and Mandarin-speaking children. Taking the use of the verb "want" ("yao" in Mandarin) as an example, English-speaking children could generally imitate it at 11 months, while Mandarin-speaking children could only regularly imitate their parents' words and phrases after the age of 1; by 16 months, 70% of the children could imitate or use the verb, and over 50% could name objects (as used in the study). Although the percentage of Mandarin-speaking children who could imitate or use the verb was lower compared to English-speaking children, the overall developmental trend was similar between the two groups [39].

IQ is a product of the complex interaction between genetics and the environment. Intelligence is no longer viewed as solely determined by genes or experiences, as it is recognized that genes can influence experiences, which can in turn affect gene expression [9]. Yuyan Mao's longitudinal follow-up study of infants and toddlers [40] revealed that children raised in different family environments showed similar developmental processes regarding copy-drawing skills, possibly due to their similar innate abilities. Conversely, the development of drawing skills may vary considerably for children in the same daycare center or classroom where living conditions and educational opportunities were similar. The age at which children started drawing a certain shape could differ by three to four months, suggesting the influence of different innate abilities [40]. Yuyan Mao believed that for a child, the environment and education play a dominant role, but the impact of innate abilities should not be disregarded, as the two facets interact with each other [40]. Western and Asian societies have distinct cultural differences, such as Chinese children using chopsticks instead of knives and forks [41]. Statistical data published in the GMDS Manual by Boyle and others showed significant differences in the average scores for the motor subscale, with non-white children scoring nearly 6 points higher [42]. Therefore, clear cultural mismatch arises when assessing the developmental level of local children using foreign developmental scales, and without revision, it is difficult to eliminate the influence of regional differences, customs, socioeconomic factors, and cultural backgrounds.

2.9.2 Environmental Impact on Child Developmental Rate

2.9.2.1 Impact of Living Environments on Self-Care Abilities

The independent development of self-care abilities in infants and young children, including self-feeding, indicating the need to urinate and defecate, using the toilet, and managing cleanliness after using the toilet, is closely related to the maturation of the nervous system and the daily environmental conditions provided by caregivers. For instance, the ability to indicate urination or use the toilet without wetting the pants during the daytime are related to socioeconomic development, and parents' stance on child-rearing (e.g., when to start toilet training) also significantly influences children's self-care abilities. Infant Jianqiang mentioned above is a good case in point. He had worn diapers from birth and received no toilet training until the age of 30 months. After that, he stopped wearing diapers during the daytime and was trained to express the need to urinate by saying "pee-pee." Initially, Jianqiang only said it after urinating. Then, there were several instances that he became engrossed in play and forgot to say it, resulting in wetting his pants. Approximately one month later, he was able to indicate the urge to urinate by saying "pee-pee." At 33 months of age, he could take off his pants and urinate by himself, although occasionally he would urinate outside the toilet or on his pants and shoes due to inaccurate positioning. Data from a follow-up study conducted in the early 1980s [37] showed that 85% of infants and toddlers then were able to indicate urination or use a chamber pot by the age of 18 months, with the youngest being 11 months old. Disposable diapers were not yet available in China back then, and infants and toddlers mostly wore split crotch pants. Some parents started training their babies to urinate very early after birth, even seeking patterns by observing their facial expressions and other behaviors. In the United States, toilet training is also considered a reflection of an individual's independent living skills. Though lacking a uniform timing for it, data showed that in 1957, 92% of its 18-month-olds had received toilet training [9]; in 1999, however, 25% of its children received training at 18 months old, 60% at age 3, and 2% were still not trained at age 4 [9, 43]; most 18- to 24-month-olds had exhibited signs of being ready for toilet training, but some children might not be ready until the age of 30 months or older [44–46]. With the emergence and popularization of disposable diapers, both Chinese and American children have shown a delayed start of indicating urination during the day. Studies conducted in both countries revealed that toilet training for children has been pushed back by more than a year or even longer. Children's ability to indicate the urge to urinate during the day is influenced by factors such as economic development, changes in social and cultural environments, and the timing of toilet training. Piaget believed that the social environment affects children's psychological development rate, and self-care is an adaptive ability that individuals demonstrate in relation to nature and society. The use of disposable diapers has delayed the time when parents start toilet training for children, posing significant challenges for revising scales.

2.9.2.2 Impact of Inadequate Responsive Caregiving on Infant Development

A severely deprived and restricted environment can hinder brain development [9]. Taking one of my pediatric patients as an example: an 8-month-old daughter, brought by her father for a routine check-up, was noticed not making eye contact with others when being teased and not responding when her name was called during the examination. When the father was asked to recall the baby's behavior during feeding at home (formula-fed or bottle-fed), he hesitated for a moment before answering, "It seems like she didn't look at people either." Through communication with the baby's father, it was discovered that both parents were IT professionals, and they did not engage in much conversation between themselves. The father admitted that he rarely spoke to the baby at home and seldom interacted or played with her. Most of the time, the child would lie down and play by herself, and the caregivers often fed her while looking at the computer. The father was then advised to observe the baby at home for a week, and he reached the conclusion after referring to relevant online materials that the baby indeed had communication issues.

A week later, the parents came to the clinic to seek assistance (without bringing the child). They were provided with professional intervention guidance and practical training methods to be employed at home. Regular visits to professional institutions for training in parenting and caregiving were also recommended. At age 2, the father brought his little daughter to the clinic to express gratitude. Guided by her father, the girl smiled at me and sweetly said, "Hello, Grandma." The father added, "I brought my child here to thank you. You provided us with such great professional help. After more than a year of effort, our child's development and communication skills have reached normal standards."

Multiple factors interact to influence child development. During critical periods of brain growth, timely responsiveness and interaction from caregivers are crucial in infant caregiving. Even if adverse factors exist during these critical periods, brain function can be significantly improved by eliminating the unfavorable influences and offering multiple environmental stimuli [2]. The plasticity of the brain in early life gives infants an opportunity for compensation and catch-up growth, while favorable external environments are vital facilitators helping them restore normal development.

2.9.2.3 Impact of Early Screen Exposure on Infant and Toddler Development

Technological advancements have greatly facilitated people's life but also changed their behaviors. The exposure to electronic screens, for example, is a pressing issue posed to us. With the prevalence of electronic information technology and video platforms, early screen exposure in young children has become a global concern [47]. In recent years, cases of developmental delays in infants and toddlers due to excessive screen exposure are frequently encountered in pediatric clinics. Research has shown that the daily screen exposure time for children <18 months of age is 0.3 hours, while that for 18- to 36-month-old children is 1.2 hours [48]. Additionally, a survey was conducted on 357 children aged 0–36 months who visited developmental-behavioral clinics and rehabilitation centers, and 237 of them underwent developmental assessments using the Erxin Scales. In the age group of 0 to <18 months ($n = 62$), the median screen exposure time was 0.4 (0, 8.0) hours per day, while in the age group of 18–36 months ($n = 175$), the median was 3.0 (0, 12.5) hours. The Kruskal–Wallis test revealed a statistically significant difference between the two age groups ($\chi^2 = 72.807$, $p < 0.001$), with the older group featured by longer screen exposure time. When dividing the children based on their overall DQs, the group with DQ $\geq$ 80 ($n = 70$) had a median screen exposure time of 0.5 (0, 11.0) hours per day, while that with DQ < 80 ($n = 167$) had a median screen exposure time of 3.0 (0, 12.5) hours. Likewise, a significant difference between the two DQ groups was found ($\chi^2 = 48.959$, $p < 0.001$). Covariance analysis, after controlling for the effect of age, showed that DQ was influenced by screen exposure time (F = 1.623, $p = 0.032$), with those exposed to screens for longer durations having lower DQs.

Further analysis of 236 children' risk index on the Erxin Scales' Communication Warning Behavior Subscale showed that the median risk index for the group with DQ $\geq$ 80 ($n = 69$) was 0 (0, 24), while that for the group with DQ < 80 ($n = 167$) was 28.0 (0, 85); the two groups were also characterized by a statistically significant difference ($\chi^2 = 112.726$, $p < 0.001$). Comparing the risk indices categorized into four levels based on the norms with the two DQ groups, the overall chi-square test showed statistical significance ($x^2 = 138.618$, $p < 0.001$). Among these 236 children, those with lower DQs had significantly higher risk indices for communication warning behaviors (as the risk index increased, the number of cases in the DQ < 80 group increased, while that in the DQ $\geq$ 80 group decreased). Moreover, there was a positive correlation between the risk index of communication warning behaviors on the Erxin Scales and screen exposure time, with a correlation coefficient of 0.435.

A study published in JAMA [49] found an association between increased screen-based media use in preschool children, compared to the guidelines provided by the American Academy of Pediatrics (AAP), and lower microstructural integrity of brain white matter tracts that support language and emergent literacy skills. Other research has suggested that excessive and early screen exposure can lead to increased risks of delayed language development, marginal intelligence, and intellectual disability [50]. Multiple studies conducted in the United States [51–54] have shown that infants aged 7 to 16 months who watched educational programs (e.g., Baby Einstein) had poorer language skills and a smaller vocabulary compared to those who watched them less frequently. For developing individuals with plastic brains, exposure to detrimental factors such as excessive screen exposure in early childhood, including the use of smartphones and other electronic screens, can exert negative effects. On one hand, the natural environment for communication between children and caregivers will be disrupted, leading to reduced interaction time. In severe cases, children may be exposed to screens for more than 10 hours per day, which can dramatically impact their normal cognitive, language, and social development. On the other hand, the children will receive no daily language input and communication from caregivers, and they cannot interact with screen characters; living in a virtual world for a long time will even make them struggle to differentiate between screen images and reality. Since the environment and experiences can shape or alter brain function [2], plastic brains are likely to undergo changes in unfavorable conditions. Prolonged exposure to screen-related detrimental factors may modify brain structures and alter brain function in a way that hinders normal child development, slowing down developmental milestones or even resulting in developmental delays. Nonetheless, improvements or catch-up trends have been observed during follow-up visits in children who had experienced slow development and prolonged screen exposure after they were no longer exposed to electronic screens and the caregivers started to focus on improving their social environment, including language input. It can hence be inferred that adverse social environment impacts children's developmental rate, while a long-term lack of normal language input affects their cognitive development.

2.10 Representative Scales in Developing Countries

2.10.1 Characteristics and Advantages of the Erxin Scales

2.10.1.1 An Indigenous Measure

Compared to physical growth, neuropsychological development is more complex to investigate. Well-known Western scales such as GDS and BSID have explored the developmental patterns of children via longitudinal tracking and were formulated based on these patterns [55]. The Erxin Scales, derived from research data on the developmental levels of normal healthy children in China, was developed on the basis of the developmental behaviors and activity patterns of children from non-Western, developing countries with traditional cultural backgrounds. Drawing on the classic theory of cognitive development and neurodevelopmental maturity, it incorporated the theoretical foundations, psychometric research methods, and developmental milestones from foreign scales. Starting from the follow-up visits of newborns in 1980, longitudinal tracking studies were conducted to investigate the developmental patterns of Chinese children. After a decade of refinement, a nationally standardized child development scales was established and named the Erxin Scales. From 2005 to 2016, following international conventions, the scales were meticulously reviewed, modified, and supplemented by establishing an item pool, conducting item analysis and screening, along with other procedures. Standardization was then carried out on representative samples of the population throughout the country. Undoubtedly, the Erxin Scales was developed under highly standardized conditions, and its revision strictly followed the prescribed process, adopting unified item operation methods and scoring criteria. Psychometric analyses also demonstrate that the scale has high discriminability, reliability, as well as content validity and construct validity. In comparison to the classic foreign measure GDS, the Erxin Scales is not only rooted in local cultural backgrounds but also featured by simplified scoring system and ease of operation. To date, nearly ten thousand people nationwide have been trained in using its revised version, and clinical departments of pediatric health, developmental and behavioral pediatrics, and pediatric neurology in over 600 hospitals have employed the scale. Such extensive clinical use has thoroughly validated the effectiveness, research quality, and cumulative effects of the Erxin Scales. The development and utilization of this scale has spanned nearly half a century (a decade from 1980 to 1990 for devising the scale, and another decade from 2005 to 2016 for completing its revision), making it a collaborative endeavor of two to three generations. Currently, no other scales in China can match this long-standing contribution.

From the perspective of scale application, the Erxin Scales demonstrates clear content construction, clarified and concise criteria for passing the test items, ease of operation, and suitability for observation. It can meet the diagnostic and screening needs in pediatric clinical practice in developing countries. Its contribution to scientific research is also comparable to that of foreign scales, and relevant research papers will be published in several specialized journals [56, 57].

As an assessment tool, the Erxin Scales is a valuable decision-making aid in psychological research, and constitutes a necessary option driven by social demand. Child assessment not only evaluates the psychological development of children, but also provides parental education and on-site demonstrations. Assessing and identifying developmental imbalance and delays in early childhood enable the parents to gain insights into the gaps between the assessment results in different domains and the quantified norms, as well as between their children's activity levels and those of specific age groups. This helps parents understand the need to establish more channels for sensory stimulation during the rapid development period so as to compensate for developmental delays and promote better neuropsychological growth in children. The evaluation provided by the scales can also serve as a baseline value for clinical assessment and rehabilitation training. Through dynamic assessment, training goals can be adjusted and training plans be modified to align more closely with the actual developmental levels of children. This is beneficial for children's rehabilitation and the evaluation of rehabilitation outcomes. In a nutshell, the Erxin Scales plays an irreplaceable role in the fields of maternal and child healthcare, early childhood development promotion, and rehabilitation work.

2.10.1.2   Advantages of the Revised Scale

Theoretical learning throughout the entire development process of the Erxin Scales enables the research team to actively keep up with the latest academic advancements. In recent years, increased prevalence of ASD has made the early screening, detection, and intervention a shared pursuit among experts. Most screening scales nowadays are filled out by parents, but they often overestimate or misjudge the abilities of their children, resulting in missed opportunities for early diagnosis. Additionally, advancements in information technology and smartphones, though greatly facilitating people's life, has changed their communication and behavior patterns. There has been an increase in human-machine dialogue in the social environment, and caregivers and children have significantly less spontaneous interaction due to unintentional "misbehavior," as a result of which challenges have been posed to infant care models. These issues were taken into consideration during the scale's revision. The Erxin Scale keeps pace with the times, providing the test takers with the DQs for both the overall scale and the subscales associated respectively with gross motor, fine motor, adaptability, language, and social behavior (independent living skills and social interaction abilities) based on data. In addition to the high proportion (18.4%) of new items in the social behavior domain, a subscale for observing child communication warning behaviors and the according risk index assessment were innovatively included to synchronize with the developmental scale. This provides assistance in the early clinical screening and diagnosis of ASD, developmental delays, language disorders, and other neurodevelopmental disorders. Unlike GDS's closely interconnected operational items, most of the test items in the Erxin Scales are relatively independent. The purpose is to guide and expand caregivers' ability to transform certain testing tools into toys and thus increase the fun involved in the test. With the family as the core, it promotes the development of children's abilities and enhances their capacity to apply past experiences (plays and games) to solve new problems.

In clinical practice, it is common to encounter infants and toddlers who exhibit relatively delayed cognitive, communication, and language development, but do not show significant atypical ASD characteristics in the gross motor domain. Due to a lack of early parental attention, it is difficult to obtain timely professional assessments, leading to cases of missed or delayed diagnosis. The application of the revised Erxin Scale in clinical settings allows for the early detection of developmental delays or imbalances in specific domains, thus enhancing clinical discriminative potential. It enables parents to realize in a timely manner that the increased human-machine interaction, decreased parent-child interaction, and the growing relational distance may cause poor social interaction skills or delays in some developmental domains of children. The scale thus serves as a reminder and encouragement for parents to increase effective communication and interaction with their children, avoiding unintentional negative impact that may arise from "careless mistakes" during childcare. More importantly, it raises social awareness of ASD risk prevention, which holds vital practical significance for infants and toddlers and is a strength of the Erxin Scale.

In terms of developmental assessment, foreign scales like the DDST often use classifications such as normal, abnormal, and suspicious levels. However, in China, people generally do not prefer such broad categorizations, showing regional cultural differences and a lack of compatibility. In Chinese cultural beliefs, there is a greater preference for evaluation results that indicate the degree of deviation from the average level, such as explaining the corresponding mental age (developmental age) of a child at the current stage. Therefore, the Erxin Scale does not use terms like abnormal or suspicious to qualitatively classify children's developmental levels after evaluation. Instead, it provides DQs and mental ages while using neutral terms such as good, average, below average, and low to express the developmental levels. It also provides percentile data for DQs at different main test ages, introducing a more intuitive quantitative reference range that better aligns with Chinese culture and is easier to accept.

2.10.1.3 Scale Management

After revision, the test data of the scale were computer-managed, with the test items digitized. Upon completion of the test, the data will be entered into a computer system, which automatically generates an assessment report, providing the average mental ages as well as overall and subscale DQs. Each assessment report is accompanied by a set of prompts regarding cognitive developmental behaviors expected to occur in children within 3 to 6 months following their developmental age or mental age. Individualized developmental recommendations and intervention guidance are provided to children at different developmental levels, aiming to facilitate the assessor's interpretation of test results and to provide parental education on informative matters. The revised scale meets the assessment needs of various professionals involved in child health care, pediatric medicine, and early intervention, and supports clinical and research work. Furthermore, it serves as a valuable reference and systematic teaching material for the training of developmental and behavioral pediatricians. The application and promotion of the Erxin Scales have risen to the national level. On August 2022, the NHC issued a notification (Maternal and Child Affairs of the NHC Office [2022] No. 12) [58], designating the documentation for the Erxin Scale as the assessment tool providing guidelines on ASD screening and intervention services (trial). This has enhanced the societal impact of the scale and signifies the review and recognition of it by national experts. The publication of this English version aims to introduce the development and revision process of the Erxin Scales to the international community and showcase the child developmental assessment and diagnostic scale with indigenous intellectual property rights from the largest developing country.

2.10.2 Learning from International Scales

The trajectory of human growth, from infancy to childhood and adolescence, and eventually to adulthood and parenthood, continues to follow predictable patterns [9]. According to Piaget, children share similar stages, trends, and outcomes of development, with the environment influencing the rate of their cognitive development. Infant development exhibits common characteristics, following patterns of progression from head to toe, from proximal to distal, and from simple to complex. The development of different systems is independent and occurs at varying rates. Behaviors that reflect the maturity of neuropsychological development include gross motor skills (e.g., lifting the head, sitting, standing, walking), fine motor skills (e.g., grasping and holding objects, using fingers to pick and pinch), adaptive abilities (e.g., searching behavior, building with blocks), sensory perception skills (e.g., responding to sounds, displaying social smiles, recognizing unfamiliar individuals), and language skills, all of which conform to universal human developmental patterns. Therefore, renowned Western developmental scales share similarities or even identical observation and evaluation methods or content for early development of neuropsychological maturity. The administration of the test items involving milestone assessments may exhibit only subtle differences in the description of passing criteria. The fact that China is a non-Western developing country with a large population, extensive geographic range, and diverse ethnic customs makes it necessary to develop a child assessment tool suitable for a wide research background. With a focus on meeting clinical needs and accurately assessing child development, the Erxin Scales manages to incorporate relatively independent test items that cover various life scenarios, while ensuring simplicity and ease of observation in their execution. The content of the items is universal, with the measurement tools being both commonly used in daily life and distinctive enough to effectively elicit target behavioral characteristics in children during testing. The passing criteria for the items are precisely and concisely articulated, easy to understand and remember. The majority of the items are based on the theory of cognitive development, demonstrating an age-related developmental sequence. Nevertheless, to address various practical challenges, some items are unrelated to the cognitive development theory, such as those assessing the natural state of the hand or excessive thumb adduction, which are associated with abnormal postures resulting from brain damage. The purpose of including such items is to enhance the scale's sensitivity to brain injuries, facilitating the screening or diagnosis of deviations or abnormalities in early infant development.

GDS as a classic developmental scale was first devised in 1925. It provided a standardized procedure for observing and evaluating infant developmental behaviors and was the first infant developmental scale in the world [9, 18]. Nearly all subsequent infant tests have borrowed certain items from this scale [9, 18], including BSID [59]. In terms of the Erxin Scales, its test items were mostly self-designed based on follow-up observations of infant behavior. However, to align with international standards, longitudinal observations of the infants were conducted using methods similar or identical to those employed by renowned Western scales [40]. The development of the scale has obtained invaluable insights from previous literature on Chinese child development [60–62], and also from the milestone items entailed in GDS (e.g., actively observing the surrounding environment, controlling the head when pulled up), BSID (e.g., turning a book page by page, imitating drawing a circle, going up and down stairs, identifying gender), and DDST (e.g., babbling, pointing to body parts, jumping with the feet together, throwing a ball over the shoulder, spontaneous scribble, and building a bridge with building blocks). The Erxin Scale's main test ages within age 3 cover seven out of eight key ages proposed by Gesell; although the age of 52 weeks (13 months) is not included, the main test ages of 12 months and 15 months are close to it. The determination of the main test ages in the Erxin Scales accords with the monitoring practices of child growth and development. Physical developmental assessments are also provided at these test ages, facilitating multidimensional measurements and interpretation of results. Furthermore, this revision has incorporated information regarding signs of child developmental progress provided by the U.S. Centers for Disease Control and Prevention (CDC) [63] and drawn inspiration from the ways of indicating developmental delays at differed stages and the failure to reach some milestones in infants and toddlers. In addition, the design of test items for children aged 3 and above has made reference to the Stanford-Binet Intelligence Scale: Fifth Edition (SB5), including its time concept, backward counting, and rectangle building [4]. The Erxin Scale is not isolated from international scales, and its evaluation of child development considers both the national context and international standards, laying the foundation for cross-cultural exchange concerning the scale.

2.10.3 Feasibility of Applying the Erxin Scales in Non-Western Countries

2.10.3.1 Accelerated Updates of Well-Known Western Scales
Rapid socioeconomic development has triggered accelerated updates of well-known scales in developed Western countries. For example, BSID is currently in its third edition (BSID-III), which comprises five parts:

Cognitive Scale, Language Scale, Motor Scale, Social-Emotional Scale, and the ABAS-II. Compared to BSID-II composed of the Mental Scale, Motor Scale, and Infant Behavior Record, this newly updated version is featured by enriched information, expanded content, and a more complex scoring system. From the perspective of neuroscience research, BSID is a highly valuable tool for assessing infant and toddler development. In 2011, the Gesell Institute released the psychometric data from a three-year study involving 1287 children aged 3 to 6 years nationwide, and named the revised scale GDO-R (Gesell Developmental Observation-Revised). Since data on 7- to 9-year-olds were not included in the study, the updated measures for children aged 3 to 6 years were reviewed by a panel of nationally recognized U.S. experts and were approved to serve as a standard assessment scale. It is evident that these updated developmental scales are more comprehensive, suitable for application in developed countries. However, they may not be entirely appropriate for other populations [9, 64], especially those from underdeveloped countries and regions.

2.10.3.2 Scarcity of Developmental Scales for Underdeveloped Countries and Regions

Non-Western underdeveloped countries and regions face similar challenges as China. Firstly, it is increasingly difficult to introduce and revise constantly updated scales from developed Western countries owing to constraints in human resources, materials, and funding. Secondly, previously introduced scales have become outdated, with certain test contents, formats, and scoring methods no longer compatible with current social development. The clinical application of outdated versions may also encounter issues of inappropriateness. All of the above places today's underdeveloped countries and regions in a dilemma caused by inconvenient modification, updating, and utilization of Western developmental scales.

At this juncture, there is a pressing need for a standardized and mature child developmental scale that is suitable for clinical use and originates from countries or regions with similar developmental backgrounds. However, it should be noted that children's neuropsychological and behavioral development differs from their physical growth, and developing corresponding scales requires a multidisciplinary team comprising professionals from pediatrics, neurology, psychology, public health, and psychometrics. They need to collaborate closely and adhere to standardized psychometric procedures throughout the process, including project design, establishment of multicenter research team, sampling, standardization on representative samples, analysis of psychometric data, scientific verification, reliability and validity tests, and subsequent validation in practical application. The entire process necessitates strict quality control, expert judgment, and careful deliberation. Due to the complexity and lengthy process of scale development, there is a scarcity of influential child developmental scales based on local cultural background in non-Western underdeveloped countries.

2.10.3.3 Extensibility and Universality of the Erxin Scales

The Erxin Scales draws heavily upon Piaget's classic theory of cognitive development and takes milestones of child development as important references. It is formulated according to the characteristics of child developmental stages and shares the theoretical foundation and research framework with internationally renowned scales. Regarding development patterns, differences in developmental rates and domains of strength indeed exist among children from different countries and regions. However, there is an overall development consistency from the perspective of developmental psychology. The fundamental principles of the Erxin Scales align more with the characteristics of developing countries, where developmental delays are more common because of such factors as poorer nutrition in children as well as lower socioeconomic status and education levels among caregivers. Instead of labeling children as suspicious or abnormal, the Erxin Scales adopts a developmental perspective to guide and promote their future growth. This is in accord with the emphasis on social fairness and mutual benefit in Chinese culture. Additionally, child development exhibits strong plasticity, and developmental delays can be compensated for by catch-up growth. In view of this, DQs and reference percentiles are available in the assessment report, which goes beyond qualitative categorization and views children's current developmental levels from an objective and developmental standpoint, providing feasible and effective suggestions and intervention measures to optimize child development. This is also in line with the beliefs of CIP regarding child development. The Erxin Scales shares similarities with international scales while also having distinct Chinese characteristics. Its assessment result focuses on depicting the current developmental level of children and regards it as a stage of the entire developmental process. It delineates the developmental space left for the children based on a comprehensive assessment and comparison with typical child development, and considers how to promote further growth by identifying areas of developmental deficiency and deviation through the assessment.

The development and revision of the Erxin Scales are rooted in China's context and incorporate the national conditions of developing countries. Over the course of several decades, it has been continuously improved. The entire research process (technical roadmap) constitutes a comprehensive and scientific scale study that covers aspects such as quality control, validity, reliability, and representativeness, demonstrating the originality, cultural adaptability, and generalizability of the scale. This research process is analogous to the dynamic development and updates of BSID and GDS. As globalization deepens, China's assistance to other developing countries is multifaceted. The test methods and tools used in this scale are more friendly and appealing to developing countries. For instance, the environmental changes encountered by children in Africa and China due to their rapid progress have commonalities or similarities: both facing technological advancements, social changes, and updates in educational concepts and commonly used items (such as the growing popularity of coloring books). The scales cover the age range from 27 days to 6 years and is developed and revised based on a large sample of participants from China. It provides a set of norms that represent the average performance of child development in developing countries. Therefore, compared to other classic international scales such as BSID, GDS, DDST, and GMDS, the Erxin Scales is believed to have greater extensibility and universality.

Early childhood development determines not only individual developmental potential but also the competitiveness of human capital at the national level. A study in China [65] pointed out that there are differences in early childhood development among different regions and also among different populations within the same region, and special attention should be paid to low-income populations and those with lower maternal education levels. Likewise, the United Nations held a special summit on development issues in September 2015, shifting from the Millennium Development Goals to the Sustainable Development Goals, and emphasizing the necessity to stress the needs of the least developed countries, landlocked developing countries, and small-island developing states. It also highlighted the integration of ambitious global development goals with development indicators tailored to specific national circumstances, thereby promoting the realization of the sustainable development goals. Exploring international comparability based on Erxin Scales developed by a developing country and promoting relevant support policies and financial investment are highly illuminating for monitoring global early childhood development.

REFERENCES

1 Gesell, A. (1946). The ontogenesis of infant behavior. In L. Carmichael (Ed.), *Manual of child psychology* (pp. 295–331). Wiley. https://doi.org/10.1037/10756-006
2 Jiang, Z. F., Shen, K. L., Shen, Y., & Zhu, F. T. (2015). *Practical pediatrics* (8th ed., pp. 66–77, 2565). People's Medical Publishing House.
3 Liu, X. Y., Chen, R. H., & Zhao, Z. Y. (2011). *Child health care* (4th ed.). Jiangsu Science and Technology Press.
4 Zhang, J. J., & Gao, Z. M. (1989). *Children intelligence test and training*. Science and Technology Press.
5 Dobbing, J., & Sands, J. (1973). Quantitative growth and development of human brain. *Archives of Disease in Childhood, 48*, 757–767.
6 Wei, J. K., Li, K. Q., & Gao, S. Q. (2002). *Modern children's Psychobehavioral Disorders*. People's Military Medical Press.
7 Liu, X. Y., & Chen, R. H. (2005). *Child health care* (3rd ed.). Jiangsu Science and Technology Press.
8 Batshaw, M. L., Pellegrino, L., & Roizen, N. J. (2007). *Children with disabilities* (6th ed.). Brokes.
9 Feldman, R. S. (2013). *Developmental psychology: The lifelong development of human beings* (6th ed., Y. J. Su & D. Zou, Trans.). World Book Publishing Company.
10 Accardo, P. J., Accardo, J. A., & Capute, A. J. (2008). A neurodevelopmental perspective on the continuum of developmental disabilities. In P. J. Accardo (Ed.), *Capute and Accardo's Neurodevelopmental disabilities in infancy and childhood* (3rd ed., pp. 3–26). Brooks Publishing Baltimore.
11 Hooks, B., & Chen, C. (2008). Vision triggers an experience–dependent sensitive period at the retinogeniculate synapse. *The Journal of Neuroscience, 28*, 4807–4817.
12 Armstrong, J., Hutchinson, I., Laing, D., et al. (2006). Facial electromyography: Responses of children to odor and taste stimuli. *Chemical Senses, 32*, 611–621.
13 Tao, G. T. (1999). *Child and adolescent psychiatry*. Jiangsu Science and Technology Press.
14 Zhang, S. C. (2018). *Speciesology*. Hatian Publishing House.

15 Gilmore, C. K., & Spelke, E. S. (2008). Children's understanding of the relationship between addition and subtraction. *Cognition, 107*, 932–945.
16 Donlan, C. (1998). *The development of mathematical skills*. Psychology Press.
17 Reynolds, C. R., Livingston, R., & Willson, V. (2015). *Measurement and assessment in education* (2nd ed.). Science Press.
18 Chen, S. J. (1994). *Psychometrics*. Time Culture Publishing Company.
19 Zheng, R. C., Cai Y. H., & Zhou, Y. Q. (1998). *Psychometrics*. People's Education Press.
20 Eduardo, E. (2009). Cognitive plasticity and cortical modules. *Current Directions in Psychological science, 18*(3), 153–158.
21 Stiles, J., Moses, P., & Paul, B. M. (2009). The longitudinal study of spatial cognitive development in children with pre- or perinatal focal brain injury: Evidence for cognitive compensation and for the emergence of alternative profiles of brain organization. In S. G. Lomber & J. J. Eggermont (Eds.), *Reprogramming the cerebral cortex: Plasticity following central and peripheral lesions*. Oxford University Press.
22 Lomber, S. G., & Eggermont, J. (2006). *Reprogramming the cerebral cortex: Plasticity following central and peripheral lesions*. Oxford University Press.
23 Vanlierde, A., Renier, L., & De Volder, A. G. (2008). Brain plasticity and multisensory experience in early blind individuals. In J. J. Rieser, D. H. Ashmead, F. F. Ebner, & A. L. Corn (Eds.), *Blindness and brain plasticity in navigation and object perception* (pp.67–83). Lawrence Erlbaum.
24 Liu, X. H., & Li, X. M. (2002). *Pediatric behavioral medicine*. Military Medical Science Press.
25 Yi, S. R., Luo, X. R., Yang, Z. W., et al. (1993). The revising of the Bayley Scales of Infant Development (BSID) in China. *Chinese Journal of Clinical Psychology, 2*, 71–75.
26 Yang, Y. F. (2016). *Rating scales for children's developmental behavior and mental health*. People's Medical Publishing House.
27 Gesell Institute of Child Development(2012).*The Gesell Developmental Observation-Revised*. https://cdn.shopify.com/s/files/1/2018/7551/files/2012-Gesell-Executive-Summary.pdf?7155388513235440535
28 Zhang, X. L., Li, J. P., Qin, M. J., et al. (1994). The revise of Gesell Development Scale on 3.5–6 years of age in Beijing. *Chinese Journal of Clinical Psychology, 3*, 148–150.
29 Huntley, M. (1996). *The griffiths mental developmental scales manual from birth to two years*. Association for Research in Infant and Child Development.
30 Tso, W. W. Y., Wong, V. C. N., Xia, X., et al. (2018). The Griffiths Development Scales–Chinese (GDS–C): A cross-cultural comparison of developmental trajectories between Chinese and British children. *Child: Care, Health and Development, 44*(3), 378–383.

31 Fan, C. R. (1988). *CDCC infant intelligence development scale test manual*. Unity Press.
32 Johnson, J. H., & Goldman, J. (1990). *Developmental assessment in clinical child psychology: A handbook*. Pergamon Press.
33 Aylward, G. P., & Verhulst, S. J. (2010). Predictive utility of the Bayley Infant Neurodevelopmental Screener (BINS) risk status classifications: Clinical interpretation and application. *Developmental Medicine & Child Neurology, 42*(01), 25–31.
34 Xu, S. S., Huang, H., Zhang, J. S., et al. (2011). Research on the applicability of Bayley Scales of Infant and Toddler Development-Third Edition to assess the development of infants and toddlers in Shanghai. *Chinese Journal of Child Health Care, 19*(1), 30–32.
35 Li, S. J., Zhang, J. J., Huang, H. M., et al. (2022). Consistency study of Griffiths mental development scales-Chinese version and Gesell developmental schedules in the developmental evaluation of infants with bacterial meningitis. *Beijing Medical Journal, 44*(6), 510–512.
36 Qu, C. y., & Sun, X. b. y. (2010). A comparative study on the mental development of 308 hearing-impaired children and 473 normal-hearing children 0-3 years old. *Chinese Scientific Journal of Hearing and Speech Rehabilitation* (5), 15–18.
37 Mao, Y. y., & Zhou, Z. F. (1986). A follow-up study on the intellectual development of children from birth to 36 months. *Acta Psychologica Sinica, 3*(2), 248–254.
38 Lin, C. S., & Chiu, C. H. (2014). Adaptation of the Chinese edition of the CSBS-DP: A cross-cultural comparison of prelinguistic development between Taiwanese and American toddlers. *Research in Developmental Disabilities, 35*(5), 1042–1050.
39 Tardif, T. (2008). *Chinese communicative development inventories: User's guide and manual* (Mandarin and Cantonese versions). Peking University Medical Press.
40 Mao, Y. Y., & Zhou, Z. F. (1986). A follow–up study on the intellectual development of children from birth to 36 months (1). *Acta Psychologica Sinica, 2*, 113–122.
41 Wong, S., Chan, K., Wong, V., & Wong, W. (2002). Use of chopsticks in Chinese children. *Child Care, Health and Development, 28*(2), 157–161.
42 Boyle, C. A., Boulet, S., Schieve, L. A., Cohen, R. A., Blumberg, S. J., Yeargin-Allsopp, M., et al. (2011). Trends in the prevalence of developmental disabilities in us children, 1997–2008. *Pediatrics, 127*(6), 1034–1042.
43 Vermandel, A., Kampen, M. V., Gorp, C. V., & Wyndaele, J. (2008). How to toilet train healthy children? A review of the literature. *Neurourology and Urodynamics, 27*, 162–166.

44 Dietz, W. H., & Stern, L. (1999). *American academy of pediatrics guide to your child's nutrition: Making peace at the table and building healthy eating habits for life*. Villard.
45 Belsky, J. (2006). Early child care and early child development: Major findings of the NICHD Study of Early Child Care. *European Journal of Developmental Psychology, 3*(1), 95–110.
46 Fritz, G., Rockney, R., et al. (2004). Practice parameter for the assessment and treatment of children and adolescents with enuresis. *Journal of the American Academy of Child & Adolescent Psychiatry, 43*(12), 1540–1550.
47 Christakis, D. A. (2014). Interactive media use at younger than the age of 2 years: Time to rethink the American Academy of Pediatrics guideline? *JAMA Pediatrics, 168*(5), 399–400.
48 Xu, Q., Wang, J. H., Zhang, L. L., et al. (2021). Research on the status and risk factors of screen exposure in children under three years of age. *Chinese Journal of Pediatrics, 59*(10), 841–846.
49 Hutton, J. S., Dudley, J., Horowitz-Kraus, T., DeWitt, T., & Holland, S. K. (2020). Associations between screen-based media use and brain white matter integrity in preschool-aged children. *JAMA Pediatrics, 174*(1), e193869.
50 Cao, H., Xie, L. L., Yin, X. G., et al. (2016). Influence of Television exposure and sleep problems on intelligence development at 18 months. *Chinese Journal of Child Health Care, 24*(3), 282–285.
51 Zimmerman, F. J., Christakis, D. A., & Meltzoff, A. N. (2007). Associations between media viewing and language development in children under age 2 years. *The Journal of Pediatrics, 151*(4), 364–368.
52 Zimmerman, F. J., & Christakis, D. A. (2007). Associations between content types of early media exposure and subsequent attentional problems. *Pediatrics, 120*(5), 986–992.
53 Robb, M. B., Richert, R. A., & Wartella, E. A. (2009). Just a talking book? Word learning from watching baby videos. *The British Journal of Developmental Psychology, 27*(Pt 1), 27–45.
54 Roseberry, S., Hirsh-Pasek, K., Parish-Morris, J., & Golinkoff, R. M. (2009). Live action: Can young children learn verbs from video? *Child Development, 80*(5), 1360–1375.
55 Brooks, J., & Weinraub, M. (1976). *A history of infant intelligence testing*. Springer.
56 Zhang, L. L., Li, X. F., Li, S., Jin, N., & Jin, C. H. (2022). The characteristics of vocabulary and phrase acquisition in Mandarin-exposed children with autism spectrum disorder in Beijing. *Chinese Journal of Practical Pediatrics, 37*(15), 1161–1166.
57 Li, H. H., Feng, J. Y., Wang, B., Zhang, Y., Wang, C. X., & Jia, F. Y. (2019). Comparison of the children neuropsychological and behavior scale and the griffiths mental development scales when assessing the development

of children with autism. *Psychology Research and Behavior Management, 12*, 973–981.
58 National Health Commission of the People's Republic of China. (2022). *Notice on the issuance of the Guidelines for Screening and Intervention Services for Autism Spectrum Disorder in Children Aged 0–6 (Trial)*. Maternal and Child Affairs of the National Health Commission Office, No. [2022]12, 2022, 8.
59 Guo, S. C. (1989). *Child health care*. People's Medical Publishing House.
60 Fan, C. R., & Zhou, Z. F. (1983). Research on intelligent development of children from birth to 6 years old. *Acta Psychologica Sinica, 4*, 429–444.
61 Song, J., & Zhu, Y. M. (1981). *Developmental assessment of children's intelligence*. Shanghai Scientific & Technical Publishers.
62 Li, H. T. (1981). Intelligence development of children in the first three years of life. *Educational Research, 11*, 69–73.
63 Centers for Disease Control and Prevention (CDC). (2005). *Learn the Signs, act Early Campaign*. https://www.cdc.gov/ncbddd/actearly/index.html
64 Flanagan, D. P., & Harrison, P. L. (2005). *Contemporary intellectual assessment: Theories, tests, and issues*. The Guilford Press.
65 Zhang, Y., Kang, L., Zhao, J., et al. (2021). Assessing the inequality of early child development in China—A population-based study. *The Lancet Regional Health. Western Pacific, 14*, 100221.

CHAPTER 3

Development and Revision of the Erxin Scales

3.1 Background of the Erxin Scales

Neuropsychological assessment in infants and young children is an essential aspect of evaluating their overall well-being. Developmental scales serve as important tools for assessing child neuropsychological development. Before the emergence of Erxin Scales, commonly used developmental scales for children in China were mostly derived from Western sources. Due to cultural differences, using non-standardized foreign scales might not accurately and comprehensively reflect the developmental characteristics of Chinese children, leading to compromised validity. Foreign scales are continually refined during their use [1–3], approximately undergoing revisions every 20–30 years. The BSID, first published in 1969, underwent two revisions in 1993 and 2006, respectively. In China, the revision of the original BSID was initiated in 1990 and completed in 1992 [4]. Although the scale was commonly used by Chinese scholars in scientific research, its limited age range (2–30 months) and training constraints had hindered its widespread clinical application. The well-known GDS (1974 edition) was introduced and revised in Beijing and Shanghai [5], but nationwide normative studies were not conducted, and the introduced version was also outdated [5–7]. The introduction and standardization of foreign scales require time, and it is likely that a revised edition is published as soon as the standardization work of a scale has just completed. To keep pace, continuous introduction and indigenous revision of foreign scales would be necessary. However, owing to limited human and financial resources as well as copyright restrictions, it was difficult to introduce and revise foreign scales. This showcased the vital necessity of developing an assessment tool aligned with the characteristics of Chinese children's psychological development. Proudly, under the leadership of CIP and in collaboration with IPCAS, an indigenous research project was launched in the early 1980s to develop the Erxin Scales for child development.

In the early 1980s, CIP initiated the development of the Erxin Scales based on the original data obtained from 60 healthy newborns born in the Beijing Fu Xing Hospital. Specifically, regular household visits, starting from once a month to once every 2–3 months after the age of 1 year, were conducted to collect the infants' developmental-behavioral data. The neuropsychological development of early childhood was observed and recorded through longitudinal tracking, spanning a period of three and a half years. Test items were designed and compiled based on the developmental patterns and behavioral characteristics of the participants [8]. And they were further refined through cross-sectional validation involving 1,275 children aged 0–4 years, resulting in China's first developmental scale for 0- to 3-year-old children. In 1985, a nationwide collaborative multicenter research team was established across 12 cities, including Beijing, Tianjin, Shanghai, Wuhan, Kunming, Fuzhou, Changchun, Baotou, Kaifeng, Zhengzhou, Guiyang, and Lanzhou. A total of 13,868 children aged 0–3 years from the 12 cities were included for standardization. Additionally, a sample of 1,185 children aged 4–5 years were added to extend the age range covered by the scale to 5 years and to obtain nationwide normative data. Finally, the 177-item neuropsychological and behavior scale for 0- to 4-year-olds, known as the Erxin Scales, was formed, which filled the gap in China's diagnostic scales for child development [6]. The Erxin Scales comprehensively evaluates the neuropsychological developmental level of infants and young children in five domains (or attributes): gross motor, fine motor, adaptability, language, and social behavior. It provides accurate measurement information on deviations, delays, and imbalance in early childhood development. The standardized Erxin Scales has become the most widely used assessment tool in pediatric and child healthcare practices nationwide [9, 10]. By the end of 2021, there were over 400 published articles in China with "Erxin Scales" as the main subject, including representative empirical research from Shanghai, Jilin, Guangdong, and other regions [11–13]. The extensive and long-term application of the scale in pediatric disciplines adequately proves its validity. Furthermore, to meet the needs of child healthcare work, supplementary test items were added in 1997, attempting to extend the age range of the Erxin Scales. However, these items were not standardized nationwide.

3.2 Necessity for Scales Revision

Over the 30 years of the Erxin Scales' application, significant changes had occurred in children's living and growth environment. For instance, most picture books and other publications for children were colorized. As a result, the previously used black-and-white line drawings in the measurement tools became somewhat abstract, and certain test instruments rarely seen or used. Children thus often exhibited unfamiliarity, distractibility, and poor coordination during assessments. Besides, the scale had a limited number of items that assess neuroreflexes and muscle tone in younger infants, thereby affecting the accurate evaluation of their motor and perception. Constant societal evolutions made the original scale no longer fully suit the needs of contemporary children, especially in providing a comprehensive and authentic reflection of the development of younger infants. Moreover, the added items aimed at extending the age range from 5 to 6 years lacked standardization on representative samples, thus affecting the diagnostic validity of the scale. All of this made it essential to improve the test content of the scales, replace inappropriate measurement tools, and incorporate measurement information adapted to social changes, highlighting the necessity of revising the Erxin Scales following international conventions.

3.3 Grants from the Government and Professional Organizations

Entrusted by Zhenmin Gao and Jiajian Zhang, the primary developers of the original Erxin Scales, Chunhua Jin from the Child Health Department of CIP formed a team in 2005 to prepare for the scale revision work. Under the guidance of Dr. Gao and Dr. Zhang, the team reviewed the instructions for operating the scale, established the revision procedures and principles, adjusted the scale structure, refined the original items, and standardized all measurement tools. Then, a preliminary pool for new items was established, the main test ages were determined, testing and statistical analysis of the primary item pool were conducted, and finally the dimensions and weights of the scale were established, resulting in the revised Erxin Scales. This work was supported by grants from the Capital Medical Development Research Fund (No. 2009-1047) in 2009 and the National Science and Technology Pillar Program during the Twelfth Five-Year Plan Period (No. 2012BAI03B00, No. 2012BAI03B01) in 2012. To expand the functionality of the scale and incorporate research on child developmental behaviors, funding was granted by Beijing Disabled Persons' Federation and Beijing Shouer Liqiao Children's Hospital in 2014 and 2015 to add a new subscale for children's communication warning behaviors. At this point, the initial scale revision plan was completed, with the addition of an ASD screening tool that was synchronized with developmental assessment and observed and interviewed by professionals. This enables the scale to not only identify children suspected of developmental delays in the early stages but also screen for ASD risks.

3.4 Formulation and Implementation of the Technical Roadmap for Scales Revision

3.4.1 Formulation of the Technical Roadmap for Scales Revision

Psychological tests or developmental assessments are systematic processes that collect information through standardized procedures. Scale revision is a specialized and research-intensive task that requires long-term, interdisciplinary collaboration. The revision of child developmental scales is even more complex, and it is crucial to establish a strict quality control system that covers the entire process. In other words, to ensure the reliability and validity of the scale, the formulation of a technical roadmap for scale revision is essential at the outset to anticipate potential issues that may arise at each step and provide guidance on how to address them. The technical roadmap serves as a guiding framework for the scale revision process and standardizes the workflow for each step, ensuring that the operational procedures adhere to the technical routes specified in psychometrics. Progress can only be made if each step follows the roadmap's prescribed sequence, guaranteeing that all processes and item selections comply with the technical specifications and requirements of psychometrics. Under the guidance of the original scale developers, the technical advisory panel discussed and formulated the basic technical roadmap for scale revision, as depicted in Fig. 3.1.

Preliminary preparation (clarify revision theories and principles), project application, and formulation of technical roadmap

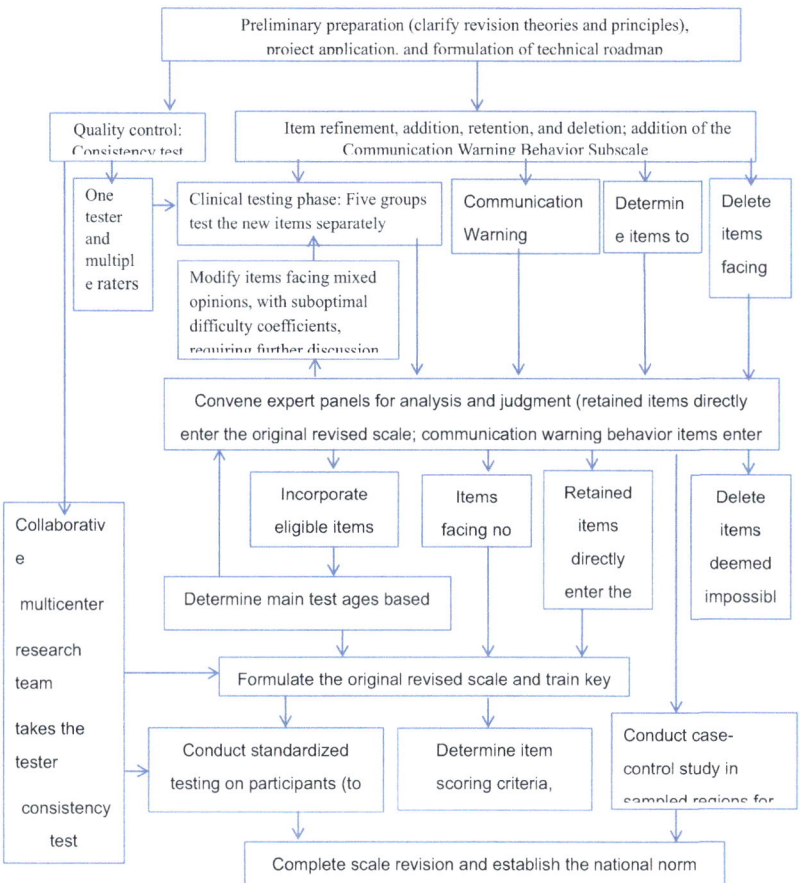

Fig. 3.1 Technical roadmap for scales revision

3.4.2 Item Management and Quality Control

Standardized tests are managed, scored, and interpreted in a professional manner. Following the guidance of the original scale developers, the established principles for designing new items in the Erxin Scales prioritized the inclusion of clinically observable, easily operable items with clearly defined criteria. A comprehensive technical roadmap for the entire revision process was developed based on these principles, and all revision procedures were ensured to follow the steps and quality control requirements outlined in the roadmap. Within the quality control system implemented according to the technical roadmap, each vital link was subject to expert validation. Over ten panel discussion sessions involving top experts in relevant fields from across the country were held to ensure the standardization of item selection.

(1) **Scrutinizing the original scale items**

A preliminary review of the original scale items was conducted, and screening criteria were established. Out of the 177 items with national norms (0–4 years), 131 were deemed valid and did not require revision, 38 needed modifications, and 8 were deleted. Experts discussed the issues raised regarding item modification and suggested treating the modified items as new ones (one panel discussion).

(2) **Adding the clinical testing phase**

A clinical testing phase was added for the newly designed items, and those met the clinical testing requirements were included in the item pool, ensuring the stability of the testing phase in later stages. The advisory panel of experts requested treating all test items for children aged 4 to 6 as new ones because this age group witnesses a transition in cognitive growth. Each item was included in the item pool after the completion of a comprehensive operational procedure (the clinical testing of new items and the determination of main test ages were reported to the experts, and five panel discussions were held).

(3) **Handling issues during the item testing phase**

Certain issues emerged from item testing, such as a well-designed item not meeting the criteria for inclusion in the item pool, or the behavior requiring an excessively long time or being difficult to observe despite the satisfactory pass rate of the item. Some new items might still yield unsatisfactory results after multiple rounds of clinical testing. These issues were discussed face-to-face by experts, with solutions proposed before devising the original revised version (three sessions).

(4) **Devising the original revised scale**
Multiple face-to-face consultations were held with the experts to solicit their opinions (three sessions). In specific, 232 items were removed while establishing the item pool (one session); among the 247 items that survived the item testing phase, 127 were deleted while devising the original revised version, leaving a total of 120 items. Some special situations arose during item testing management. For example, modification suggestions were offered by experts concerning a supplementary item for main test ages because of the unsatisfactory results in multiple rounds of clinical testing (e.g., the item regarding fiddling with bell tongue), and the item was deemed unnecessary for further testing and supposed to be directly incorporated into the original revised scales (one session). After the completion of the initial revision, nationwide sampling was carried out and a collaborative multicenter research team was established across the sampled regions. Personnel were trained in testing methods to ensure specific quality control for the national representative sample (expert discussion results: experts were selected to participate in the whole testing process, providing supervision and quality control) (one session).

(5) **Adding the communication disorder index**
To enhance the scale's capacity for screening for developmental disorders and ASD risks in particular, experts of the field were invited to discuss the research methods, item selection, and reference thresholds for the newly added Communication Warning Behavior Subscale (2 sessions).

(6) **Evaluating the psychological characteristics of the scale**
The normative data were reviewed meticulously, followed by in-depth discussion among experts (2 sessions). After the completion of the revision, the scale underwent expert reviews and project acceptance (1 session).

3.4.3 Proposals for patent application

Experts suggested applying for patents on the new items which originally assess cognitive growth (e.g., those employing novel methods). As a result, the tool kit used for assessing children's shape cognition, the analog test suite, and the multifunctional doll obtained the utility model patent certificates.

3.5 PRELIMINARY PREPARATION

3.5.1 Determination of Scale Revision Principles

(1) **Establishing the scale structure**

Based on Piaget's theory of child cognitive development [14] and drawing on the literature reviewed [15–22], the overall structure of the scale was established. Behaviors or actions reflecting neuropsychological characteristics were proposed and the measurement information was enriched to promote understanding of various developmental domains in children. The scales intended to assess child development in terms of five attributes, including gross motor, fine motor, adaptive/cognitive skills, language, and social behavior. In the meanwhile, negative behaviors and social-emotional aspects disproportionate to children's age were also included in the assessment content, with evaluation indices added. Through observation and/or inquiry, behaviors failing to match children's age or vastly different from ordinary behaviors were captured. In combination with developmental levels, a more comprehensive picture of various behavioral manifestations in child development was obtained, enabling the identification of early signs of developmental delays or other suspected neurodevelopmental disorders in children. This facilitates follow-up visits and timely intervention, promoting the clinical application of the scale.

From a cognitive development perspective, the order of developmental milestones is important for infants and children under 3 years old, but it becomes less prominent for older children. In view of this, new items should focus on visual thinking, logical thinking, cognition, language expression, calculation, judgment, and executive functions. In addition to considering various factors mentioned above, the adaptability of the scale and other environmental influences should also be taken into account. China has a vast territory with significant regional and linguistic differences. Therefore, new items also tried to avoid or minimize the influence of living environment, customs, and language, and to enhance the feasibility of applying the scale to children from ethnic minorities.

(2) **Longitudinally observing child developmental behaviors**

To accurately and reliably reflect children's developmental levels, longitudinal observations and regular records of the developmental behaviors and living situations of seven children (two observed from birth to 2 years old, and five from birth to 4 years old) were made in the early stage, so as to explore the items and structure of the scale. While reviewing the original scale items, it was found that the age at which infants know the color red significantly advanced as a result of economic development, improved living conditions, and education levels. Most typically developing children know the color red at around 21–24 months of age. Among the seven children observed longitudinally, five of them knew the color red at 21 months of age, and by the age of 30 months, almost all of the children knew the color red and even knew two or more colors. Consequently, the item assessing knowledge of the color red, which was originally set at 30 months of age, was moved forward to 21 months of age. The item which asked 21-month-olds to place round building blocks in upright (forward) and inverted (backward) templates is another case in point. Previous assessment indicated a very low pass rate for the item at 21 months of age. Among the seven observed children, only one passed this item at 21 months of age, but four of them passed by 24 months of age. Therefore, the main test age for this item (i.e., Put the round building blocks into the inverted template correctly) was moved from 21 to 24 months, and all subsequent template-related items were moved backward by one main test age segment.

(3) **Emphasizing past application experience**

The literature probing into the application of the Erxin Scales was consulted, and importance was placed on drawing on previous application experience. Relevant evaluation personnel were invited to exchange their application experiences, and spot checks on the assessors were made based on the instruction manual to ensure the standardization of scale administration.

(4) **Avoiding lengthiness**
The addition of new test items aimed to assess cognitive and sensory development while also considering social communication and interactive behaviors with others. The goal of adding new items was to measure children's development both extensively and profoundly, while avoiding lengthiness.
(5) **Increasing a new assessment domain**
A new domain, namely the Communication Warning Behavior Subscale, was increased during the revision. This facilitated the scale's screening for deviations, delays, and imbalance in early child development, and also enhanced its ability to identify ASD risks.

3.5.2 Clarification of Scale Structure and Domain Attribution

To make the scale structure and domain attribution reasonable, the test items were reorganized and repositioned, and their attribution was determined according to the original scales' five dimensions (subscales) corresponding to the five domains or attributes. To go into detail, the items involving gross motor skills related to maintaining bodily postures or whole-body movements, such as rolling, sitting, crawling, standing, walking, running, throwing, and jumping, including neck and waist muscles used to control and maintain body balance, were classified under the gross motor domain. The items related to fine motor skills involving small muscle movements of the hands and fingers, such as grasping and pinching, were categorized under the fine motor domain. Those concerning the abilities related to coordinating hand and eye movements while manipulating objects, or actions requiring visual perception coordination, such as attempting to grasp a toy by changing body posture, drawing, and stacking building blocks, were classified under the adaptability domain; items assessing adaptability in children aged 3 and above focused on problem-solving skills, including perception, attention, memory, and thinking processes involved in information processing. The language domain comprised items associated with verbal and nonverbal activities related to language pronunciation, expression, and comprehension, such as visual perception, auditory perception, and body language including postures and gestures. Lastly, the social behavior domain was composed of items involving interaction and communication with others, such as eye contact, vocalization, laughter, and other social games (social communication skills), as well as activities related to daily self-care (independent living skills) such as buttoning clothes and tying shoelaces. The newly added domain of communication warning behaviors retained the structural characteristics of the original scales.

3.5.3   Principles for Determining Main Test Ages

The main test ages were determined based on children's birthdate and the measurement date, calculated as children's chronological age and expressed in months (with 30 days defined as one month). The Erxin Scales consist of 28 age segments (or main test ages). The age segment closest to but younger than the chronological age would be automatically selected as the main test age by the computer. The design of new test items was based on the cognitive development theory and also on accumulated clinical experience. The grouping of new items by main test ages was guided by the fact that children below the main test age tend to show a lower pass rate, while those above the main test age tend to show a higher pass rate. The pass rate for items in a developmental scale should increase with age, meaning that the number of individuals passing the items should progressively increase as a function of age. Regarding the Erxin Scales, the pass rates of items for main test ages were controlled within the 50–75% range as per the original scales, while those for items in the item pool generally ranged from 20 to 90%. The main test ages, operational methods, and passing criteria were established through repeated clinical testing and subsequent item testing. The pass rates of adjacent age segments as well as the main test ages were taken into account in decision-making. The item testing data were submitted to a panel of experts, who evaluated the candidates for main test ages and made suggestions about item inclusion based on the purpose of the supplementary test items and theoretical foundations. The inclusion of items also relied on factors analysis of the participants and the results of confirmatory factor analysis.

3.5.4 *Principles for Determining Scale Dimensions and Item Weights*

The developmental assessment section of the scale consists of five dimensions or subscales (domains or attributes): gross motor, fine motor, adaptability, language, and social behavior, with equal weights assigned to each dimension. And each dimension comprises one or two test items, with each item assigned an equal weight. The weight assigned to each dimension for the main test ages within the age ranges of under 1 year, 1–3 years, and 3–6 years is 1 point, 3 points, and 6 points, respectively. For example, if each domain for the main test ages under 1 year contains two test items, then the weight of each item would be 50%, resulting in 0.5 points for each; on the other hand, if there is only one item for the domain, it would have a weight of 100%, resulting in 1 point. Similarly, for the age ranges of 1–3 years and 3–6 years, each dimension follows an equal weight distribution for the items.

For the newly added Communication Warning Behavior Subscale, the weights were determined based on the research results of the Erxin Scales revision project entitled "Exploration of Indicators of Autism Spectrum Disorder in Infancy and Early Childhood" funded by the Beijing Disabled Persons' Federation.

3.5.5 *Examination of the Original Scale Items*

The operational and observational methods for each item in the original scale were examined, including assessing whether the wording of the instructions accurately conveys the intended purpose of the items. The items requiring supplementation, modification, or deletion were identified, along with the justifications.

(1) **Item retention**

The items in the original scales, which were designed reasonably, aligned with the corresponding age-related developmental levels, less susceptible to deviations in test administrators' understanding, and demonstrated good stability, were retained without the need for further clinical validation or testing.

(2) **Item modification**

Feedback from experienced assessors was sought to enhance the descriptions of the instructions. Additional details were provided for statements deemed overly simplistic, and modifications were made to statements that might lead to ambiguity, ensuring a more precise expression of the intended purpose of the items and hence more specific and meticulous operational procedures. For example, for the item "Hold object with both hands to stand up," the original instruction was described simply as "Place the child beside the bed rail in a standing position. The criterion is to support the entire body weight with both hands on the rail, maintain the standing position for 5 seconds or more, and avoid leaning the chest against the rail." By comparison, the revised instruction is as follows: "Place the infant on the bed and assist the infant in gripping the bed rail with both hands, assuming a standing position without the chest leaning against the rail. Observe the infant. The criterion is to support the body weight with both hands on the rail and maintain the standing position for 5 seconds or more." Noteworthily, specific prompts were added to guide the assessor in adhering to the criterion, emphasizing that the chest should not lean against the bed rail and that the body should maintain stability even in the event of slight swaying, without the risk of falling. Another example is the item "Identify four colors." In the original scales, the four-color picture was arranged horizontally in the order of red, yellow, blue, and green, which often led to the recitation of the sequence without actually identifying the colors. In the revision, the four-color picture was modified to be arranged in a circular pattern, with each color occupying a quarter of the circle. This change was made to avoid potential difficulty caused by the horizontal arrangement in making accurate judgment. Considering the impact of socioeconomic development and education on children, adjustments were made to certain items, such as "Know numbers," the main test age for which was lowered from 60 to 54 months. Similar cases were treated as modified items which underwent retesting.

There is another notable aspect to mention. In the past, the inclusion of items in the scale required a pass rate of 50–75%. However, during item testing in the revision process, it was found that children's fine motor skills, such as unbuttoning, buttoning, and using chopsticks to pick up peanuts, were generally lower in pass rates compared to when the original scale was developed. A typical example is the task of using chopsticks to pick up peanuts, which only achieved a pass rate of 45–48% during the item testing phase. How should we handle the issue of low pass rates for fine motor skills in children? Should we lower the threshold? Regarding this critical issue, the original scale developers and revision consultants Jiajian Zhang and Zhenmin Gao were asked for their opinions, and an expert panel was convened. However, all of them disagreed with the idea of lowering the threshold, because this would impact children's development. It was recommended that no changes be made if the pass rates reach the levels during the item testing phase after the national normative research. This principle was followed in the later analysis of normative data, and some experts also suggested strengthening parental education and emphasizing the cultivation of children's fine motor skills.

(3) **Item deletion**

The items lacking characteristic manifestations of neuropsychological development, being overly simple or excessively difficult, or redundant within the same domain were considered for deletion. For example, the question "How many pieces are there when you cut an apple?" was considered too simple for typically developing 48-month-olds, with a pass rate exceeding 95%, and therefore it was deleted. With the changing times, wallets are rarely used nowadays, and stamps are no longer a daily necessity.

Therefore, questions such as "What would you do if you found a wallet?" and "What should you stick on the envelope when sending a letter?" were proposed for deletion, and the expert panel unanimously agreed to remove similar items as mentioned above.

3.5.6 *Increase of Supplementary Items and Extension of Applicable Age Range up to 6 Years*

One of the reasons for adding new test items was to address the insufficiency existed in the original scales. Specifically, relatively few test items were incorporated in the original scale for infants. Especially if an infant younger than 3 months exhibited suboptimal performance in one item, his/her DQ would be significantly lower than the actual developmental level. Continuous observations revealed considerable fluctuations. To rectify this, supplementary items were introduced, such as "Tilt and raise the head when lying prone" at 1 month of age, "Thumb separates when tapped lightly" and "Smile spontaneously" at 2 months of age, which improved the stability of the scale. There was no normative data for the age range from 66 to 84 months in the original scales. In this revision, most of the items were modified and treated as new ones requiring clinical testing and item testing.

3.6 Implementation of Item Testing

3.6.1 Pass Rates for Modified Items During Clinical Testing

The items modified from the original scale required testing, and a multi-level scoring system was adopted to validate the pass rates at the main test ages. For example, regarding the item "Understand adult facial expressions" at the age of 8 months, the assessor or the parent praises or reprimands the infant and observes the infant's reaction. A score of 0 indicates no understanding, while a score of 1 indicates the infant's display of excitement or distress, among other reactions. The pass rates for this item at 8 months of age and adjacent ages are shown in Table 3.1, and the age of 8 months (with a pass rate of 68.9%) was determined as a main test age according to the principles. Another example is the item "Hold onto the railing to squat down and pick something up" for the age of 11 months. The assessor assists the infant in standing while holding onto a railing without leaning against it. A toy is placed near the infant's feet, and the infant is encouraged to squat down and pick it up. A score of 0 indicates the infant (1) cannot squat down or (2) cannot stand up again after squatting down. A score of 1 indicates that the infant uses one hand to hold onto the railing while squatting down, picks up the toy with the other hand, and is able to stand up again with some slight body sway but not falling. Moreover, a score of 2 indicates that the infant uses one hand to hold onto the railing while squatting down, picks up the toy with the other hand, is able to stand up again with coordinated movements, and does not sway. The rates for a score of 2 for this item at the ages of 11, 12, and 15 months are 22.6%, 50.4%, and 90.6%, respectively. If the scores of 1 and 2 are combined, the pass rates become 47.6%, 74.4%, and 97.3%, respectively. Although both 11 and 12 months could be considered as the main test age for this item, the former (with a pass rate of 47.6%) was adopted in accordance with the original scale. Infants' rates for achieving scores of 1 and 2 at different month ages are shown in Table 3.2.

Table 3.1 Number of participants and pass rates for the item "Understand adult facial expressions" (n%)

Test age (month)	0 point	1 point	Number of participants
5	48 (92.3)	4 (7.7)	52
6	97 (82.2)	21 (17.8)	118
7	56 (53.8)	48 (46.2)	104
8*	33 (31.1)	73 (68.9)	106
9	10 (10.1)	89 (89.9)	99
10	15 (15.6)	81 (84.4)	96
11	1 (1.7)	59 (98.3)	60
12	1 (1.7)	58 (98.3)	59

* Determined main test age

Table 3.2 Number of participants and pass rates for the item "Hold onto the railing to squat down and pick something up" (n%)

Test age (month)	0 point	1 point	2 points	1 point and 2 points combined	Number of participants
7	21 (100)	0	0	0	21
8	46 (100)	0	0	0	46
9	86 (91.5)	5 (5.3)	3 (3.2)	8 (8.5)	94
10	79 (79.8)	11 (11.1)	9 (9.1)	20 (20.2)	99
11*	44 (52.4)	21 (25.0)	19 (22.6)	40 (47.6)	84
12△	33 (25.6)	31 (24.0)	65 (50.4)	96 (74.4)	129
15	2 (2.7)	5 (6.7)	68 (90.6)	73 (97.3)	75
18	8 (0)	0	8 (100.0)	8 (100.0)	8

3.7 Determination of Main Test Ages for New Items

(1) **Pass rates for target-age items**

The items supplemented to a certain age were considered target-age items, primarily determined by their pass rates at the corresponding age. In some special cases, the pass rates of the adjacent age groups were also considered. For example, the items "Tilt and raise the head when lying prone" and "Watch black-and-white targets" for the age of 1 month, "Thumb separates when tapped lightly" and "Smile spontaneously" for 2 months, as well as "Make protective action" and "Engage in joint attention" for older ages were all supplementary items. Additionally, the item "Describe the picture contents" was a substitute for extended ages. Generally, when the pass rate of new items arranged in descending order of age was closest to 50–75% (or at least within 40–80%), the corresponding age would be selected as the main test age for the item. Upon the determination of the main test age, the operational and scoring methods for that item were established accordingly. When determining the main test age, the pass rates of the item for adjacent ages should also be taken into account.

(2) **Determining main test ages based on scores**

Supplementary items underwent continuous modifications through item testing and repeated assessments during the establishment of the item pool. For example, for the new item "Make protective action," the pass rates based on scores are shown in Table 3.3. The 9, 10, and 11 months were all potential main test ages for the item. Nevertheless, the age of 10 months was selected considering that this item examines the parachute reflex and focuses on the timing of its occurrence, and that a normal infant should exhibit this reflex at around 9–10 months of age. Moreover, a minimum threshold was set at a score of 1. By combining scores of 1 (presence of a reflex) and 2 (standard bilateral extension of forearms), it was observed that only a very small number of infants beyond 11 months of age had not exhibited this reflex. This item can serve as a milestone in the development of the nervous system and as a watershed in determining the presence of brain damage in infants. If an infant beyond the main test age still fails to pass this test item, it should raise concerns about possible brain and nerve damage in the infant.

Table 3.4 shows the pass rates based on scores for the item "Engage in joint attention." The pass rates with 1 point (strong attraction required) at the ages of 11, 12, and 15 months are 52.9%, 53.8%, and 42.1%, respectively. All these three age segments were potential main test ages for the item. After combining scores of 1 and 2 (slight attraction required), the pass rates become 63.5%, 90.8%, and 96.8%, respectively. It was decided after discussion that 12 months would be the main test age,

Table 3.3 Number of participants and pass rates for the item "Make protective action" (n%)

Test age (month)	0 point	1 point	2 points	1 point and 2 points combined	Number of participants
6	13 (100)	0 (0)	0 (0)	0 (0)	13
7	44 (69.8)	8 (12.7)	11 (17.5)	19 (30.2)	63
8	72 (72.7)	15 (15.2)	12 (12.1)	27 (27.3)	99
9 △	32 (32.0)	31 (31.0)	37 (37.0)	68 (68.0)	100
10*	22 (22.2)	26 (26.3)	51 (51.5)	77 (77.8)	99
11 △	3 (3.6)	12 (14.3)	69 (82.1)	81 (96.4)	84
12	2 (1.9)	1 (1.0)	102 (97.1)	103 (98.1)	105
15	0 (0)	2 (14.3)	12 (85.7)	14 (100)	14

*Determined main test age; △ candidate main test age

with a minimum threshold set at a score of 1. The main reasons for this decision are twofold. Firstly, if infants at this age do not engage in joint attention, the item "Fail to look in the direction pointed by others" would be included as a scoring item in the Communication Warning Behavior Subscale. Secondly, the pass rate for the item at 11 months is 63.5% after combining the scores of 1 and 2. Although this also aligns with the principle of determining main test ages, selecting 12 months as the main test age is more logical considering the consistency between ages before and after the item and across different domains.

For the item "Describe the picture contents" at ages of 72 and 78 months, the requirement is to describe the contents of the pictures. In view of the national applicability related to region, environment, and language, a multi-level scoring system was used to assess language expression and summarization abilities. Lower levels of language expression and summarization do not require perfection, but rather relevance to the topic. The main test ages were determined based on the pass rates for each age. Tables 3.5 and 3.6 present the scoring and pass rates for the items "Describe the picture contents" at 72 months and "Summarize the theme of pictures" at 78 months, respectively.

The clinical testing results at the main test age of 72 months are shown in Table 3.5. A score of 1 indicates the ability to correctly describe the contents of three pictures but without understanding the themes, while a score of 2 indicates understanding the themes in addition to correctly

3 DEVELOPMENT AND REVISION OF THE ERXIN SCALES

Table 3.4 Number of participants and pass rates for the item "Engage in joint attention" (n%)

Test age (month)	0 point	1 point	2 points	1 point and 2 points combined	Number of participants
8	29 (74.4)	7 (17.9)	3 (7.7)	10 (25.6)	39
9	49 (75.4)	11 (16.9)	5 (7.7)	16 (24.6)	65
10	51 (56.0)	31 (34.1)	9 (9.9)	40 (44.0)	91
11△	31 (36.5)	45 (52.9)	9 (10.6)	54 (63.5)	85
12*	11 (9.2)	64 (53.8)	44 (37.0)	108 (90.8)	119
15△	3 (3.2)	40 (42.1)	52 (54.7)	92 (96.8)	95
18	2 (2.1)	33 (34.0)	62 (63.9)	95 (97.9)	97
21	0 (4.3)	2 (14.3)	12 (85.7)	14 (100)	14
24	0 (0)	2 (16.7)	10 (83.3)	12 (100.0)	12

*Determined main test age; △ candidate main test age

Table 3.5 Number of participants and pass rates for the item "Describe the picture contents" (n%)

Test age (month)	0 point	1 point for describing pictures	2 points for describing pictures and understanding the themes	1 point and 2 points combined	Number of participants
36	21 (100.0)	0 (0.0)	0 (0.0)	0 (0)	21
42	67 (97.1)	0 (0.0)	2 (2.9)	2 (2.9)	69
48	93 (95.9)	1 (1.0)	3 (3.1)	4 (4.1)	97
54	93 (86.9)	10 (9.4)	4 (3.7)	14 (13.1)	107
60	90 (76.9)	5 (4.3)	22 (18.8)	27 (23.1)	117
66△	63 (59.5)	10 (9.4)	33 (31.1)	43 (40.5)	106
72*	29 (27.9)	29 (27.9)	46 (44.2)	75 (72.1)	104
78△	11 (11.5)	15 (15.6)	70 (72.9)	85 (88.5)	96
84	15 (17.8)	5 (6.0)	64 (76.2)	69 (82.2)	84

*Determined main test age; △ candidate main test age

Table 3.6 Number of participants and pass rates for the item "Summarize the theme of pictures" (n%)

Test age (month)	1 point for describing pictures	2 points for describing pictures and understanding the themes	3 points for understanding and articulating the themes accurately	Number of participants
48	50 (53.8)	25 (26.9)	18 (19.3)	93
54	44 (47.3)	28 (30.1)	21 (22.6)	93
60	22 (24.4)	25 (27.8)	43 (47.8)	90
66	21 (33.3)	17 (27.0)	25 (39.7)	63
72	12 (38.7)	4 (12.9)	15 (48.4)	31
78*	3 (23.1)	4 (30.8)	6 (46.1)	13
84	4 (26.7)	0 (0.0)	11 (73.3)	15

*Determined main test age

describing the contents (though probably with imprecise expressions). The table shows that 66, 72, and 78 months were all potential main test ages. Nonetheless, by combining scores of 1 and 2 and setting a minimum threshold at 1, it was more appropriate to select 72 months as the main test age, with a pass rate of 72.1%.

Table 3.6 presents the clinical testing results at the main test age of 78 months. A score of 1 indicates the ability to correctly describe the contents of three pictures but without understanding the themes, a score of 2 indicates the ability to describe the content of each picture and understand the theme (though probably with imprecise expressions), and a score of 3 indicates the ability to accurately state the themes.

It can be seen from the pass rates exhibited in Tables 3.5 and 3.6 that a score of 2 was observed in both sets of tests. In Table 3.5, the pass rates with a score of 2 for 72 and 78 months are 44.2% and 72.9%, respectively; while in Table 3.6, the pass rate for 78 months is 30.8%, but that with a score of 3 is 46.1%.

On this basis, the expert panel decided to select the criterion for a score of 2 (i.e., being able to describe pictures and understand the themes) as the standard for the age of 78 months, making it the main test age for this item.

3 DEVELOPMENT AND REVISION OF THE ERXIN SCALES   81

(3) **Determining main test ages based on item pass trends**
Some test items contain multiple questions to be answered, necessitating continuous testing across multiple age groups. The number and percentage of correct answers were recorded for each age group, and through observation and analysis of the trends, the main test ages were determined. For instance, for a test item where children aged 30–42 months are shown a card with 24 color pictures, the percentages of pictures with names correctly stated by the children are presented in Table 3.7, and the trends are illustrated in Fig. 3.2. Based on the observed trends, stating the names of 10 (10/24) and 14 (14/24) pictures was set as the threshold for the main test ages of 30 months and 36 months, respectively.

Furthermore, for a test item assessing adaptability where children aged 42–54 months are required to identify the damaged or missing parts in six pictures on a card, the percentages of the parts (including the demonstrated one) correctly identified by children at different ages are presented in Table 3.8, and the trends are illustrated in Fig. 3.3. Identifying 3 and 4 damaged or missing parts was set as the threshold for the main test ages of 48 months and 54 months, respectively.

Another example is the spot-the-difference test item, which involves finding out 10 differences in a set of pictures. The item was administered to children aged 48 months to 84 months. The percentages of differences spotted by children are presented in Table 3.9, and the trends are depicted in Fig. 3.4. Based on the observed trends, the item was included in the assessment for ages of 48, 60, and 72 months. The threshold for these main test ages was set at finding out 3, 5, and 7 differences, respectively.

Table 3.7 Percentages (%) of pictures with names correctly stated by children at ages of 30, 36, and 42 months

Test age (month)	9	10	11	12	13	14	15
30*	70.1	65.1	48.9	41.9	37.2	25.6	14.0
36*	90.0	87.5	80.0	77.5	65.0	52.5	35.0
42	100	100	97.4	92.3	87.2	66.7	64.1

*Determined main test age

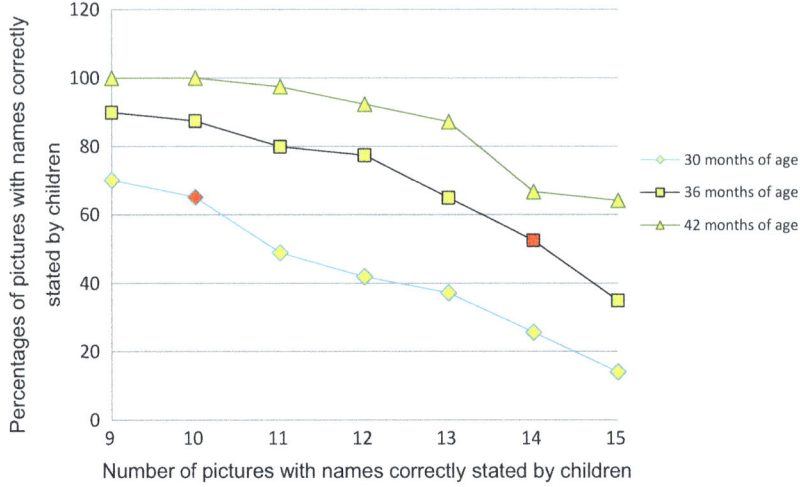

Fig. 3.2 Percentage trends of pictures with names correctly stated by children at ages of 30, 36, and 42 months

Table 3.8 Percentages (%) of damaged or missing parts correctly identified by children at ages of 42, 48, and 54 months

Test age (month)	2	3	4	5	6
42	71.1	44.7	31.6	13.2	2.6
48*	81.6	60.5	44.7	10.5	0
54*	93.0	83.7	55.8	32.6	2.3

*Determined main test age

3.7.1 Establishment of a Preliminary Pool for New Items

(1) **Establishing a preliminary pool for new items amid constant revision**

After designing the new test items and their operational procedures, the healthcare professionals in the revision team formed five testing groups to test children at the expected main test ages and at least four adjacent (two before and two after) ages. Observations and operational procedures were refined based on feedback from doctors and nurses regarding the test process and results,

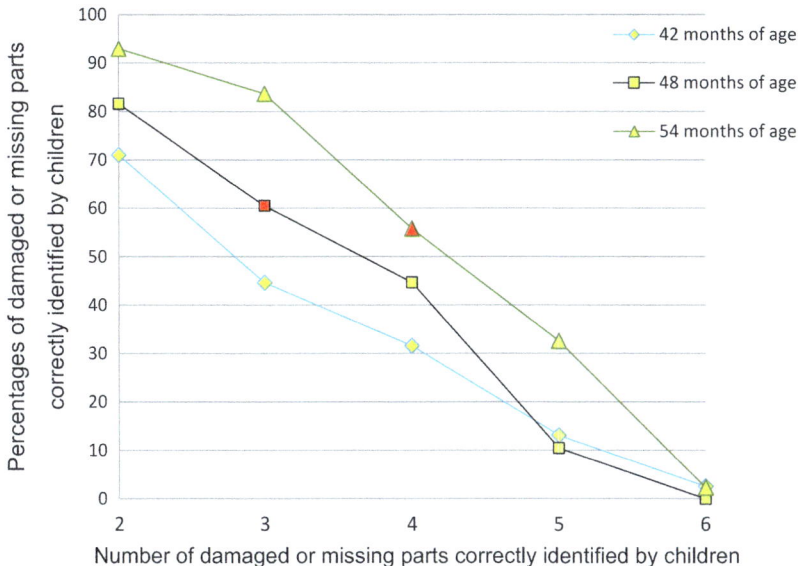

Fig. 3.3 Percentage trends of damaged or missing parts correctly identified by children at ages of 42, 48, and 54 months

Table 3.9 Percentage (%) of differences spotted by children aged 48 months to 84 months

Test age (month)	The number of differences spotted by children									
	1	2	3	4	5	6	7	8	9	10
48*	80.0	67.5	48.1	30.2	22.5	7.5	6.5	0	0	0
54	93.2	90.05	88.7	74.5	50.1	28.5	7.6	1.8	0	0
60*	96.5	96.5	91.8	87.5	48.8	32.1	14.9	4.5	0	0
66	100	95.3	73.5	68.5	68.5	45	20.8	8.9	1.8	0
72*	100	98.5	98.7	93.2	76.5	59.3	45.4	15.9	2.3	0
78	100	98.5	97.3	92.5	90.7	75.7	34.5	17.6	7.5	0.5
84	100	99.8	99.8	99.5	93.5	60.4	43.5	28.5	1.5	4.5

*Determined main test age

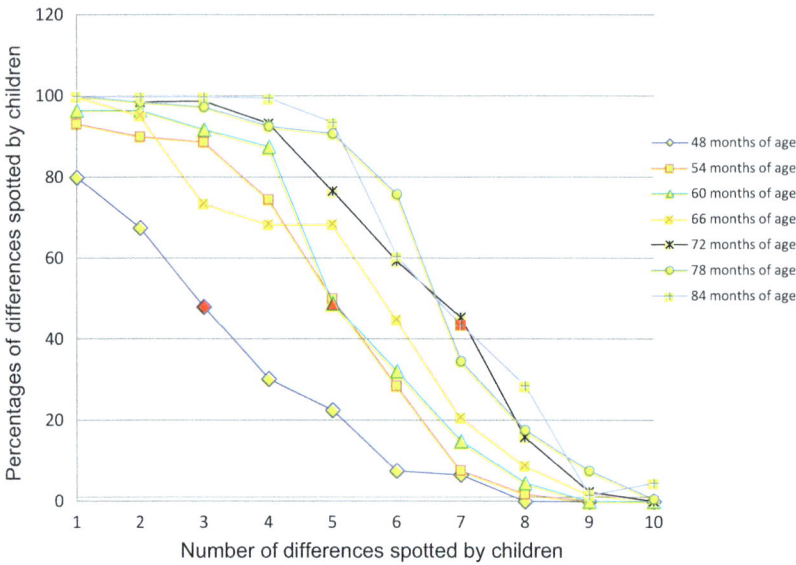

Fig. 3.4 Trends of the percentages of differences spotted by children aged 48 months to 84 months

and clinical testing was conducted to determine the most appropriate main test ages. Some items required repeated clinical testing and multiple modifications, and each modification could not be immediately tested. To ensure consistency in test administration, a "washout period" of at least one month was provided for the operators to avoid the interference or carryover of previous operations. After the tests, a particular item should be discarded only when all participating operators agree that it is difficult to observe. Some items, despite being designed to achieve the intended objectives perfectly, may not be suitable for inclusion in the scale due to prolonged assessment time that does not allow for immediate behavioral responses. A good case in point is the test item which involves inserting wooden blocks with different shapes (triangles, circles, trapezoids, pentagons) into corresponding holes in a box. In the test, children aged 18 to 24 months were encouraged to insert the blocks into the corresponding holes as the operator demonstrated, but they needed to explore and match the shapes to successfully insert the blocks. The test for this item required at least half an hour or even longer to elicit the intended behavior. Although the test was designed craftily to assess cognitive abilities, it was not suitable for use in a scale due to the prolonged period of time required. Likewise, traditional Chinese puzzle games like the tangram were also discarded owing to similar reasons.

The items with creative design and clear measurement objectives but failing to achieve perfect fluency due to flaws during testing were modified. The similarity item for 54-month-olds is an example which initially involved presenting children with shape templates consisting of circles, squares, and triangles, as well as square and circular buttons, and asking them to classify on their own. After the operational method was developed, the item was tested among children at ages of 54, 60, 66, and 72 months. However, the initial testing failed to capture children's interest due to loosely structured and purposeless design, thus not achieving the intended goal of assessing cognitive abilities. Furthermore, the buttons used in the test were ordinary, large buttons commonly found on clothing, the square ones were not perfect squares, and the shape templates were inconsistent in color. Through continuous refinement of the operational method during the testing phase, it was ultimately revised to presenting different combinations of shape templates in two separate sessions, requiring children to classify them and articulate their reasoning. After subsequent clinical testing, the main test age for the item was finally determined to be 54 months. To capture children's interest, the shape templates were uniformly redesigned in red, and specific molds were used for production according to design requirements. The tools used in this operation have applied for a utility model patent.

(2) **Distribution of new items across domains**

Among the 497 new items added to various domains or attributes for developmental assessment, 232 of them were discarded during the constant revision while establishing the item pool, leaving 247 items entering the preparatory testing phase. In other words, only 51.6% of the test items in the pool were retained for further testing. The deletion and retention of new items in each domain are presented in Table 3.10.

Table 3.10 Percentages of deleted and retained new items in each domain

Domain	Number of new items	Number of deleted items (%)	Number of items entering preparatory testing phase (%)
Gross motor	80	55 (68.8)	25 (31.2)
Fine motor	110	39 (35.5)	71 (64.5)
Adaptability	73	40 (54.8)	33 (45.2)
Language	76	31 (40.8)	45 (59.2)
Social behavior	73	33 (45.2)	40 (54.8)
Communication warning behavior	67	34 (50.7)	33 (49.3)
Total	479	232 (48.4)	247 (51.6)

3.7.2 Quality Control During Scale Revision

(1) **Consistency testing**

Prior to administrating the test items, standardized training was provided to the assessors. For items that underwent multiple modifications to the operating procedures or criteria, two training sessions were conducted with an interval of at least one month. The trained assessors should achieve a high level of consistency in their understanding, observation, and operation of the test items. A consistency level of 0.9 or above was deemed acceptable for participating in item administration.

(2) **Child inclusion criteria**

Healthy children aged 0 to 7 years old (from 27 days old up to 7 years and 1.5 months old), born at full term, singleton, and without any high-risk factors (with Apgar scores of 10 at 1 and 5 minutes) were included in the study.

(3) **Child exclusion criteria**

Preterm infants, infants with Apgar scores less than 8 at 1 and 5 minutes, with a history of significant asphyxia or pathological jaundice, or with confirmed neurological developmental abnormalities were excluded from the study. Additionally, those with acute or chronic infectious diseases within the past month were also excluded.

(4) **Age grouping rules**

For children aged under 1 year, each month constituted one segment, resulting in a total of 12 segments. For children aged

1–3 years, segments were formed every 3 months, resulting in 8 segments. For children aged 3–5 years, segments were formed every 6 months, resulting in 4 segments. The assessment scale was extended up to 6 years of age, with an additional 4 age segments formed every 6 months. The main test ages for the extended age range were 66, 72, 78, and 84 months. Consequently, there were a total of 28 age segments for the entire scales.

(5) **Measurement time windows**

a. **Different time windows for different age groups:** For infants aged 1–3 months, the time window was set as 3 days before and after the exact month age. For example, for a 2-month-old infant, the window would be from day 57 to day 63. For infants aged 4–11 months, the time window was set as 7 days before and after the exact month age. For example, for a 4-month-old infant, the window would be from day 113 to day 127. For infants aged 12 months, the time window was set as 7 days before and 15 days after the exact month age. For children aged 15–35 months, the time window was set as 15 days before and after the exact month age. For example, the window would be from month 14.5 to month 15.5 for a 15-month-old toddler. For children aged 36 months, the time window was set as 15 days before and 45 days after the exact month age. For children aged 42–84 months, the time window was set as 45 days before and after the exact month age. For example, for a 48-month-old child, the window would be from month 46.5 to month 49.5.

b. **Starting time of measurement:** In the normative research of the original scales, one month was equated with 30 days, and the time window for infants under 1 year old was set as 15 days before and after the exact month age, with the starting time of measurement set as 15 days after birth. To make the main test ages better reflect the chronological ages of normally developing children especially during infancy, the revised Erxin Scales also considered one month as 30 days, with those within 28 days after birth categorized as newborns. However, the normative research time window for infants within 3 months of age was shortened to 3 days before and after the exact month age, with a lower limit of 27 days. Therefore, the revised Erxin Scales set the starting time of measurement as 27 days after birth. Due to the narrowed time window for normative research, the starting time of measurement for each main test age was shifted backwards by 12 days for infants within 3 months of age, and by 8 days for infants aged 4–12 months. For children older than 1 year, the time windows for the main test ages remained the same as in the original scales.

c. **Prescribing time windows for the standardized scale:** The participants were strictly assessed according to the time window requirements for the age groups, so as to make the participants in the group closer to the chronological age of the corresponding population. By establishing this time window protocol for various age groups, it laid the foundation for future studies on premature infants.

It should be noted that time window was a method used in the normative research. In clinical practice, however, test ages were still calculated by equating a month with 30 days, without considering the time window issue from the standardization research stage.

(6) **Rules for retaining or deleting new items after testing**

For items after testing, either newly added or modified from the original scale, the test results and pass rates were required to be submitted to a panel of experts for detailed discussion. Items with reasonable operation methods and clear theories would be retained, otherwise they would be deleted. The retained items were included in the original revised scales and then tested on representative samples.

3.7.3 Formation of the Original Revised Scales

(1) **Retention and deletion of items in the item pool**

During the iterative modifications while establishing the item pool, 232 out of the 479 newly added test items were discarded, and 247 (51.6%) entered the next stage, namely the preparatory testing phase. Among the initially retained 247 items, 127 (51.4%) of them were deleted after further testing, thereby leaving only 120 items (48.6%) entering the original revised scale. Moreover, from the deleted items five new ones were derived and agreed to be included in the original revised scale by the expert panel. By this point, the original revised scale was devised.

(2) **Distribution of new items across domains in the original revised scales**

In the 0- to 4-year part of the scale, 8 out of the original 177 items were removed, and 52 new items were added, resulting in a total of 221 items in this age range for the original revised scales. For the extended age range from 5 to 6 years, 40 items were added, making a total of 92 new items across the original five domains of the scales. Additionally, 33 new items were added to the Communication Warning Behavior Subscale. Taken together, there were 125 new items in the original revised scales. The distribution of newly added items across domains is shown in Table 3.11.

(3) **Modified items in the original scale across domains**

Among the 177 items in the 0- to 4-year part of the original scales (with national norms), 131 (74.0%) required no modifications, 38 (21.5%) needed improvements, and 8 (4.5%) were deleted. The distribution of modified items across domains is shown in Table 3.11.

(4) **Determination of scoring and testing methods**

The characteristics of child development determine the testing methods of developmental scales. Child development progresses continuously and gradually, with each level of achievement building upon the previous level. Changes occur in distinct processes or

Table 3.11 Distribution of modified and newly added items across domains in the original revised scales

Domain	Items modified from the original scale (%)	Newly added items (%)
Gross motor	3 (7.9)	17 (13.6)
Fine motor	7 (18.4)	19 (15.2)
Adaptability	11 (28.9)	16 (12.8)
Language	12 (31.6)	17 (13.6)
Social behavior	5 (13.2)	23 (18.4)
Communication warning behavior		33 (26.4)
Total	38	125

stages, and behaviors and developmental processes differ qualitatively across different stages [23]. In the revision process, a multi-level scoring method was employed during the testing phase of new items, with the pass rate being the main reference for item retention or deletion. Nonetheless, dichotomous scoring was adopted for the original revised scale formed, and the main test ages, operations, and passing criteria were determined. During the standardization research, each test item was also scored dichotomously, indicating pass or fail. Testing rules for the scale were as follows. Testing begins with the corresponding item based on each child's chronological age and the main test age (selecting the younger main test age corresponding to the chronological age). After finishing the testing for the main test age, two age segments earlier (in the direction of ages younger than the main test age) must be tested. If the child passes the items in a domain for two consecutive age segments, passes would be assumed for all previous items in that domain; otherwise, testing continues backwards until the child passes the items in a domain for two consecutive age segments. Then, testing proceeds in the opposite direction (ages older than the main test age), and in each domain, testing continues until the child fails the items in a domain for two consecutive age segments. The Communication Warning Behavior Subscale adopted a cumulative scoring rule: All items before the main test age need to be observed or inquired; after the main test age, inquiry regarding the domain stops if two consecutive items receive negative responses.

3.8 Standardization of Measurement Tools

3.8.1 Selection of Measurement Tools

In this revision, all tools used in the assessment were standardized. The research funding was efficiently allocated to optimize the testing tools for the original scales and determine their materials, texture, color, size, and specifications. Safety, aesthetics, durability, ease of use, and ease of cleaning and disinfection were also taken into account.

3.8.2 Collaborative Production of Testing Pictures

All pictures used in the assessment were originally produced. Firstly, children's developmental milestones, behavioral patterns, everyday life knowledge, as well as the key aspects and challenges to be reflected in the assessment were described in written form by developmental behavior specialists. Medical professionals or nurses good at drawing also contributed hand-drawn sketches to the descriptions. Joint discussions about the picture contents were then held with child artists who were hired specifically for this purpose. The aim was to create pictures that strike a balance between professional representation and child-friendly aesthetics, meeting the requirements of professional assessment. Out of the original set of 16 pictures, 9 were retained, 3 were removed, and 4 were replaced with color pictures as determined through discussions among experts. The newly designed pictures included 62 color illustrations.

3.8.3 Accessibility of play materials

Play materials from everyday objects familiar to children were used for testing to facilitate children's cognitive and socio-emotional development. When selecting item-specific materials, their accessibility in the home environment was considered. For example, activities such as reacting to the figure in the mirror, removing cup, and pouring water without spilling could be easily conducted in various home settings.

3.8.4 Novelty and operability of new measurement tools

The selection of measurement tools focused on objects or play materials that are appealing to children to enhance their interest and motivation. New measurement tools, including black-and-white targets, latches, hats, scissors, test-specific paper, screws and nuts, balls with rope, and multifunctional dolls, were designed to demonstrate both novelty and operability. Specifically designed or custom-made tools include special brass bells, mirrors, red balls, four-color picture cards, and templates with similar shapes. The types of measurement tools increased from the original 40 to 54.

3.8.5 Replacement of Measurement Tools

(1) **Safety and convenience**

Considering the safety and ease of organization, certain measurement tools were replaced. For example, transparent glass bottles were replaced with equally sized transparent plastic bottles to avoid safety issues associated with glass breakage. In specific cases, such as the "shake and gaze at the rattle drum" task, the use of sheepskin rattle drum proved challenging for infants with weak physical strength or premature babies who were unable to lift and shake them. This hindered observation and differentiation, thus affecting assessment results. To address this, the operation remained unchanged, but the rattle drum was replaced with a bell stick.

(2) **Specific match between testing tools and instructions**

Each scales have its specific testing tools, operational methods, and passing criteria, which should not be arbitrarily changed or replaced. The measurement tools used for the Erxin Scales were specifically matched with the corresponding instructions. During the standardization research for scale usage, instances were observed where evaluators used alternative or similar tools for Erxin Scales tests. This affected the consistency in operations and the validity of scale usage. It is emphasized that dedicated tools matching the Erxin Scales instructions should be used, and arbitrary replacements be avoided.

3.9 RESEARCH SAMPLE AND SAMPLING CRITERIA

Based on the revision time of the scale, 2010 national census data were referred to when determining the ratio of children aged 0–1, 1–4, and 5–9, and a 1:1 gender ratio was adopted, employing a stratified cluster random sampling method. Theoretically 2,520 individuals were supposed to be sampled in Beijing. However, in effect 2,779 children aged 0–7 participated in the assessment, with 1,468 boys (52.8%) and 1,311 girls (47.2%), resulting in a 1.1:1 male-to-female ratio. Fathers, mothers, and guardians with a bachelor's degree or above accounted for 51.7%, 48.3%, and 41.5%, respectively. The national sampling followed the same criteria as Beijing, with a theoretical sample size of 5,880 individuals and an actual participation of 6,173 individuals, including 3,155 males (51.1%) and 3,018 females (48.9%). As a result, the theoretical size for the national and Beijing samples combined was 8,400 individuals, with an actual participation of 8,952 individuals, including 4,623 males (51.6%) and 4,329 females (48.4%).

The determination of new items in the Communication Warning Behavior Subscale was based on a case–control study conducted in the areas where the Erxin Scales were revised nationwide. At the completion of the scale revision, the total number of children involved in the sampling and the case–control study was 9,796.

REFERENCES

1 Bayley, N. (1993). *Bayley scales of infant development* (2nd ed.). The Psychological, Corporation.
2 Bayley, N. (2006). *Bayley scales of infant and toddler development* (3rd ed.). Technical manual. Harcourt Assessment.
3 Soares, M., & McCrimmon, A. (2013). Test review: Wechsler preschool and primary scale of intelligence, fourth edition: Canadian. *Canadian Journal of School Psychology, 28*(4), 345–345.
4 Yi, S. R., Luo, X. R., Yang, Z. W., et al. (1993). The revising of the Bayley Scales of Infant Development (BSID) in China. *Chinese Journal of Clinical Psychology, 2*, 71–75.
5 Zhang, X. L., Li, J. P., Qin, M. J., et al. (1994). The revise of Gesell Development Scale on 3.5–6 years of age in Beijing. *Chinese Journal of Clinical Psychology, 3*, 148–150.
6 Zhang, J. J., Gao, Z. M., Xue, H., et al. (1997). The study of developmental diagnostic scale of children aged 0–4 years. *Chinese Journal of Child Health Care, 3*, 144–147.
7 Gesell, A. L., Amatruda, C. S., Knobloch, H., & Pasamanick, B. (1975). *Gesell and Amatruda's Developmental diagnosis: The evaluation and management of normal and abnormal neuropsychologic development in infancy and early childhood*. Harper & Row Publishers.
8 Xue, H., Mao, Y. Y., Zhang, C. R., et al. (1986). An attempt to develop a neurodevelopmental scale for children aged 0–3 years by combining vertical and horizontal examination. *Chinese Journal of Medicine, 66*(2), 70–74.
9 Jian, Z. F., Zhang, G. H., Zeng, Y. X., et al. (2013). Research on the correlation between Alberta infant motor scale and the motion field of 0–6-year-old pediatric examination table of neuropsychological development. *Chinese Journal of Child Health Care, 21*(12), 1327–1329.

10 Long, F., Chen, Y. B., Wang, Y. L., et al. (2010). Evaluation of the intellectual development status of transported premature infants by Neonatal behavioral neurometry combined with the Erxin Scale. *Chinese Journal of Neonatology, 25*(1), 20–23.
11 Feng, L. Y., Zheng, M. S., Liu, X. Y., et al. (1997). Study on mental development on children in urban and rural of Shanghai. *Shanghai Journal of Preventive Medicine, 9*(11), 496–498.
12 Yang, X. Z., Yang, G. X., Zhang, C. M., et al. (1992). A preliminary study on the child heart mental development scale for 0–3-year-olds. *Maternal and Child Health Care of China, 7*(4), 51–53.
13 Pan, H. N., Chen, S. M., Wu, Y. L., et al. (2007). Analysis of clinical test results of neuropsychological development examination table in 1200 children. *Maternal and Child Health Care of China, 22*(10), 1337–1340.
14 Piaget, J. (1981). *Principles of genetic epistemology* (X. D. Wang, Trans.). The Commercial Press.
15 Tardif, T. (2008). *Chinese communicative development inventories: User's guide and manual (Mandarin and Cantonese versions)*. Peking University Medical Press.
16 Amiel-Tison, C., & Gosselin, J. (2001). *Neurological development from birth to six years: Guide for examination and evaluation*. Johns Hopkins University Press.
17 Allen, D. A., Rapin, I., & Wiznitzer, M. (1998). Communication disorders of preschool children: The physician's responsibility. *Journal of Developmental and Behavioral Pediatrics, 9*(3), 164–170.
18 Charman, T., Drew, A., Baird, C., & Baird, G. (2003). Measuring early language development in preschool children with autism spectrum disorder using the MacArthur communicative development inventory (Infant Form). *Journal of Child Language, 30*(1), 213–236.
19 Jing, J. (2003). The neural mechanism of speech and language disorders in children. *Chinese Journal of Child Health Care, 11*(5), 323–327.
20 Liang, W. L., Hao, B., Wang, S., et al. (2001). The study of chinese language and communicative development-word part. *Chinese Journal of Child Health Care, 5*, 295–297.
21 Jin, X. M., Ma, J., Zhang, Y. W., et al. (2009). A preliminary study on development of the Chinese children's first 50 words. *Chinese Journal of Evidence-Based Pediatrics, 4*(3), 301–305.
22 Jin, X. M. (2003). Speech training for speech-language development and hearing impairment. *Journal of Clinical Pediatrics, 21*(12), 820–823.
23 Feldman, R. S. (2013). *Developmental psychology: The lifelong development of human beings* (6th ed.) (Y. J, Su & D. Zou, Trans.). World Book Publishing Company.

CHAPTER 4

Psychometric Analysis of the Erxin Scales

4.1 Difficulty Distribution of Items Across Domains

Difficulty coefficient, which represents pass rate, is crucial for assessing the difficulty level of items in child developmental scales. Ideally, the difficulty coefficients of items in a psychological scale should follow a normal distribution centered around 0.5. In the case of developmental scales, however, the test items are usually slightly easier, so that the children being assessed will be interested, confident, and cooperative, thus facilitating smooth administration of the test. To reach a moderate difficulty level with balanced proportion of easy and difficult items, during the initial item testing phase of scale revision, items with difficulty coefficients ranging from 0.25 to 0.9 ought to be retained, while those with difficulty coefficients below 0.25 or above 0.9 should be eliminated or reduced to a small portion. The difficulty coefficients of items in the five domains all approximated a normal distribution, with an average difficulty of 0.65 ± 0.21. The difficulty levels were consistent across domains, indicating a solid internal structure.

Among the items in the five attributes (excluding those related to communication warning behaviors), 70.9% (185/261) had a difficulty coefficient within the range of 0.2 to 0.8, leaving 76 falling outside the range. Specifically, items with a difficulty coefficient less than 0.2 accounted for 2.3% (6/261), while those exceeding 0.8 accounted for

© The Author(s), under exclusive license to Springer Nature
Singapore Pte Ltd. 2024
C. Jin et al., *Erxin Scales: Child Developmental Scale of China*,
https://doi.org/10.1007/978-981-99-9997-2_4

Table 4.1 Difficulty coefficients and composition ratio of test items in the five attributes for children ages 0 to 6 years old

Domain/Attribute	Difficulty coefficient $M \pm SD$ ($\overline{X} \pm s$)	Distribution of difficulty coefficients (number of items %)			Total
		< 0.2	0.2–0.8	> 0.8	
Gross motor	0.67 ± 0.17	0 (0)	35 (70.0)	15 (30.0)	50
Fine motor	0.55 ± 0.22	3 (5.8)	43 (82.7)	6 (11.5)	52
Adaptability	0.66 ± 0.20	1 (1.8)	37 (67.3)	17 (30.9)	55
Language	0.70 ± 0.18	0 (0)	38 (73.1)	14 (26.9)	52
Social behavior	0.70 ± 0.20	2 (3.9)	32 (61.5)	18 (34.6)	52
Total	0.65 ± 0.21	6 (2.3)	185 (70.9)	70 (26.8)	261

26.8% (70/261). Further, among those with a difficulty coefficient exceeding 0.8, approximately one-third (24 items) were for assessing infants under 6 months old, and one-sixth (12 items) were distributed among the 42- and 48-month age groups. The remaining 34 items were scattered across different age groups. The difficulty coefficient distribution of items across the five attributes is shown in Table 4.1.

4.2 Item Discrimination

The overall DQs of the participating children were ranked based on their chronological age, and the upper and lower 27% of the children were selected for chi-square tests. By calculating the critical ratio (CR) or cut-off value for the main test ages of each test item, a significance level of $p < 0.05$ was adopted to evaluate the discriminative or distinguishing ability of each item. If an item yielded a p-value below 0.05, it was considered to have high discriminability and was deemed suitable for the corresponding age group. Out of the 261 items in the gross motor, fine motor, adaptability, language, and social behavior domains of the original revised scale, 259 (99.2%) demonstrated discriminability ($p < 0.05$). As for the two items lacking discriminability at the main test age ($p > 0.05$), one was "Walk up the stairs with support from the wall" at 21 months, and the other was "What is your surname?" at 60 months. However, both items showed statistical significance ($p < 0.05$) at the age segment earlier than the corresponding main test age, namely at 18 months and 54 months, respectively [1]. Considering that test items should be administered in the

Table 4.2 Composition ratio of correlation between test items and month age in each attribute

Correlation strength*	Number of items in each attribute (%)					Total
	Gross motor	Fine motor	Adaptability	Language	Social behavior	
Strong	35(70.0%)	32(61.5%)	26(47.3%)	21(38.9%)	16(32.0%)	130(49.8%)
Moderate	15(30%)	16(30.8%)	27(49.1%)	29(53.7%)	28(56.0%)	115(44.1%)
Weak	0	4(7.7%)	2(3.6%)	4(7.4%)	6(12.0%)	16(6.1%)

*$r \geq 0.7$: strong correlation, $0.5 < r < 0.7$: moderate correlation, $r < 0.5$: weak correlation

two adjacent age segments before and after the main test age, these two items were retained.

4.3 Correlation Between Test Items and Month Age

The scale items were arranged in ascending order of difficulty according to month age and categorized structurally. Correlation existed between the pass rate of test items and the month ages in the gross motor, fine motor, adaptability, language, and social behavior domains, with the exception of Item #4 ("Natural state of hands" in fine motor domain at 1 month of age) [2]. Among them, 49.8% (130/261) exhibited a strong correlation ($r \geq 0.7$), while 44.1% (115/261) showed a moderate correlation ($0.5 < r < 0.7$) (See Table 4.2).

4.4 Reliability Tests

4.4.1 Inter-Rater Reliability

The Kendall's coefficient of concordance concerning DQs for both the overall scale and the five domains ranged from 0.98 to 1.

4.4.2 Homogeneity Reliability

The internal consistency (Cronbach's α) coefficient of the overall scales were determined based on the main test ages of the items. The participants were divided into 28 age segments, and the coefficients of the

Table 4.3 Homogeneity reliability coefficients of the overall scale for each main test age

Main test age	N	Standardized Cronbach's α	Number of items	Main test age	N	Standardized Cronbach's α	Number of items
1 month	164	0.892	20	21 months	229	0.887	26
2 months	183	0.954	29	24 months	220	0.890	28
3 months	197	0.940	30	27 months	211	0.895	27
4 months	216	0.946	28	30 months	213	0.882	28
5 months	201	0.938	29	33 months	233	0.850	27
6 months	289	0.915	28	36 months	220	0.886	28
7 months	286	0.910	28	42 months	243	0.906	29
8 months	260	0.882	27	48 months	293	0.899	30
9 months	270	0.868	28	54 months	324	0.875	29
10 months	249	0.882	26	60 months	330	0.861	29
11 months	225	0.892	26	66 months	324	0.873	29
12 months	245	0.910	26	72 months	304	0.898	30
15 months	270	0.921	25	78 months	283	0.905	30
18 months	241	0.883	26	84 months	181	0.877	20

overall internal consistency for all age groups were above 0.85 (see Table 4.3). For the five domain-specific subscales, 91.4% (128/140) of the items gained a Cronbach's α of 0.60 or higher at the main test ages. Specifically, the percentages for the gross motor, fine motor, adaptability, language, and social behavior domains were 96.4%, 92.9%, 96.4%, 89.3%, and 82.1%, respectively (see Table 4.4).

4.4.3 Split-Half Reliability

After conducting an independent equivalent split of the data, the overall scale still demonstrated satisfactory psychometric properties, with the Cronbach's α of the two parts reaching or approaching 0.80 at the main test ages. The Spearman-Brown coefficients of the two parts reached 0.80 at 27 main test ages, as shown in Table 4.5. For the gross motor, fine motor, adaptability, language, and social behavior subscales, after applying the Spearman-Brown correction, the split-half reliability coefficients were 100%, 85.7% (24/28), 92.9% (26/28), 92.9% (26/28), and 82.1% (23/28), respectively, with an average of 90.7% (127/140), as shown in Table 4.6. It is worth noting that only the adaptability subscale showed a low split-half reliability coefficient of 0.333 at 84 months of age.

Table 4.4 Homogeneity reliability coefficients of the subscales for each main test age

Main test age	Standardized Cronbach's α				
	Gross motor	Fine motor	Adaptability	Language	Social behavior
1 month	0.830	**0.485**	0.754	0.723	0.829
2 months	0.894	0.657	0.892	0.843	0.856
3 months	0.881	0.744	0.849	0.714	0.695
4 months	0.885	0.867	0.699	0.673	0.749
5 months	0.779	0.842	0.812	0.720	0.717
6 months	0.763	0.752	0.825	**0.507**	0.568
7 months	0.725	0.753	0.786	0.555	0.621
8 months	0.746	0.810	0.675	0.624	**0.470**
9 months	0.803	0.810	**0.545**	0.672	**0.441**
10 months	0.818	0.775	0.636	0.743	0.574
11 months	0.827	0.742	0.619	0.736	0.628
12 months	0.908	0.732	0.724	0.756	0.597
15 months	0.814	0.696	0.781	0.833	0.555
18 months	0.678	0.610	0.662	0.781	0.552
21 months	**0.534**	0.677	0.683	0.784	0.713
24 months	0.744	0.639	0.695	0.813	0.695
27 months	0.769	0.646	0.717	0.800	0.655
30 months	0.743	**0.539**	0.640	0.745	0.684
33 months	0.598	0.573	0.646	0.655	0.630
36 months	0.694	0.603	0.739	0.755	0.718
42 months	0.807	0.732	0.775	0.707	0.715
48 months	0.823	0.722	0.717	0.628	0.657
54 months	0.798	0.664	0.754	**0.539**	**0.475**
60 months	0.798	0.664	0.754	**0.539**	**0.475**
66 months	0.711	0.704	0.636	0.557	0.611
72 months	0.797	0.630	0.633	0.721	0.700
78 months	0.840	0.671	0.651	0.742	0.608
84 months	0.818	0.703	0.574	0.572	**0.501**

4.4.4 Test–Retest Reliability

The test–retest reliability was assessed for two age groups, 0–4 years and 4–6 years. For the age group of 0–4 years [3], the test–retest reliability correlation coefficient was 0.971 for the overall scales, and 0.902, 0.903, 0.900, 0.939, and 0.955 for the gross motor, fine motor, adaptability, language, and social behavior subscales, respectively (see Table 4.7). For the age group of 4–6 years [4], all the subscales achieved a reliability

Table 4.5 Split-half reliability coefficients of the overall scale for each main test age

Main test age	N	Cronbach's α				Spearman-Brown coefficient
		Part 1		Part 2		
		Value	Number of items	Value	Number of items	
1 month	164	0.82	10	0.77	10	0.917
2 months	183	0.92	15	0.91	15	0.968
3 months	197	0.89	15	0.88	15	0.956
4 months	216	0.90	15	0.91	15	0.962
5 months	201	0.89	15	0.89	15	0.950
6 months	289	0.84	15	0.85	15	0.937
7 months	286	0.81	15	0.87	15	0.925
8 months	260	0.81	15	0.80	15	0.902
9 months	270	0.82	15	0.76	15	0.922
10 months	249	0.82	15	0.79	15	0.943
11 months	225	0.82	15	0.82	15	0.940
12 months	245	0.86	15	0.83	15	0.952
15 months	270	0.87	15	0.87	15	0.963
18 months	241	0.79	15	0.82	15	0.924
21 months	229	0.81	15	0.80	15	0.933
24 months	220	0.81	15	0.80	15	0.932
27 months	211	0.82	15	0.82	15	0.934
30 months	213	0.81	15	0.79	15	0.893
33 months	233	**0.71**	15	0.76	15	0.890
36 months	220	0.78	15	0.79	15	0.896
42 months	243	0.83	15	0.83	15	0.914
48 months	293	0.82	15	0.78	15	0.914
54 months	324	0.77	15	**0.73**	15	0.895
60 months	330	0.81	15	**0.73**	15	**0.742**
66 months	324	0.81	15	0.79	15	**0.774**
72 months	304	0.84	15	0.84	15	0.806
78 months	283	0.87	15	0.82	15	0.809
84 months	181	0.84	15	0.76	15	0.786

coefficient above 0.8 except for the gross motor domain, which had a coefficient of 0.78 (see Table 4.8).

4 PSYCHOMETRIC ANALYSIS OF THE ERXIN SCALES 101

Table 4.6   Split-half reliability coefficients of the subscales for each main test age

Main test age	Gross motor	Fine motor	Adaptability	Language	Social behavior
1 month	0.757	**0.501**	0.741	0.612	0.882
2 months	0.865	0.709	0.915	0.901	0.921
3 months	0.862	0.750	0.853	0.811	0.831
4 months	0.882	0.861	0.729	0.900	0.778
5 months	0.777	0.880	0.835	0.874	0.637
6 months	0.710	0.793	0.824	0.856	**0.528**
7 months	0.686	0.626	0.767	0.794	0.690
8 months	0.729	0.602	0.672	0.821	0.836
9 months	0.798	0.784	0.620	0.809	0.894
10 months	0.819	0.929	0.718	0.886	0.770
11 months	0.876	0.950	0.772	0.804	0.748
12 months	0.958	0.874	0.872	0.741	0.724
15 months	0.982	0.782	0.903	0.822	0.716
18 months	0.903	0.761	0.644	0.738	0.769
21 months	0.846	0.867	0.585	0.849	0.737
24 months	0.922	0.865	0.642	0.848	0.704
27 months	0.982	0.867	0.605	0.801	0.662
30 months	0.979	**0.496**	0.567	0.769	0.668
33 months	1.000	0.560	0.618	0.686	0.570
36 months	0.935	**0.546**	0.586	0.760	0.674
42 months	0.873	**0.539**	0.726	0.769	0.729
48 months	0.787	0.661	0.664	0.710	0.614
54 months	0.734	0.681	0.633	0.562	0.801
60 months	0.723	0.658	0.718	**0.458**	0.782
66 months	0.792	0.637	0.646	0.588	**0.545**
72 months	0.771	0.647	0.668	0.636	**0.544**
78 months	0.744	0.721	**0.561**	0.603	**0.529**
84 months	0.710	0.663	**0.333**	**0.542**	**0.515**

Table 4.7   Test–retest reliability coefficients for the 0–4 years age group (n = 101) ($\overline{X} \pm s$)

Item	First test	Second test	Correlation coefficient
Gross motor DQ	105 ± 15	106 ± 15	0.902
Fine motor DQ	95 ± 14	96 ± 14	0.903
Adaptability DQ	100 ± 17	102 ± 17	0.900
Language DQ	102 ± 17	102 ± 18	0.939
Social behavior DQ	103 ± 21	103 ± 20	0.955
Overall DQ	101 ± 14	102 ± 14	0.971

Table 4.8 Test–retest reliability coefficients for the 4–6 years age group (n = 30) ($\overline{X} \pm s$)

Item	First test	Second test	Correlation coefficient
Gross motor DQ	120 ± 11	120 ± 11	0.78
Fine motor DQ	107 ± 10	108 ± 9	0.84
Adaptability DQ	117 ± 13	120 ± 12	0.89
Language DQ	119 ± 12	119 ± 10	0.89
Social behavior DQ	127 ± 16	127 ± 15	0.94
Overall DQ	118 ± 7	119 ± 7	0.90

4.5 Correlation with Criterion Scales

The correlation of the Erxin Scales with GDS and WPPSI-Rs was tested to assess the criterion-related validity. For the age group of 0–3 years (under 4 years), 101 children sampled from Beijing and another 124 children sampled across the country were included. Each child underwent assessment respectively using the revised Erxin Scales and GDS within a maximum interval of 15 days. The correlation coefficients between the Erxin Scales overall DQ and the GDS adaptability DQ were 0.637 for Beijing and 0.570 nationwide, indicating a moderate correlation. For the age group of 4–6 years, 30 children from Beijing and 74 children nationwide underwent assessment respectively using the revised Erxin Scales and WPPSI-R within a maximum interval of 30 days. The correlation coefficients between the Erxin Scales overall DQ and the WPPSI-R full-scale IQ were 0.78 for Beijing and 0.66 nationwide, indicating a moderate to high correlation. See Table 4.9 for the correlation with GDS and WPPSI-R regarding their assessment results.

4.6 Factor Analysis

The items for different main test ages were combined into nine subsets starting from 1 month of age. Specifically, the nine subsets were created for the following age ranges: 1–3 months, 4–6 months, 7–9 months, 10–12 months, 15–21 months, 24–30 months, 33–42 months, 48–60 months, and 66–84 months. Except for the last subset which had a sample size of 780 individuals and 40 items (see Section 5.5 of Chapter 5 for detailed analysis), the sample sizes for the other subsets ranged from 325 to 406 individuals, and the number of items ranged from 27 to 30.

Table 4.9 Correlation of the revised Erxin Scales with GDS and WPPSI-R ($\overline{X} \pm s$)

Age group	Region	Item	$\overline{X} \pm s$	N	Pearson correlation
4–6 years	Beijing	Erxin Scales overall DQ	107 ± 12	30	0.78
		WPPSI-R full scale IQ	105 ± 16		
	Nationwide	Erxin Scales overall DQ	107 ± 10	74	0.66
		WPPSI-R full scale IQ	110 ± 13		
0–3 years	Beijing	Erxin Scales overall DQ	98 ± 10	101	0.64
		GDS adaptability DQ	91 ± 11		
	Nationwide	Erxin Scales overall DQ	97 ± 7	124	0.57
		GDS adaptability DQ	95 ± 10		

The suitability for factor analysis was assessed using Kaiser–Meyer–Olkin (KMO) measure and Bartlett's test of sphericity. The KMO values of the subsets ranged from 0.932 to 0.976, indicating high internal consistency of the scale. All developmental scales should have their items arranged in ascending order of difficulty. However, the first and last items may have limited expansion, and the corresponding data obtained may be affected and not easily meet the statistical requirements. In view of this, the first subset of the scale was analyzed first to examine if it met the statistical requirements, and the factor analysis results are shown in Table 4.10. We could see that the scale had good construct validity and thus was suitable for factor analysis. The cumulative variance explained by the extracted five factors (with eigenvalues greater than 1 after rotation) accounted for 66.878% of the total variance, and the average communality of the items was 0.669. The horizontal columns in the table list the loadings of the standardized items on each extracted factor, while the vertical columns list the loadings of the items on a specific extracted factor. The dimensions of the scale were named to match the extracted factors, and three of them could be essentially represented by "gross motor," "adaptability," and "language," consistent with the established terminology in the industry. However, the fine motor items with loadings greater than 0.5 were dispersed across different factors, with 50% overlapping with the adaptability factor. Social behavior items were concentrated in Factors 1 and 2, and items with loadings close to 0.5 overlapped with the factors of language and adaptability. Despite this, it is still feasible to name them based on the existing nomenclature from a developmental perspective, given the difficulty in differentiating the mutually influenced and promoted sensory perception skills of infants [1]. The same method was used to analyze the other eight subsets, which achieved better match between the extracted factors and each domain compared with the first subset. Due to the large amount of data and the repetitive nature of the analysis for the eight subsets, only the analysis results for the 1–3 months subset are listed in Table 4.10.

4.7 Confirmatory Factor Analysis

To further validate the fit between the conceptual model and the actual data, confirmatory factor analysis ought to be conducted separately for the nine subsets identified during factor analysis. Considering the characteristics of the developmental scale and the basic requirements for sample size in confirmatory factor analysis, every two adjacent age segments were combined (e.g., 1 month and 2 months, 2 months and 3 months), and the combined age groups were analyzed in sequence. The analysis parameters for the combined age groups are shown in Table 4.11. The Comparative Fit Index (CFI) and the Non-Normed Fit Index (NNFI) were both greater than 0.9 (closer to 1 is better), and the Root Mean Square Error of Approximation (RMSEA) was mostly below 0.08 (smaller is better), with a maximum of 0.10. This indicates that the five-dimensional structure of the scale, corresponding to the five attributes, was sound [1]. To ensure the integrity and coherence of the analysis process, a separate confirmatory factor analysis was conducted for the first subset (1–3 months) mentioned above, the results of which are listed in the first row of Table 4.11. The model fit indices generated by the analysis are presented in Fig. 4.1, where n signifies the number of items in the analyzed data, the letters following n signify the domains or attributes (a for gross motor, b for fine motor, c for adaptability, d for language, and e for social behavior), the numbers before the underscore signify the sequential number of the items in each domain, and the numbers after the

Table 4.10 Factor loadings matrix after rotation and the match with scale domains for items assessing infants aged 1–3 months

Domain/ Attribute	Item	Percentage of variance explained by eigenvalues	Cumulative percentage explained	Factor 1	2	3	4	5	Communality
Adaptability	#25 Watch toy on the front of the chest immediately			0.836	0.221	0.249	0.153	0.008	0.834
Social behavior	#29 Actively observe the surrounding environment			0.831	0.207	0.230	0.130	−0.015	0.804
Social behavior	#28 Laugh when seeing people			0.816	0.235	0.200	0.135	−0.050	0.782
Adaptability	#26 Eyes and head turn 180° following the red ball			0.805	0.143	0.126	0.160	0.012	0.710
Fine motor	#23 Hold the bell stick for 30 s			0.782	0.205	0.212	0.112	−0.024	0.712
Adaptability	#16 Eyes turn up and down following the red ball			0.697	0.404	0.116	0.236	0.058	0.722
Language	#18 Make complex reactions to sounds			0.640	0.497	0.175	0.130	0.016	0.705

(continued)

Table 4.10 (continued)

Domain/ Attribute	Item	Percentage of variance explained by eigenvalues	Cumulative percentage explained	Factor					Communality
				1	2	3	4	5	
Fine motor	#24 Put hands together			0.636	0.228	0.146	−0.108	0.100	0.500
Gross motor	#22 Head raising 45° when lying prone			0.609	0.024	0.405	0.233	−0.051	0.592
Adaptability	#6 Cross the midline with eyes following the red ball			0.605	0.202	0.103	0.475	0.277	0.720
Adaptability	#15 Watch the big toy immediately			0.599	0.478	0.194	0.316	−0.036	0.725
Gross motor	#21 Head upright when held straight			0.543	0.046	0.455	0.240	−0.065	0.566
Fine motor	#13 Hold the bell stick for a moment	27.663	27.663	0.542	0.394	0.404	0.001	−0.110	0.624

4 PSYCHOMETRIC ANALYSIS OF THE ERXIN SCALES 107

Domain/ Attribute	Item	Percentage of variance explained by eigenvalues	Cumulative percentage explained	Factor 1	2	3	4	5	Communality
Adaptability	#5 Watch black-and-white target			0.240	0.689	−0.0002	0.329	−0.006	0.641
Social behavior	#19 Smile spontaneously R			0.097	0.664	0.219	0.152	0.031	0.522
Language	#17 Pronounce "a," "o," "e" or other consonants			0.535	0.617	0.110	0.183	−0.102	0.722
Language	#27 Laugh out loud R			0.524	0.601	0.056	−0.017	0.005	0.639
Fine motor	#14 Thumb separates when tapped lightly			0.124	0.584	0.265	−0.046	0.166	0.457
Social behavior	#20 Respond when being teased			0.499	0.548	0.295	0.199	−0.132	0.692
Language	#8 Respond to sound	15.041	42.703	0.352	0.508	0.173	0.130	0.165	0.456

(continued)

Table 4.10 (continued)

Domain/Attribute	Item	Percentage of variance explained by eigenvalues	Cumulative percentage explained	Factor					Communality
				1	2	3	4	5	
Gross motor	#2 Tilt and raise the head when lying prone			0.153	0.179	0.827	0.029	0.050	0.743
Gross motor	#12 Head lifted off the bed when lying prone			0.444	0.141	0.776	0.093	−0.063	0.831
Gross motor	#11 Head upright for a moment when sitting up by pulled the wrists			0.536	0.236	0.654	0.190	−0.102	0.817
Gross motor	#1 Head upright for a moment when sitting upright with shoulders supported by the tester	11.996	54.699	0.234	0.276	0.653	0.176	0.097	0.598

Domain/Attribute	Item	Percentage of variance explained by eigenvalues	Cumulative percentage explained	Factor 1	2	3	4	5	Communality
Fine motor	#3 Clench a fist when touching the palm			0.110	0.021	0.061	0.658	0.058	0.453
Social behavior	#10 Eyes track people who move around			0.249	0.363	0.211	0.647	0.097	0.667
Social behavior	#9 Stare at the speaker	8.031	62.730	0.241	0.513	0.158	0.600	−0.154	0.730
Fine motor	#4 Natural state of hands			−0.068	0.234	0.122	0.248	0.786	0.753
Language	#7 Make small guttural sound R	4.147	66.878	−0.078	0.269	0.371	0.369	−0.570	0.678
	Eigenvalue			8.022	4.362	3.479	2.329	1.203	

underscore signify the main test age in months. The fit indices suggest a sound five-factor structure.

Based on the discrimination index of the items, the characteristics of the developmental scale, and the results of factor analysis and confirmatory factor analysis, the following criteria for item deletion were determined: Items with factor loadings below 0.3 in two consecutive combined age groups were deleted (e.g., Item #4 "Natural state of hands"); items with factor loadings low in one group but not in the other were retained (e.g., Item #3 "Clench a fist when touching the palm"). After removing Items #3 and #4, the fit indices generated by the software are shown in Fig. 4.1. We can see that the RMSEA and χ^2 values decreased (a smaller χ^2 value indicates a better model fit when the degree of freedom (df) remains unchanged), indicating a better model fit and the superiority of their deletion over retention. However, the retention of Items #3 and #4 would also be statistically acceptable and hence done considering the limitations faced by the initial items of development scales and the continuity of clinical assessments. Item #7 ("Make small guttural sound"), with the minimum negative loading in the factor analysis, had high loadings in two consecutive combined age groups and thus was retained. Additionally, the 48–84 months subset (encompassing items for infants aged 4–6 years) had a larger sample size than required and higher χ^2 values. Although its CFI and NNFI were above 0.9, further subgroup analyses were necessary. The analyses for the age groups of 48–54 months and 54–60 months are presented in Table 4.11. Taking 66, 72, and 78 months as one subset and 78 and 84 months as another for analysis, all item factor loadings met the statistical requirements, with a minimum value above 0.3. The corresponding parameters are listed in the last two rows of Table 4.11. To facilitate understanding, the model fit indices for the 66–78 months subset are presented in Fig. 4.2. Among them, Item #257 "Know one's own zodiac sign" had a low factor loading, and its deletion improved the model fit (although this item was retained in the 54–66 months subset where its factor loading of 0.3 was within the acceptable range). The analysis of model fit data showed that CFI and NNFI were above 0.90, and RMSEA values were mostly below 0.080 (those for the age groups of 1–2 months and 11–12 months were slightly above 0.08 but still below 0.10). The factor loadings of items might only be low in one of the two consecutive subsets (combined age groups), which was determined by the necessity of continuous item testing across multiple age segments in the developmental scale. The good fit between

Table 4.11 Specific parameters of model fit for each combined age group

Combined month age group	X^2	df	X^2/df	CFI	NNFI	RMSEA
1–3	756.0	309	2.45	0.97	0.97	0.095
1 and 2	331.8	142	2.34	0.92	0.90	0.098
2 and 3	261.4	142	1.84	0.98	0.98	0.067
3 and 4	204.7	94	2.17	0.93	0.91	0.077
4 and 5	263.1	142	1.85	0.98	0.97	0.073
5 and 6	214.2	142	1.51	0.98	0.97	0.049
6 and 7	757.9	314	2.41	0.96	0.95	0.070
7 and 8	944.9	340	2.78	0.94	0.93	0.079
8 and 9	792.5	314	2.52	0.92	0.91	0.077
9 and 10	631.5	242	2.60	0.90	0.89	0.078
10 and 11	647.7	265	2.44	0.94	0.94	0.071
11 and 12	861.1	314	2.74	0.91	0.90	0.089
12 and 15	607.0	265	2.29	0.95	0.95	0.073
15 and 18	635.2	265	2.40	0.96	0.96	0.076
18 and 21	612.6	289	2.12	0.94	0.93	0.068
21 and 24	550.9	289	1.90	0.95	0.94	0.062
24 and 27	532.2	289	1.84	0.95	0.94	0.062
27 and 30	497.2	314	1.84	0.95	0.94	0.053
30 and 33	627.5	314	1.84	0.93	0.92	0.069
33 and 36	382.5	242	1.58	0.94	0.93	0.050

(continued)

Table 4.11 (continued)

Combined month age group	X^2	df	X^2/df	CFI	NNFI	RMSEA
36 and 42	706.2	289	2.44	0.91	0.90	0.082
42 and 48	975.6	367	2.66	0.92	0.91	0.083
48 and 54	767.7	314	2.66	0.93	0.92	0.071
54 and 60	771.7	367	2.10	0.93	0.93	0.059
48–84	21518.2	2136	10.07	0.97	0.93	0.094
66–78	1157.9	367	2.14	0.91	0.90	0.084
78–84	279.4	141	2.14	0.95	0.94	0.074

Chi-square = 1157.41, df = 367, P-value = 0.000, RMSEA = 0.084

4 PSYCHOMETRIC ANALYSIS OF THE ERXIN SCALES 113

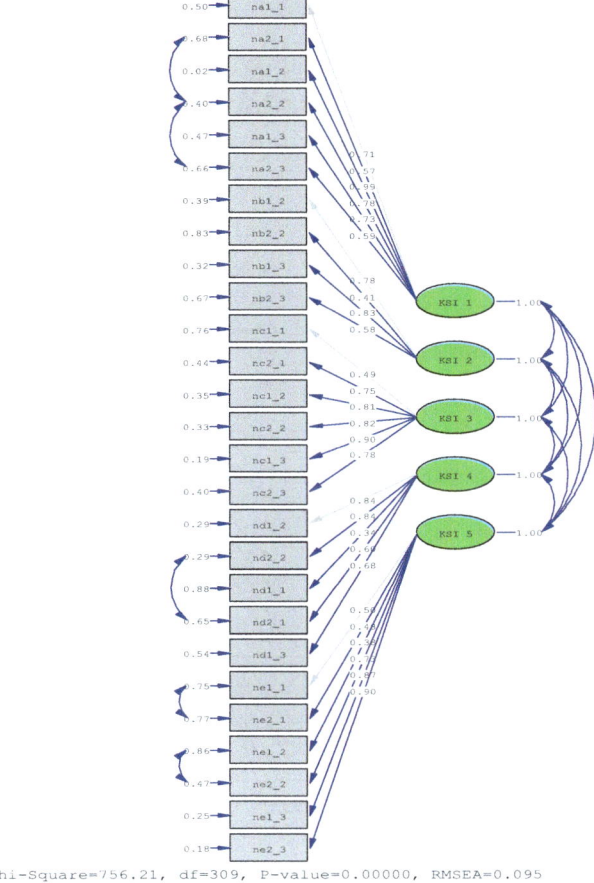

Fig. 4.1 Model fit indices for the 1–3 months subset (excluding Items #3 and #4 at 1 month)

the theoretical model and the actual data reflected the great construct validity of the five-dimensional structure of the developmental scale. Due to the large amount of data, graphs illustrating the model fit indices for other combined age groups are omitted.

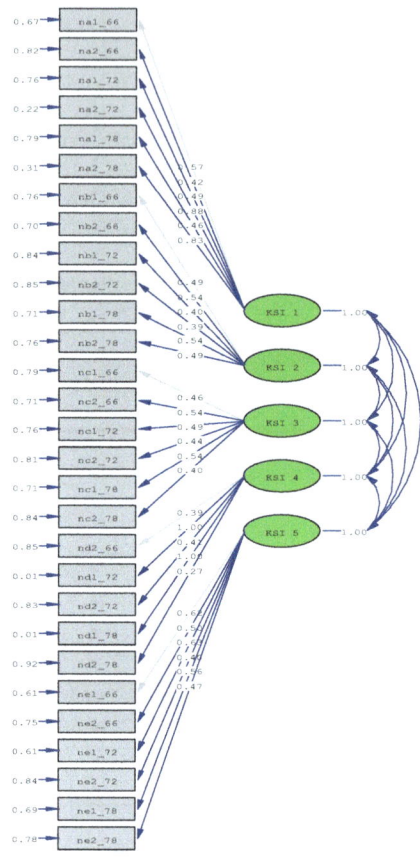

Chi-square=1157.41, df=367, P-value=0.000, RMSEA=0.084

Fig. 4.2 Model fit indices for the 66–78 months subset (excluding Item #257 at 66 months)

References

1. Jin, C. H., Li, R. L., Zhang, L. L., et al. (2014). Revision and validity of China Child Development Scale. *Chinese Journal of Child Health Care, 22*(12), 1242–1246.
2. Jin, C. H., Zhang, L. L., Zhang, Y., et al. (2015). Correlation analysis of the testing items of revised "China Developmental Scale for Children" and

month age. *Chinese Journal of Child Health Care, 23*(1), 21–23.
3 Zhang, L. L., Jin, C. H., Li, R. L., et al. (2015). Reliability of China development scale for children aged 0–4 years in Beijing. *Chinese Journal of Child Health Care, 23*(6), 573–576.
4 Li, R. L., Jin, C. H., Zhang, L. L., et al. (2015). Psychometric analysis of the "China Development Scale for Children" (aged 4–6 years old). *Chinese Journal of Child Health Care, 23*(9), 934–936.

CHAPTER 5

Application Value of the Erxin Scales

5.1 Developing Child Assessment Scales: an Essential Requirement for Progress

China has always placed great emphasis on the physical development of children. Since 1975, national survey on children's physical development has been conducted every 10 years in nine provinces and cities. To date, there have been five surveys, which not only provide insights into the developmental, nutritional, and health status of children in different regions of China and their changing trends but also contribute to the improvement of the evaluation system for children's physical development. As a result, children's physical development and nutritional status have been effectively ensured. With the continuous progress of the society, certain previously overlooked psychological and behavioral problems in children have gradually become prominent. People started to realize that deviations or abnormalities in children's psychological and behavioral development are not easily detected by parents and non-professionals. There has also been a lack of systematic assessment tools, often leading to missed opportunities for early detection and intervention, placing significant mental and financial burdens on families with children affected by these disorders. Up to now, existing medical capabilities cannot solely rely on instrument-based examinations or test data indicators to provide early diagnosis for certain neurological developmental disorders such as developmental delay, ASD, and language disorders.

© The Author(s), under exclusive license to Springer Nature Singapore Pte Ltd. 2024
C. Jin et al., *Erxin Scales: Child Developmental Scale of China*,
https://doi.org/10.1007/978-981-99-9997-2_5

There is also no reliable evidence for the definitive improvement or treatment of these conditions through the use of specific medications. The early symptoms of developmental disorders often overlap with manifestations of delayed child growth and immature development. This highlights the significance of evaluating and monitoring the psychological and behavioral development of children in early stages.

Infants and young children neurobehavioral development is a dynamic and complex process that might be characterized by rapid progression, relative slowness, or even regression. Different races exhibit different developmental trajectories, and even within the same race, differences in cognitive abilities (e.g., memory, categorization, and visual discrimination) as well as motor skills exist due to cultural backgrounds and varying levels of education. The developmental process and pace of children in China differ from those of children in other countries. In a study by Chen Jiaying [1], it was found that children in Shanghai lagged behind American children by 4–10 months in tasks such as "preparing for meals," "putting on a T-shirt," and "using a fork and spoon"; nevertheless, they were ahead by 4–8 months in tasks such as "imitating drawing" and "drawing mouth shapes." In terms of language development, Shanghai children exhibited delayed speech, with only about half of them consciously calling their parents by "mama" or "baba" at the age of 1 year, while American children achieved this milestone at 9 months. However, Shanghai children caught up with American peers at the age of 18–20 months, and since then their language abilities progressed rapidly, surpassing American children at the age of 2.5 years. Additionally, Chinese children were 3–5 months ahead of American children in tasks such as "naming one color" and "counting wooden blocks" on average, while their development of independent sitting, standing, and walking was comparatively delayed by 1–2 months. These differences indicate a striking cultural mismatch arising from the influence of regional factors, customs, socioeconomic conditions, and cultural backgrounds when using foreign assessment scales.

Developing a practical and operational developmental scale is a challenging task, requiring a high level of expertise and involving stringent requirements, complex operations, and a prolonged research cycle. Foreign countries have made earlier progress in this line of inquiry, with a wealth of research on child psychological and behavioral development conducted. For example, BSID and GDS, developed after the publication of the Binet-Simon Intelligence Scales, have been adopted by various countries since their publication. However, the use of non-standardized international scales may not ensure fair comparability among children from different countries and fail to accurately reflect their actual developmental levels. In China, commonly used diagnostic tools mostly originated from foreign mature scales which were based on the developmental patterns of their local children. Therefore, researching and developing an assessment scale suitable for Chinese children's psychological and behavioral development is an essential requirement for progress.

5.2 High Content Validity

The validity of a scale primarily reflects the degree of conformity between actual measurements and expected results. Low validity makes it difficult to achieve the intended purpose of the assessment and can even lead to misjudgments in clinical settings. Assessing content validity of a scale is complicated, and some researchers argue that it is difficult to explore from a mathematical perspective and provide a mathematical definition. Content validity relies to some extent on expert judgment [2]. The Erxin Scales, based on longitudinal observation and cross-sectional validation, was standardized on representative samples, satisfying the basic requirements for content validity from the very beginning of its development. This psychometric property was also emphasized throughout the scale revision process. At each stage, experts were invited to evaluate the items and provide necessary modification suggestions. They also addressed various issues regarding the scale's content validity from technical perspectives, effectively contributing to the validity research [2]. To enhance content validity, including criterion-related validity, and improve clinical discrimination and predictive ability, specific items for identifying brain and neurological impairments were added to the Erxin Scales, and the measurement time window for assessing infants under 1 year old was shortened. During the revision, consistent training was provided to evaluators, and only those achieving a consistency level of 0.9 or above were allowed to participate in assessment administration. The average difficulty coefficient of newly added and modified items was 0.64, indicating an appropriate level of item difficulty slightly skewed toward being easy, which is consistent with the characteristics of a developmental scale and helps children complete the tests. Testing tools were optimized by eliminating distractions (e.g., using a specially designed unframed mirror) and designing items that better capture children's interest (e.g., replacing black-and-white pictures with colored ones). These are all essential steps for ensuring a high content validity. Moreover, the measurement content and operation details were modified based on feedback and the pass rates of corresponding age groups during the clinical validation stage. During item testing, the difficulty coefficient, i.e., the pass rate of items, served as a reference for experts to judge whether to retain or delete the items, reflecting the essence of content validity of the scale.

The continuous updates of electronic products exert both direct and indirect impact on children's socialization [3]. The increase in screen time and human–machine interaction [4] has led people to overlook the important role of interpersonal interactions in child development. In this revision of the scale, the most significant addition was made in the domain of interpersonal communication. A revision team led by clinical experts in developmental behavior was formed, which also involved the original scale developers as consultants and specialists from clinical, developmental pediatrics, child psychology, and public health fields. Based on the theory of cognitive development and neurodevelopmental maturity, original items as well as the testing tools were modified or supplemented with new ones. Observing the developmental levels of children of different ages and referring to longitudinal follow-up data, a progressive approach was adopted to continuously address the issues related to the scale's content validity. The revision process was conceptualized based on the original scales, starting from the design of test items, repeated modifications through clinical validation, and the establishment of a preliminary item pool, to the addition of items associated with communication warning behaviors, and then to subsequent case–control studies in the sampled regions. Throughout each step in the process, experts were involved in for judgment and validation. All of this demonstrates the high content validity of the scale.

5.3 High Discriminability of the Newly Revised Scale Items

The fundamental requirement for the revision of a diagnostic scale is to have reliable and accurate foundational data. Scale items developed for the assessment of neuropsychological and behavioral development should possess statistically significant discriminability (CR). Each item should also demonstrate clinical differentiation and discriminative power. Only items with high discriminability can truly reflect the developmental maturity of the assessed children and showcase their ability to discriminate the levels of the subjects. This is one piece of evidence for the construct validity of the scale. Each item in the scale can be considered an independent test. The items in the revised scale with significant discriminability accounted for 99.2% of the total. It is evident that the items successfully measured the intended characteristics, fulfilled the assessment purpose, and thereby demonstrated the high discriminability of the newly revised scales.

5.4　Close Correlation Between Scale Items and Month Age

The original test items of the Erxin Scales were developed based on the developmental sequence of infants and young children, with developmental levels arranged from low to high. The purpose was to identify children with developmental deviations, imbalance, and delays. The current revision followed the same research path, with additional items designed based on years of clinical experience and observation of developmental behaviors in children. The items were arranged according to the difficulty levels in different domains by statistically analyzing their pass rates at different ages. The correlation between item difficulty and month age further contributed to the factor analysis, providing evidence for the construct validity of the scale. Items showing a moderate or high correlation with age accounted for 93.9% of the total, with those showing high correlation occupying 49.8%; all the gross motor items showed a moderate or high correlation with age, indicating their close link. Items with a low correlation accounted for 6.1%, with a minimum coefficient of 0.387. These items were primarily associated with social behaviors, suggesting that children's behavior is influenced by their living environment. Analysis also revealed that only Item #4 ("Natural state of hands") had a weak correlation with age, and its factor loadings were also low during the factor analysis and confirmatory factor analysis, indicating that it could be discarded. However, it was decided to retain the item because of its clinical value reflected from its purpose to observe brain and neurological damage in newborns and younger infants.

5.5 HIGH INTERNAL CONSISTENCY OF THE SCALES

Reliability is a key indicator for assessing the consistency and stability of a scale. Scales with high reliability are deemed more solid and persuasive. The revised Erxin Scales were featured by both high test–retest reliability and inter-rater reliability. The Cronbach's α (internal consistency coefficient) of the overall scale for the 28 main test ages ranged from 0.850 to 0.954. Regarding the subscale items, 96.4% of the gross motor items (27/28), 92.9% of the fine motor items (26/28), 96.4% of the adaptability items (27/28), 89.3% of the language items (25/28), and 82.1% of the social behavior items (23/28) achieved a Cronbach's α of 0.6 or above (with an average of 91.4%).

Further analysis was conducted separately for the assessment data on children below and above 4 years old. In the age group of 0–4 years, the gross motor, fine motor, adaptability, language, and social behavior items with a Cronbach's α coefficient of 0.6 or above accounted for 95.8%, 91.7%, 95.8%, 87.5%, and 83.3%, respectively. A Cronbach's α coefficient greater than 0.6 for the subscales would be acceptable [5]. Though some domains' Cronbach's α coefficients were below 0.6, they were still higher than or comparable to those for the original scale domains (e.g., the coefficient for the Fine Motor Subscale at 1 month of age was 0.485, higher than that for the original subscale), indicating higher reliability of the revised scales [6]. As regards the items for the age group of 4–6 years, the overall internal consistency was all above 0.8. Analysis was also carried out to examine the internal consistency for various combined age groups in different domains. When considering the age groups of 48–60 months and 54–66 months, a consistency value below 0.6 was found for the language and social behavior domains. Following the measurement rules of the developmental scale, the assessment of children over 4 years old involved items from at least five consecutive age groups. Adjusting the combined age groups and analyzing according to the 42–60 months and 66–84 months subsets, the internal consistency of each domain was close to or above 0.7 [7], indicating higher reliability of the extended portion of the scale for the 4–6 years age group.

Judging from the scale's split-half reliability, the Cronbach's α for the two parts of the scale at the main test ages reached or approached 0.8, meeting the psychometric requirements. After corrected using the Spearman-Brown formula, the split-half reliability coefficients for the overall scale ranged from 0.806 to 0.968 at all main test ages except for the 60, 66, and 84 months, which had a coefficient of 0.742, 0.774, and 0.786, respectively. The items of the five subscales (gross motor, fine motor, adaptability, language, and social behavior) with a split-half reliability coefficient reaching 0.5 or above accounted for 99.3% (139/140) of the total. Only the split-half reliability at 84 months was relatively low, but it was acceptable considering that it occurred at the end of a subscale.

5.6 Solid Scale Structure as Revealed by Factor Analysis

For psychological scales to achieve the intended assessment goal and be widely used, high validity is yet another vital prerequisite which also serves as one of the key indicators of successful scale revision. However, validity has a broad and complex meaning, lacking specific model for its measurement [2]. The evaluation of content validity relies to some extent on experiential judgment, while that of construct validity requires the use of mathematical models [2, 8]. The resulting data need to be analyzed, studied, and evaluated by relevant experts with professional explanations provided. Factor analysis is a latent structure analysis method proposed by psychologist Charles Spearman in 1904. It transforms complexly intertwined variables into a smaller number of factors, groups variables based on their correlations, and explores the underlying patterns among scale items. Through factor analysis, factor loadings of each item and their correlation with the extracted factors can be identified, with a larger loading indicative of a closer relationship between the item and the factor.

From the factor analysis model of the 1–3 months subset, some items loaded high on a certain factor and low on other factors, while some others exhibited similar loadings on multiple factors. For example, Items #21 and #22 had loadings of 0.609 and 0.543 on Factor 1 respectively, but their loadings on Factor 3, which focused primarily on gross motor skills, were 0.405 and 0.455. This implies that the two items could be named according to either Factor 1 or Factor 3. Likewise, Items #17 and #27 had loadings of 0.617 and 0.601 on Factor 2, and of 0.534 and 0.524 on Factor 1, respectively; therefore, it was acceptable to name them according to either Factor 2 or Factor 1. Via analyzing the loadings of items on extracted factors and considering the specialized intention of the items as well as their match with the five attributes, gross motor, adaptability, and language corresponded precisely to Factors 3, 1, and 2, respectively.

As mentioned earlier while introducing BSID-III, the domains included in a scale, though measured independently, are to some extent interdependent [9]. It was found 50% of the fine motor items with loadings greater than 0.5 overlapped with adaptability items, and a few items with high loadings fell into Factors 4 and 5. Social behavior items mainly loaded on Factors 1 and 2, with 33% of those with loadings greater than 0.5 on Factor 4. Children's perceptual development is both independent and overlapping, and is difficult to be separated from cognitive development entirely. The results of the factor analysis reflected this characteristic clearly. In the measurement of perceptual development in the Erxin Scales, some items measured both adaptive skills and fine motor skills, as well as language or social behaviors. The attribution of items to specific domains should also consider their primary purpose of measurement in reference to the factor analysis results.

Factor analysis theory states that items with low loadings should be deleted. However, developmental scale items are arranged in ascending order of age and developmental levels, and the testing methods differ from those of adult psychological scales. To ensure the coherence and operability of scale administration, the match between the loadings of extracted factors and the test items ought to be fully weighed. Despite the overlap of the extracted factors with multiple domains, the five dimensions of the scale and their names followed the conventions without violating the premise of factor analysis. As expected, five factors were extracted for the mathematical model via factor analysis, and the five-factor structure explained an adequate amount of the variance while being sufficiently independent of each other to fulfill their respective measurement purposes. This further justified and supported the naming and structure of the five domains or subscales, including gross motor, fine motor, adaptability, language, and social behavior.

Factor analysis is an intermediate means to achieve a goal and can only explain the structure between the analyzed items; it does not necessarily reveal the essence of the phenomenon itself. Some scholars even argue that traditional techniques such as factor analysis should not be used for developmental scales [2]. To avoid excluding potentially qualified items in the development and research process [8], caution should be exercised during decision-making regarding item deletion and retention.

5.7 GOOD FIT BETWEEN CONCEPTUAL MODEL AND ACTUAL DATA

Confirmatory factor analysis provides insights into the goodness of fit between the conceptual model and actual data. By employing multiple indicators to represent the constructed model for latent variables, researchers can examine the theoretical conception and variable structure [10]. To further assess the fit between the conceptual model and the actual data, a mandatory confirmatory factor analysis was conducted on the five-dimensional Erxin Scales, and the corresponding structural equation data confirmed the rationality of the original scales' structure and naming [11]. The model fit indices resulted from the factor analysis of the 1–3 months subset suggested that the test items met the requirements and the factor loadings were mostly above 0.3 [12]. Developmental scales necessitate continuous item testing across consecutive age groups, and the items are both independent and interconnected. This leads to the possibility for an item to have a low factor loading in the previous age group but a comparatively high loading in the subsequent group. Retaining such items can make the assessment more targeted and continuous. If items with factor loadings below 0.3 in two consecutive age groups are deleted, the model fit of the scale would improve, and the structure be optimized. It is worth mentioning that Item #7 ("Make small guttural sound"), with the minimum negative loading in the factor analysis, had high loadings in two consecutive age groups during confirmatory factor analysis, and thus it was more appropriate to retain the item. In Fig. 5 depicting model fit indices for the 1–3 months subset, bidirectional arrows suggesting interconnections could be found between adjacent or the same-age items, indicating that the scale items were influenced by child perception development and closely related to month age. By comparison, no such bidirectional arrows could be found in Fig. 6, reflecting the independence of each item in the 4–6-year-old section of the scale.

5.8 Selection of Criterion Scales and the Criterion-Related Validity

The evaluation of the validity of a scale often requires comparing it with external standards. For this reason, the Erxin Scales were compared to GDS for items in the 0–3 years (under 4 years) age group. The correlation coefficients between the two scales were 0.64 for the Beijing sample and 0.57 for the national sample, which were higher or close to those reported in similar studies in China [13]. However, these coefficients failed to reach 0.7, possibly due to the relatively outdated version of the GDS employed. Although GDS is a widely recognized assessment tool for child development, the Beijing revised version was based on its 1974 edition, which is nearly 40 years old and has only been regionally revised without a national normative sample. In the absence of other recognized and reliable standardized scales, GDS was selected as a criterion measure. And the correlation coefficients of 0.57 and 0.64 indicated both the success of the revision and the need for updated versions of developmental scales introduced into China [14–16]. This highlights the lag in devising developmental tools in China [17], emphasizing the urgent need for researching indigenous child developmental scales.

For items in the age group of 4–6 years, WPPSI-R was selected as the criterion scale for comparison. The Spearman correlation coefficients between the Erxin Scales overall DQ and WPPSI-R full-scale IQ were 0.78 for the Beijing sample and 0.66 for the national sample, indicating a high criterion-related validity for this part of the Erxin Scales. After obtaining the national norm, the Erxin Scales compensated to some degree for the deficiencies in developmental assessment and diagnostic measures for preschool children in China. Its 4–6-year-old section can be used as a standalone diagnostic tool and can also serve as an ideal criterion scale for the introduction of foreign instruments.

5.9 Design and Standardization of Testing Tools

Standardization of the original testing tools is crucial to ensuring the scale reliability and validity. It was observed while assessing children's cognitive abilities that the original testing tools were somewhat outdated. Scenarios that were common or frequently encountered by children in the past are now rare, and some black-and-white pictures appear abstract. Modifying the pictures to color format may potentially reduce the difficulty of assessment. In the initial stage of the revision, two picture recognition cards were designed to address the difficulty involved in picture use. One card contained 18 color pictures, which was the same quantity of black-and-white pictures in the original recognition card. The other card included an additional 6 color pictures, resulting in a total of 24 color pictures. Preliminary clinical test results indicated that the difficulty presented by the picture recognition card with 24 color pictures was similar to that of the original card with 18 black-and-white pictures (with comparable recognition rates), and it had a higher correlation with age. Therefore, it was decided to replace the original black-and-white cards with those containing 24 color pictures. Except for geometric shapes, all other pictures were modified to color format. The proposal to replace black-and-white pictures with color ones received unanimous approval from the expert panel, with particular recognition and support gained from Professor Jiannong Shi from IPCAS.

New testing tools were designed while optimizing the original ones, given the rapid development of electronic products nowadays. The objective was to guide parents in emphasizing children's hands-on abilities, and also to uphold traditional values by exploring early parenting concepts rooted in cultural heritage and ancestral traditions. By doing so, it can facilitate the revitalization of valuable skills that foster children's cognitive development in the modern era. For example, the test requiring turning over the rope serves the dual purpose of assessing children's manual dexterity and facilitating peer interaction. The tool used in the test is easily accessible, and no special environment for operation is needed. In the cognitive domain, the design of similar graphic templates reflects the fusion of traditional and contemporary elements. We believe that clever design is inspired by everyday life, and adding an element of fun to the measurement process can increase children's interest and willingness to engage. Such an approach to assessing children's cognitive abilities aligns with their logical thinking and cognitive development.

The testing tools of the scale have specific requirements, and cannot be replaced with similar artifacts. Otherwise, the scale validity would be impacted. In this revision, all tools involved in the assessment were standardized. Specialized tools were designed while considering potential interferences, such as adjusting the decibel level of a specially made brass bell sound or ensuring that mirrors had no frames. The color of the testing table (deep green or dark) was explicitly specified to avoid a lack of contrast that might cause failure to attract infants' attention during tests entailing pellets. Changes in the arrangement of the four-color card were made to prevent misrecognition based on sequence. The use of a bobble sewn with six pieces of flannelette instead of a red ball wrapped in woolen yarn made it easier to handle and clean. Zippers, screws, and scissors were utilized for assessing fine motor skills and coordination in young children, and also encouraging parents to consciously cultivate their children's hands-on abilities. In view of the lack of a unified protocol for buttoning in the original scale, outfit with uniformly sized buttons was designed for the multifunctional dolls, thereby standardizing buttoning-related operations. Moreover, a decline in children's manual dexterity was observed during this revision, reflected in the significantly decreased pass rates for tasks such as using chopsticks to pick up peanuts or tying slipknots or shoelaces compared to the 1980s. These fine motor skills are closely related to cognitive abilities. Consequently, the revision maintained the original operational requirements for these tasks without decreasing the difficulty, so as to raise awareness among peers and early childhood educators and promote parents' efforts to enhance their children's manual dexterity and self-care abilities.

Color perception is a form of visual perception. Infants are normally attracted to complex stimuli. When a baby shows disinterest or does not look at a red ball, it will be difficult to determine whether it is due to organic visual impairment or developmental issues affecting visual perception. The revised scales hence utilized black-and-white targets to elicit gaze from infants who are not interested in the red ball. This reduces clinical confusion and the likelihood of misdiagnosis. If an infant fails to show interest or look at the black-and-white targets, a referral should be made, as it can facilitate early detection of congenital cataracts and timely intervention, thereby reducing the risk of disability.

The testing tools were optimized to suit both full-term and premature infants. For example, the rattle drum was replaced with a bell stick, the size, weight, and handle thickness of which were all specified to accommodate the small hands of premature infants. Improvements and specifications were also made to the inner diameter of the bottle used for the pellet pinching tasks. These considerations form the basis for research on the application of the scale to premature infants.

The Erxin Scales have been developed to align with contemporary children's living environments. The revision, optimization, and standardization of its testing tools reflect a clever, innovative design that is in line with the characteristics of modern children, making the assessment more relevant and closely aligned with their needs.

References

1. Chen, J. Y., Wei, M., & Chen, S. M., et al. (2007). Standardization of Denver II development screening test in Shanghai and its relative factors. *Chinese Journal of Child Health Care, 15*(5), 476–478.
2. Ter Laak, J. (2000). *Psychological diagnosis* (H. C. Chen, Trans.). Chinese Language Press.
3. Yang, Y. F. (2011) Vigorously promote the development of children's sociality. *Chinese Journal of Child Health Care, 22*(3): 225–227.
4. Li, H., Wang, F. X., & Fan, Y. P., et al. (2012). The Media and infants' cognitive development. *Journal of Psychological Science, 35*(5), 1113–1118.
5. Lewis, R. A., Zhang. H. C., & Li, J. (2006). *Psychological measurement and evaluation*. Beijing Normal University Press.
6. Zhang, L. L., Jin, C. H., & Li, R. L., et al. (2015). Reliability of China development scale for children aged 0–4 years in Beijing. *Chinese Journal of Child Health Care, 23*(6), 573–576.
7. Li, R. L., Jin, C. H., & Zhang, L. L., et al. (2015). Psychometric analysis of the "China Development Scale for Children" (aged 4–6 years old). *Chinese Journal of Child Health Care, 23*(9), 934–936.
8. DeVellis, R. F. (2010). *Scale development: Theory and applications* (2nd ed.). Chongqing University Press.
9. Piñon, M. F. (2010). *Theoretical background and structure of the Bayley Scales of Infant and Toddler development* (pp. 1–28), Third Edition, Bayley-III Clinical Use and Interpretation. Academic Press.
10. Wang, Z. M. (2001). *Research methods in psychology* (2nd ed.). People's Education Press.
11. Hou, J. T., Wen, Z. L., & Cheng, Z. J. (2004). *Structural equation model and its application*. Educational Science Publishing House.
12. Hua, J., Wu, Z. C., & Gu, G. X., et al. (2012). Assessment on the validity and reliability of family environment scale on motor development for urban pre-school children. *Chinese Journal of Epidemiology, 33*(5), 464–469.
13. Sun, X. M., Ren, Y. H., & Su, Z. Y. (1996). Study on Bayley scales of infant development. *Maternal and Child Health Care of China, 1*, 51–53.
14. Yi, S. R., Luo, X. R., & Yang, Z. W., et al. (1993). The revising of the Bayley Scales of Infant Development (BSID) in China. *Chinese Journal of Clinical Psychology, 2*, 71–75.
15. Zhang, X. L., Li, J. P., & Qin, M. J., et al. (1994). The revise of gesell development Scale on 3.5-6 years of age in Beijing. *Chinese Journal of Clinical Psychology, 3*, 148–150.

16 Xu, S. S., Huang, H., & Zhang, J. S. (2010). Research and application of diagnostic developmental scales for infants. *Chinese Journal of Child Health Care, 18*(11), 859–861.
17 Jiang, F. (2014). Early childhood development: Challenges for child health care in the new era. *Chinese Journal of Child Health Care, 22*(3), 228–230.

CHAPTER 6

Research on the Communication Warning Behavior Subscale

6.1 Research Background

In recent years, there has been an increase in the prevalence of ASD, both globally and in China, as indicated by numerous reports [1–5]. ASD has become a major public health issue that profoundly affects children's well-being [3, 4]. While diagnosing classic autism is relatively straightforward, early-stage ASD can be subtle, and atypical ASD often lacks specificity, resulting in potential oversight. Particularly, even when parents notice social communication difficulties in their children, such as language, behavior, and motor impairments, they may mistakenly attribute them to temporary developmental deviations. As a consequence, medical attention would be delayed until the children struggle to adapt to kindergarten at the age of 3 or 4 [6] or even face difficulties adjusting to school life. Most children with ASD exhibit communication and behavioral issues before the age of 2.5 to 3.5 years [7, 8], but parents only become concerned when there are evident social communication barriers or significant problems. Parents of children with hidden or atypical ASD tend to overlook or deny clinical symptoms, even when their children display typical autism symptoms or meet diagnostic criteria. They often resist, refuse, or deny the diagnosis, using excuses such as "late bloomer" or "belated speech." This resistance is particularly pronounced among parents whose ASD children have relatively better abilities in tasks like reading or navigation (although not necessarily at a normal developmental level). Some

© The Author(s), under exclusive license to Springer Nature Singapore Pte Ltd. 2024
C. Jin et al., *Erxin Scales: Child Developmental Scale of China*, https://doi.org/10.1007/978-981-99-9997-2_6

parents experience conflicting emotions, lacking valid reasons to deny ASD while fearing confirmation from doctors. This ambivalence resulted from the anxious and demanding process of seeking a definitive diagnosis frequently leads to delayed intervention. Consequently, there is an urgent clinical need for research on early behavioral manifestations of ASD.

Children with ASD exhibit diverse and complex behavioral patterns, often accompanied by sensory abnormalities. They have weak integration abilities in social and emotional interactions, show little interest in engaging with peers, and struggle to adjust their behaviors in social settings. Around 45% to 75% of the affected children experience developmental delays [9]. While children with ASD share similarities with those showing intellectual and language disabilities, there are also notable differences. For example, children with intellectual developmental disorders exhibit social behaviors that align with their developmental level, while children with language disorders may have difficulties in language production and expression but typically have normal comprehension and show interest in social interactions and a desire for playmates. Clinically, it is crucial to differentiate children with ASD from those with developmental disorders to ensure early and targeted rehabilitation training. Various diagnostic criteria and systems have been provided by resources such as the Diagnostic and Statistical Manual of Mental Disorders: Fifth Edition (DSM-5), International Classification of Diseases-10th and 11th Editions (ICD-10, ICD-11), and Chinese Classification of Mental Disorders-Third Edition (CCMD-3). The abstract nature of psychiatric symptom descriptions, however, can pose challenges for non-specialist physicians in understanding and accurately applying the diagnostic criteria and terminology. Consequently, clinical diagnoses often involve the use of scales for screening or diagnosing ASD as an adjunctive tool [10–14].

Assessment scales are one of the indispensable measures for early detection of ASD, and developing effective screening or diagnostic tools constitutes a vital means for promoting early diagnosis and intervention [2]. Developed countries have been devoted to the development of autism rating scales [7]. However, owing to differences in research purposes, target populations, and language systems, the application of foreign scales for early identification of ASD is not entirely satisfactory. In China, the research on ASD started relatively late, and there is a lack of comprehensive investigation into behavioral characteristics of children with ASD from varied lenses, providing limited research data on early warning signs for parents. Although there are research reports on characteristic behaviors of children with ASD in China [15, 16], relatively few studies involve systematic observation, recording, tracking, organizing, summarizing, and compiling of ASD screening or diagnostic scale data [11, 15, 16]. Even scarce are those transforming psychiatric terminology into behavioral manifestations that parents can understand and forming scales [10]. Currently, no normative ASD screening scale has been developed in China that covers children aged 0–6 years. Some researchers believe that the development and promotion of scales can help non-professionals grasp the clinical characteristics and enhance their knowledge of ASD [5]. Early identification of ASD in children and timely and appropriate intervention can alleviate symptoms, and even enable them to integrate into normal social life. There is an urgent need to study early screening tools for ASD, increase parents' sensitivity to ASD behavioral characteristics, promote early detection, and seek timely medical attention.

Therefore, a new domain or subscale was proposed to be added to the Erxin Scales during revision to facilitate screening for ASD risks. It was named as the "Communication Warning Behavior Subscale" to avoid parents denying or responding subjectively to the questions due to fear, aversion, or resistance to ASD diagnosis. The subscale aims to accurately reflect children's social interaction behaviors, repetitive behavior patterns, and observable sensory abnormalities. It serves as a complementary tool for preliminary screening of children who may be at risk for ASD while comprehensively assessing their developmental levels.

6.2 Feasibility Analysis

During the revision of the Erxin Scales, apart from the addition of items aiming to identify brain and neurological impairments and social behaviors related to interpersonal interaction, the Communication Warning Behavior Subscale was newly developed on the basis of the five original attributes, thereby allowing for simultaneous screenings for ASD and developmental assessment. In so doing, the capabilities of the scale are expanded and validity strengthened. The researchers leading the revision of the Erxin Scales have extensive experience in pediatrics and developmental pediatrics, along with expertise in managing child rehabilitation institutions and interdisciplinary backgrounds. Their advantageous position has contributed to the exploration of early signs of ASD in children.

Through observations and interviews with parents, relatives, and caregivers of autistic children, the research team identified indicative behaviors associated with ASD, compiled and categorized the daily behavioral manifestations accordingly, and identified distinctive early behaviors that differentiate autism from normal child development. By carefully examining and verifying the complex and diverse behavioral characteristics of children with ASD, two core symptoms emerged social/communicative interaction and repetitive behavior patterns, including perceptual abnormalities. These findings contributed to the formation of a preliminary screening tool named "Primary Scale of Child Social Interaction and Activity Patterns," aligning with the two dimensions of DSM-5 and drawing from international experiences. After that, analyses of item discrimination, reliability, and validity were conducted following established procedures for scale construction, with the utilization of statistical methods such as factor analysis to select appropriate items. Overall, the technical roadmap is practical and feasible. The proposal to expand the Erxin Scales' capacity to encompass ASD screening function has received support from consultant Zhenmin Gao and gained recognition from the expert panel. Notably, guidance from experts such as Yufeng Yang, Zonghan Zhu, and Meixiang Jia has been instrumental in this endeavor.

6.3 Formation of the Subscales

Based on literature review [9, 15, 16] and expert discussions, a preliminary survey questionnaire was drafted to probe into common behavioral manifestations of autism. Additional items capturing specific atypical behaviors in children suspected of having ASD were included in the questionnaire through interviews with parents or caregivers of children already diagnosed with autism. The aim was to objectively and comprehensively capture the behavioral patterns and sensory perception states of autistic children. Referring to DSM-5 [17, 18], a 67-item checklist for child social interaction and activity patterns indicative of ASD-related atypical behaviors was formed, adopting the scoring system of the Aberrant Behavior Checklist (ABC) [19, 20]. Each behavior was assigned a score based on the severity of its impact on social communication and impaired or restricted functioning. Items of behaviors significantly impacting social interaction and demonstrating distinctive features of autism received higher scores, while general developmental behaviors received lower scores. A preliminary screening scale comprising 66 items (one item, "Like to smell, such as smelling certain things excessively," was removed because its low discrimination index ($p > 0.05$) made the experts think it would fail to differentiate between the preference for smells in normal children and excessive smelling) was used to survey parents or caregivers of children diagnosed with autism, as well as concurrently survey healthy children during routine check-ups. Some of the children were assessed with the Clancy Autism Behavior Scale (CABS) [21]. Factor analysis was employed to extract factors and explore the scale structure based on cumulative variance contribution rates, eigenvalues, and the scree plot. Items for ASD screening preselected from the item pool based on normal developmental process and expected communication behaviors for each age group were matched with the corresponding age group in the Erxin Scales. This led to a 33-item Communication Warning Behavior Subscale as an integral part of the Erxin Scale. The weights of these items were determined, and finally a case–control study was conducted in the sampled areas of the Erxin Scales to further validate the subscale.

Altogether 844 children participated in the study, including 178 autistic children and 666 healthy children. Specifically, 58 autistic and 66 healthy children were sampled from Beijing, while 120 autistic and 600 healthy children were sampled elsewhere across China. According to the statistical requirements of psychometrics, all the retained items that were included in the scale demonstrated significant discriminability ($p < 0.05$ for CR value in Chi-square test). The Cronbach's α coefficient for the subscale was 0.936 (with a corrected coefficient of 0.940). A correlation coefficient of 0.881 was obtained between the subscale and CABS, and the test–retest reliability measured by the Spearman's correlation was 0.982. Factor analysis was used to examine the construct validity of the subscale. A total of 11 factors with eigenvalues greater than 1 were extracted, and the factor loading matrix, explained variance (contribution rate), cumulative explained variance (cumulative contribution rate), and eigenvalues all reflected good construct validity. Most of the factor loadings were above 0.5, with the minimum being above 0.3. The majority of the items showed high loadings on one factor and low loadings on other factors. Some items exhibited similar loadings on two extracted factors, indicating a close internal structure of the items. The 11 extracted factors demonstrated the heterogeneity of ASD.

To obtain screening thresholds, ROC curve was plotted based on the clinical diagnosis of ASD according to DSM-5 criteria. The more convex and closer to the upper left corner the ROC curve is, the greater the test's diagnostic value. As shown in Fig. 6.1, the area under the curve (AUC) for the Communication Warning Behavior Subscale and CABS scores was 0.978 and 0.951, respectively. Both AUCs showed statistical significance ($p < 0.001$). Based on the ROC curve, multiple sets of sensitivity and 1-specificity (false positive rate) were attained. The cut-off point should be selected based on high sensitivity and specificity values as a reference for diagnosis or screening [22]. The ASD scores ranged from 29.5 to 32.5 (i.e., a cut-off point of 30–33), with a sensitivity of 0.845 and a false positive rate ranging from 0.067 to 0.090. In other words, a diagnostic/screening cut-off point of 31–32 might be more appropriate for suspected communication disorders. Referring to the data from the control group, the normative risk index of the Communication Warning Behavior Subscale was categorized as followsA score Fig. 6.1 shows less possibility of ASD; a score between 7 and 12 indicates a need for follow-up observation; a score between 12 and 30 indicates a risk of communication and interaction disorder, and a score greater than 30 indicates a high possibility of ASD.

6.4 Validity Re-evaluation of the Communication Warning Behavior Subscale

To further evaluate the discriminant validity of the revised Erxin Scales and the Communication Warning Behavior Subscale matched by main test ages, a re-evaluation of validity was conducted on the basis of the original case–control study. From 2016 to 2017, an expanded sample was collected in previously sampled region to conduct confirmatory survey involving three groups: ASD group, non-ASD group, and healthy control group. The data analysis results indicated stable evaluation of the subscale's normative index, making it suitable for assessing the risk levels of children in different developmental stages. The findings of the re-evaluation are as follows.

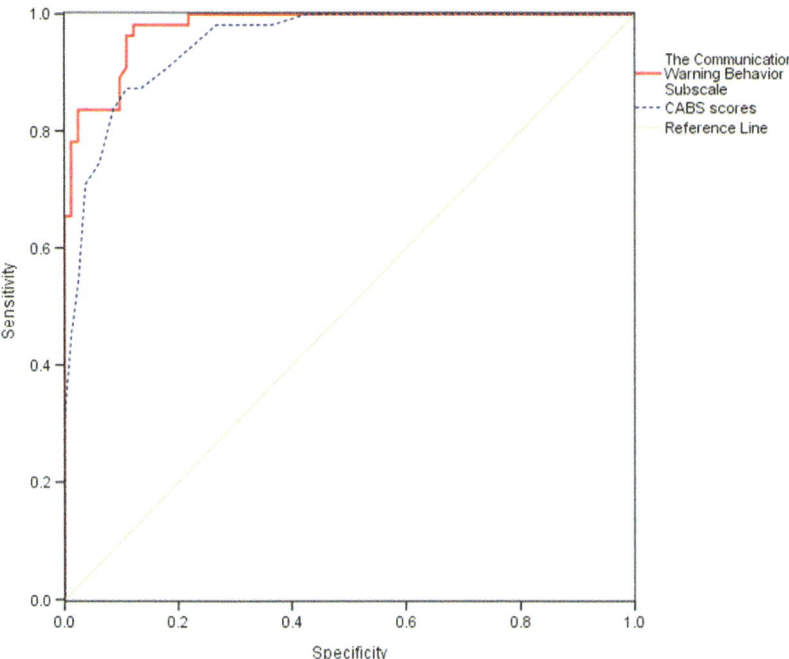

Fig. 6.1 ROC curve plotted based on DSM-5 criteria for diagnosing ASD

6.4.1 Expanding the Sample

1. Sample size and age

A total of 1,989 children were included nationwide, with 1,319 boys and 670 girls, and an average age of 3.89 ± 1.24 years (95% CI: 3.83–3.94). Among them, there were 283 cases of autism (241 boys and 42 girls) with an average age of 3.77 ± 1.22 years (95% CI: 3.63–3.91), 110 cases of developmental delays (83 boys and 27 girls) with an average age of 3.72 ± 1.51 years (95% CI: 3.44–4.01), and 1,596 cases of healthy children (995 boys and 601 girls) with an average age of 3.92 ± 1.22 years (95% CI: 3.86–3.98). The ages of the three groups were homogeneous, and the one-way analysis of variance (ANOVA) results indicated no statistically significant difference in age among the groups (F = 2.846, p = 0.058).

2. Clinical grouping

The ASD group was composed of children clinically diagnosed by doctors, receiving institutional training for three months, and then re-evaluated with a confirmed diagnosis. The non-ASD group included individuals with no ASD but neurodevelopmental disorders such as global developmental delay, intellectual disability, and language disorder. The healthy control group comprised healthy children matched by ages.

6.4.2 Plotting the ROC Curve

The ROC curve is a commonly used graphical tool in signal detection theory for selecting the optimal signal detection model and setting the optimal threshold within the same model instead of a fixed value. It has been introduced in psychology for perceptual detection of signals. The ROC curve combines sensitivity and specificity in a graphical manner to analyze their relationship. In recent years, it has been widely applied to fields of medicine, radio, biology, and forensic psychology. The area under the ROC curve can be used to evaluate the accuracy of diagnosis. By considering the trade-off between false negatives and false positives, the optimal cut-off point can be selected as a diagnostic reference. To demonstrate the discriminability of the subscale, the ROC curve was plotted based on the DSM-5 clinical diagnosis criteria for ASD, as shown in Fig. 6.2.

The AUC for the Communication Warning Behavior Subscale and the CABS scores was 0.970 (95% CI: 0.957–0.983) and 0.954 (95% confidence interval: 0.936–0.973), respectively, both being statistically significant ($p < 0.001$). The fitted curve was closer to the upper left corner, and appeared smoother compared to the that in the previous normative study of the scales.

Based on the ROC curve, multiple sets of sensitivity and false positive rate (1-specificity) were obtained, and values with high sensitivity and specificity were selected as reference diagnostic or screening cut-offs. According to Table 6.1, the sensitivity was 1.0 and the false positive rate ranged within 1.00–0.51 for scores below 7.5. For scores between 8.5 and 13.5, the sensitivity was 1.000, while the false positive rate ranged within 1.000–0.351. For scores between 14.5 and 25.5, the sensitivity ranged within 0.995–0.978, and the false positive rate ranged within

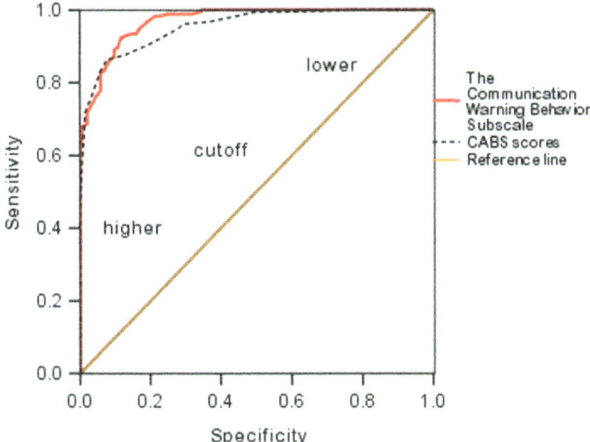

Fig. 6.2 ROC curve plotted based on the DSM-5 criteria for diagnosing ASD

0.346–0.205. For scores between 26.5 and 35.5, the sensitivity ranged within 0.967–0.913, while the false positive rate ranged within 0.190–0.107. The sensitivity for scores above 36.5 tended to decrease, while the ASD false positive rate was almost 0 for scores above 56. The analysis of the ROC curve suggested that the diagnostic cut-offs for suspected abnormalities for the Communication Warning Behavior Subscale scores within 26.5–35.5 had a sensitivity and specificity range largely overlapped with the cut-off range of 29.5–32.5 from the normative study. Moreover, a cut-off above 56 indicated a greater likelihood of ASD. These findings suggest that the expanded sample study confirmed the clinical value of the normative categorization of the revised Erxin Scales' Communication Warning Behavior Subscale.

6.4.3 Comparison of Overall DQs and Subscale Scores Among Groups

The children included in the study for validity re-evaluation, namely 59 of those (20.8%) in the ASD group, 28 (25.4%) in the non-ASD group, and 458 (28.7%) in the healthy control group, were able to complete the developmental assessment at the same time. Kruskal–Wallis test revealed significant statistical differences among the three groups in

Table 6.1 Sensitivity and 1-specificity (false positive rate) obtained from the segmented ROC curve

Diagnostic cut-offs on ROC curve	Sensitivity	False positive rate (1-Specificity)
1.5–7.5	1.000	1.000–0.522
8.5–13.5	1.000	1.000–0.351
14.5–25.5	0.995–0.978	0.346–0.205
26.5–35.5	0.967–0.913	0.190–0.107
36.5–54.5	0.908–0.652	0.098–0.005
55.5–109.5	0.630–0.000	0.000

terms of overall DQs, Communication Warning Behavior Subscale scores, and CABS scores. The ASD group had the highest scores on the Communication Warning Behavior Subscale, while the healthy control group had the lowest scores.

The non-ASD group had an average score of 29 on the Communication Warning Behavior Subscale, which overlapped with the cut-off point suggested by the ROC curve from the normative study, indicating a reasonable division of cut-off points for the scale (see Table 6.2).

Table 6.2 Comparison of Erxin scales overall DQs, communication warning behavior subscale scores, and CABS scores among the three groups

Group	Overall DQ (Number of cases) ($\bar{x} \pm s$) (95% CI)	Subscale score (Number of cases) ($\bar{x} \pm s$) (95% CI)	CABS score (Number of cases) ($\bar{x} \pm s$) (95% CI)
ASD[1]	(59) 57 + 15 (53–61)	(283) 61 + 20 (59–63)	(184)16 ± 5 (15–17)
Non-ASD[2]	(28) 61 ± 12 (56–65)	(110) 29 ± 15 (25–32)	(57) 8 ± 4 (7–9)
Healthy control[3]	(458) 94 ± 11 (93–95)	(1596) 4 ± 7 (3–4)	(164) 3 ± 3 (3–4)
X^2	206.252	1011.251	263.432
p	0.001	0.001	0.001
1:2	0.274	0.001	0.001
1:3	0.001	0.001	0.001
2:3	0.001	0.001	0.001

Table 6.3 Composition ratio of scores stratified for the three groups

Group	< 7	7–12	12–30	30–50	≥ 50	Total
	n (%)	n (%)	n (%)	n (%)	n (%)	n
ASD	0 (0.0)	0 (0.0)	18 (6.4)	66 (23.3)	199 (70.3)	283
Non-ASD	8 (7.3)	9 (8.2)	40 (36.3)	46 (41.8)	7 (6.4)	110
Healthy control	1256 (78.7)	153 (9.6)	157 (9.8)	29 (1.8)	1 (0.1)	1596
Total	1264	164	213	141	207	1989

6.4.4 Composition Ratio of Subscale Scores in Each Group

To further validate the rationality of the cut-offs and the clinical reference value of the normative categorization, the scores were stratified according to the normative cut-off values. The average scores and the diagnostic cut-offs on the ROC curve were analyzed for the ASD group, non-ASD group, and healthy control group. The stratified data for scores above 50 were added (see Table 6.3). There was a significant difference in the composition ratio of scores among the three groups ($X^2 = 1889.216$, $p < 0.001$). In the ASD group, all children scored above 12, and 93.6% had scores above 30. In the healthy control group, 78.7% had scores below 7, 88.3% had scores below 12, and only 1.9% had scores above 30. The scores of non-ASD children were concentrated within 12–50, but there was also a proportion with scores below 7, indicating that conducting ASD risk assessment along with developmental evaluation is more meaningful for clinical differential diagnosis and early identification. Further data analysis indicated that the Communication Warning Behavior Subscale had reasonable normative cut-offs for screening neurodevelopmental disorders and provided clinical reference value.

6.4.5 Factor Analysis and Scree Plot

1. Extraction of eigenvalues

Factor analysis was conducted to demonstrate the construct validity of the scales based on item analysis. Construct validity refers to the extent to which the scale measures ASD traits. For the Communication Warning Behavior Subscale, a KMO measure of 0.741 was found, indicating suitability for factor analysis. The subscale consisted of 33 items, and the component matrix (before rotation) revealed 11 factors (components) with eigenvalues greater than 1, with 57.267% of the total variance explained. Except for the item "Sleep disorders after birth" which had a factor loading below 0.3, other factor loadings on the extracted factors ranged mostly between 0.3 and 0.5, concentrated within the first extracted factor. Another factor analysis was conducted after removing the item "Sleep disturbance after birth." The component matrix after orthogonal rotation still disclosed 11 factors with eigenvalues greater than 1, with 58.269% of the total variance explained. The factor loadings showed improvement, with 78.1% (25/32) above 0.5, 18.7% (6/32) falling between 0.4 and 0.5, and only one below 0.3 (see Table 6.4).

2. Link between eigenvalues and number of components

The link between eigenvalues and the number of components were depicted in the Scatter plot shown in Fig. 6.3. The slope was relatively pronounced from components 2–10 and decreased gradually after the 9th component, nevertheless without approaching 0 even for the last component. This indicates the significant heterogeneity in symptoms among children with autism, and also suggests that the items covered by the ASD subscale should not be overly simplified. It should be noted that the Communication Warning Behavior Subscale consisted of 33 items, but the scatter plot showed only 32 items. This is because the item "Sleep disturbance after birth" was excluded from the analysis owing to its low factor loading. However, the panel of experts suggested retaining the item to provide evidence for future data analysis given that sleep problems are commonly observed in children with ASD.

6.4.6 *Internal Consistency of the Subscale and Its Correlation with the Criterion Measure*

The Communication Warning Behavior Subscale showed a correlation coefficient of 0.876 with the criterion measure of CABS. In addition, its Cronbach's α coefficient was 0.943, and the standardized value was 0.947, indicating a high level of internal consistency of the scales.

Table 6.4 Rotated component matrix for the communication warning behavior subscale

Sequential number of subscale item in Erxin Scale instruction manual	Component										
	1	2	3	4	5	6	7	8	9	10	11
240	**0.710**	0.132	0.144	0.000	0.035	0.155	−0.197	−0.008	0.025	0.164	−0.023
283	**0.673**	0.002	0.003	0.089	0.060	−0.048	−0.067	−0.042	0.261	−0.234	0.084
123	**0.598**	0.067	−0.026	0.188	0.337	0.223	0.061	−0.011	−0.065	−0.102	0.142
152	**0.576**	−0.006	0.280	0.088	−0.045	0.074	−0.129	0.050	−0.052	0.281	−0.166
84	0.007	**0.661**	0.143	0.128	−0.023	0.098	−0.178	0.001	0.001	0.224	−0.142
174	0.271	**0.648**	0.010	−0.089	0.052	0.039	0.078	0.045	0.069	−0.034	0.021
141	−0.049	**0.499**	0.001	0.161	0.163	−0.071	0.043	0.210	0.049	−0.247	−0.145
272	0.002	**0.486**	0.014	0.467	−0.042	0.094	0.195	−0.012	0.112	−0.030	0.013
22	−0.155	**0.452**	0.115	0.225	0.140	0.433	0.127	−0.024	−0.056	−0.065	0.060
161	0.334	−0.039	**0.665**	−0.027	−0.009	−0.014	0.155	0.212	0.124	0.019	0.056
43	0.211	0.105	**0.625**	0.116	0.183	0.089	0.233	−0.126	0.121	0.173	−0.096
185	−0.015	0.141	**0.591**	0.235	0.094	0.000	−0.102	0.106	−0.186	−0.005	0.259
218	−0.084	0.024	**0.556**	0.191	0.262	0.065	−0.212	−0.174	0.369	−0.140	−0.170
229	−0.098	0.398	**0.428**	0.196	0.205	0.119	−0.184	−0.137	0.134	0.241	0.120
94	0.144	0.162	0.254	**0.627**	0.014	−0.111	−0.075	0.036	0.034	−0.036	−0.003
53	0.037	0.114	0.169	**0.596**	−0.026	0.098	−0.188	0.163	−0.047	−0.062	0.026
195	0.113	−0.073	−0.025	**0.592**	0.209	0.195	0.257	−0.172	−0.067	0.339	0.082
103	0.037	−0.013	−0.044	**0.479**	0.139	0.047	0.195	0.292	0.106	0.050	−0.310
113	−0.004	−0.095	0.133	0.123	**0.794**	−0.097	−0.048	−0.058	0.097	0.132	0.077
32	0.113	0.288	0.122	−0.015	**0.567**	0.038	−0.177	0.199	0.160	−0.034	−0.042
196	0.260	0.216	0.140	−0.052	**0.559**	0.168	0.280	0.075	−0.112	−0.068	−0.110
64	0.154	0.070	0.074	−0.071	0.001	**0.824**	−0.004	0.114	0.017	−0.049	−0.060

(continued)

Table 6.4 (continued)

Sequential number of subscale item in Erxin Scale instruction manual	Component										
	1	2	3	4	5	6	7	8	9	10	11
250	0.125	0.040	−0.022	0.128	−0.012	**0.801**	−0.027	0.036	0.146	0.107	0.033
206	−0.203	−0.008	0.068	0.041	−0.024	−0.040	**0.765**	0.007	0.031	0.001	−0.086
294	−0.125	0.085	−0.082	−0.124	−0.058	0.113	**0.397**	0.288	0.083	0.327	0.152
173	−0.013	0.052	0.123	0.026	−0.026	0.162	0.046	**0.787**	−0.070	−0.021	0.032
162	0.024	0.069	−0.116	0.305	0.180	−0.063	−0.018	**0.557**	0.229	0.084	−0.001
207	0.054	0.220	0.161	0.015	−0.134	0.070	0.317	0.024	**0.672**	−0.038	−0.042
261	0.093	−0.006	0.026	−0.002	0.217	0.084	−0.096	0.071	**0.647**	0.118	0.026
184	0.027	0.000	0.074	0.024	0.058	−0.014	0.030	0.028	0.056	**0.704**	−0.084
132	0.008	−0.165	0.074	−0.042	−0.025	−0.006	−0.023	0.033	−0.037	−0.109	**0.740**
74	0.112	0.339	−0.036	0.153	0.323	0.015	−0.034	0.025	0.230	0.223	**0.434**

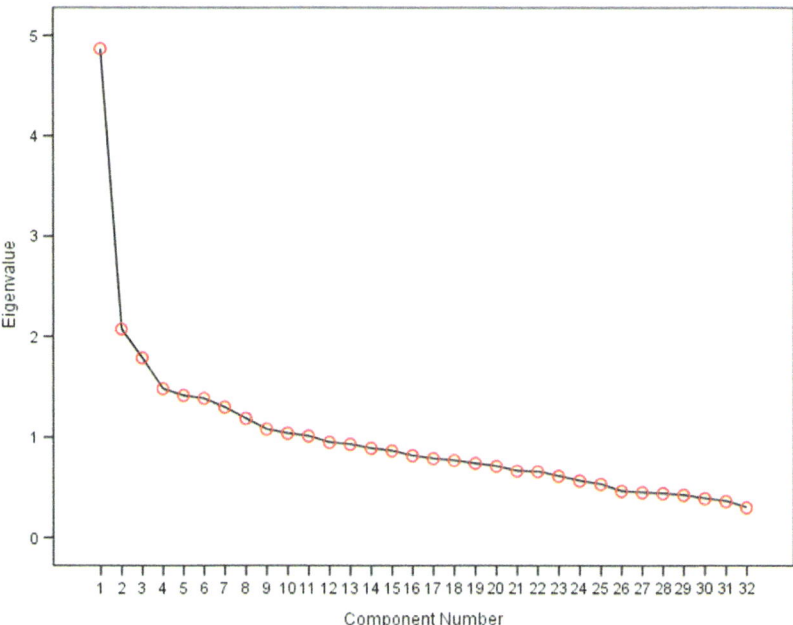

Fig. 6.3 Scatter plot depicting the link between eigenvalues and the number of components

6.5 Highlight of the Scales Revision

ASD is a complex neurodevelopmental disorder characterized by sensory abnormalities and significant heterogeneity, and is also reflected in children's psychological and behavioral development. When parents fill out screening questionnaires or scales, subjective misjudgments may arise due to their incorrect cognitive perceptions or misunderstanding of specific items, leading to an inaccurate reflection of children's communication abilities and behaviors. Parents often overestimate the levels of their children having suspected ASD. The newly developed Communication Warning Behavior Subscale differs from parent-completed screening tools. It involves on-site observation and assessment by professional evaluators, who objectively evaluate negative behaviors in children through observations and assessments of various test items related to gross and fine motor skills, adaptive abilities, language, and social behavior. Simultaneously, interviews with parents are conducted to verify the objectivity or coincidence nature of the child's behavioral manifestations. The evaluation process lasts for a minimum of 30 minutes, ensuring the reliability of the scale.

Unlike other autism screening scales, the Communication Warning Behavior Subscale incorporated in the Erxin Scale is administered synchronously with developmental assessment. By analyzing the overall and subscale DQs as well as the Communication Warning Behavior Subscale scores, the presence or absence of developmental delays and the risks of communication disorders in children could be comprehensively evaluated. This process enables parents to receive professional warnings regarding the risk of autism. The scale plays a particular guiding and demonstrative role in the early development and education of infants and toddlers.

In the face of increased autism prevalence today, the addition of the Communication Warning Behavior Subscale to the Erxin Scales as an ASD screening tool is of crucial practical significance. According to Zhenmin Gao, former director of the Urban Child Health Research Center of CIP and one of the experts in scale development, the inclusion of the communication warning behavior domain enhances the scale's capability to identify and predict ASD risks; it constitutes the greatest advancement in scale functionality and is the key highlight of the successful revision of the Erxin Scales.

References

1. Kogan, M. D., Blumberg, S. J., Schieve, L. A., Boyle, C. A., Perrin, J. M., Ghandour, R. M., Singh, G. K., Strickland, B. B., Trevathan, E., & van Dyck, P. C. (2009). Prevalence of parent–reported diagnosis of autism spectrum disorder among children in the US, 2007. *Pediatrics, 124*(5), 1395–1403.
2. Huang, L. J., Jin, Y., & Li, S. Y. (2011). Screening tools for children with autism spectrum disorder under 2 years of age: A review. *Chinese Journal of Child Health Care, 19*(10), 915–917.
3. Xu, X. (2013). Autism spectrum disorders. *Journal of Clinical Pediatrics, 31*(11), 1199–1100.
4. Zou, X. B., & Deng, H. Z. (2013). Expounding on the diagnosis criteria of autistic spectrum disorders of diagnostic and statistical manual of mental disorders-fifth edition. *DSM-V. Chinese Journal of Practical Pediatrics, 28*(8): 3.
5. Fan, Y. B., Jie, X. F., & Zou, X. B. (2008). Review on the prevalence of

autism. *Chinese Journal of Child Health Care, 16*(4), 439–440.
6. Liu, Y. J., & Jia, M. X. (2010). The retrospective analysis of the data of 144 autistic children. *China Modern Medicine, 17*(24), 193–194.
7. Rapin, I., & Tuchman, R. F. (2008). Autism: Definition, neurobiology, screening, diagnosis. *Pediatric Clinics of North America, 55*(5), 1129–1146.
8. Jing, J. (2007). Early diagnosis and early intervention of autism in children. *Chinese Journal of Child Health Care, 15*(5), 453–454.
9. Xu, X. (2013). Early screening and diagnosis of autism spectrum disorders in children. *Chinese Journal of Practical Pediatrics, 28*(8), 576–579.
10. Liu, J., Wang, Y. F., Guo, Y. Q., et al. (2004). The development of a screening checklist for childhood autism. *Chinese Mental Health Journal, 18*(6), 400–403.
11. Gong, Y. X., Liu, J., & Li, C. J., et al. (2011). Reliability and validity of the Chinese version of the Modified Checklist for Autism in Toddlers. *Chinese Mental Health Journal, 25*(6), 409–414.
12. Wu, F. Y., Xu, X., & Liu, J., et al. (2010). Study on the application of autism screening scale (CHAT–23). *Chinese Journal of Child Health Care, 18*(4), 288–291.
13. Zhong, X. Q., & Jing, J. (2010). Diagnostic value of screening autism children by Chinese edition infant and early children social development screening test. *Chinese Journal of Mental Health Care, 24*(1): 43–46.
14. Zhong, X., Li, W. J., & Liu, M. H., et al. (2012). Comparison of two behavioral rating scales for children with autism in clinical application. *Journal of Nanchang University (Medical Sciences), 52*(7), 81–83.
15. Li, A. Y., Zhang, X., & Lv, C. C, et al. (2010). Analysis of behavioral characteristics of children with autism aged 1.5 to 3 years old. *Chinese Mental Health Journal, 24*(3): 215–218.
16. Li, Y. M., Jing, J., & Zou, X. B., et al. (2009). Cognitive profile of emotional expression in young children with autism. *Chinese Journal of Evidence-Based Pediatrics, 4*(1), 23–28.
17. American Psychiatric Association. (2015). *Diagnostic and statistical manual of mental disorders: DSM–5™ (5th ed.)* (D. L. Zhang, Trans.). Peking University Press.
18. American Psychiatric Association, DSM-5 Task Force. (2013). *Diagnostic and statistical manual of mental disorders: DSM-5™ (5th ed.).* American Psychiatric Publishing, Inc.
19. Li, X. R. (1994). *Modern pediatric psychiatry.* Hunan Science and Technology Press.
20. Ma, J. H., Guo, Y. Q., & Jia, M. X., et al. (2011). Reliability and validity of the Chinese version of the Aberrant Behavior Checklist (ABC) in children with autism. *Chinese Mental Health Journal, 25*(1), 14–19.

21 Chen, Y., Chen, Z. M., & Hu, R. L., et al. (2007). Clinical application of Clancy Autism Behavior Scale. *Guangdong Medical Journal, 28*(3), 375–377.
22 Chen, P. Y. (2005). *SSPS13.0 Statistical software application tutorial.* People's Medical Publishing House.

CHAPTER 7

Data Analysis of Normative Sample for the Erxin Scales

7.1 Basic Data on the Normative Sample

7.1.1 Sampled Participants

A total of 8,952 children from across the country completed the developmental assessment in five domains and the basic data survey. After data cleaning, 38 participants with incomplete basic data or abnormal measurement information were excluded, resulting in a representative sample of 8,914 children (4,596 boys and 4,318 girls) for further analysis regarding descriptive statistics of DQs and probability density curve trends (density plot).

7.1.2 Distribution of Overall and Subscale DQs

The DQ value entailed in the Erxin Scales represents ratio IQ, and the mental age is calculated based on the number of completed items and then compared to the chronological age. The manual calculation process has been replaced with computer input, where the evaluation report is automatically generated after entering the items. The means, standard

---

The original version of the chapter has been revised: Figures and Tables have been updated. A correction to this chapter can be found at https://doi.org/10.1007/978-981-99-9997-2_11

© The Author(s), under exclusive license to Springer Nature Singapore Pte Ltd. 2024, corrected publication 2025
C. Jin et al., *Erxin Scales: Child Developmental Scale of China*, https://doi.org/10.1007/978-981-99-9997-2_7

Table 7.1 Descriptive statistics of overall and subscale DQs ($N = 8,914$)

Scales	Median	M ± SD	(95% CI)	Skewness*	Kurtosis**
Overall scale	99	99.7 ± 14.0	99.4–100.0	0.165	5.047
Subscale					
Gross motor	99	99.9 ± 17.2	99.5–100.2	0.970	6.438
Fine motor	96	96.6 ± 17.4	96.2–97.0	1.017	6.601
Adaptability	100	100.7 ± 17.1	100.3–101.0	0.884	4.599
Language	100	101.2 ± 18.4	100.9–101.6	0.215	4.990
Social behavior	100	101.4 ± 16.4	101.0–101.7	1.156	6.224

*Std. Error of Skewness = 0.026; **Std. Error of Kurtosis = 0.052

deviations, medians, and tests for normality (skewness and kurtosis) of the overall and subscale DQs obtained by the representative sample are presented in Table 7.1. The skewness value of the overall DQs was close to 0, while those of the subscale DQs were less than or close to 1. The kurtosis values were all greater than 1, indicating a concentrated data distribution [1]. The probability density curve exhibited a tall and narrow shape, resembling a normal distribution skewed slightly to the right. The subscale DQs, except for the fine motor values, had means ranging from 99 to 102 and medians from 99 to 100 (95% CI).

The mean of fine motor DQs was the smallest among all subscales, and was 3 points lower than that of the overall DQs. This discrepancy may be attributed to the revision of the scales, where the passing criteria were not adjusted for certain fine motor items with lower pass rates compared to the original scale's research data. Fine motor development is closely related to developmental maturity and the opportunities provided in daily life, and hence merits more stimulation. Restrictions on, limited exposure to, or rare engagement in hands-on activities could all potentially impact the development of a child's manual dexterity and hand-eye coordination.

7.1.3 Frequency Distribution, Histogram, and Probability Density Curve of DQs

(1) **Frequency distribution of DQs among the sampled participants**

To facilitate the investigation into the distribution of overall DQs among the sample and explore the cut-off point for developmental delay, the DQ scores were grouped with an interval of 6. Among the 8,914 children, 1.7% had DQs of 69 or below, 2.5% had DQs below 75, 4.7% had DQs below 81, while 58.4% had DQs ranging from 93 to less than 111. See Table 7.2 for the frequency distribution of overall DQs, and Fig. 7.1 for the histogram and probability density curve.

(2) **Frequency distribution of DQs among children aged 2 to 84 months**

Due to the rapid and diverse development in newborns [2], the observation and evaluation of sensory perception development in infants aged 27–33 days is influenced not only by physiological states such as sleep

Table 7.2 Frequency distribution of overall DQs among the sample of 8,914 children

Group for overall DQs	Frequency	Valid percent	Cumulative percent
<51	81	0.9	0.9
51–57	18	0.2	1.1
57–63	17	0.2	1.3
63–69	39	0.4	1.7
69–75	72	0.8	2.5
75–81	195	2.2	4.7
81–87	556	6.2	11.0
87–93	1285	14.4	25.4
93–99	1994	22.4	47.8
99–105	1988	22.3	70.1
105–111	1224	13.7	83.8
111–117	610	6.8	90.6
117–123	389	4.4	95.0
123–129	185	2.1	97.1
129–135	111	1.2	98.3
135–141	78	0.9	99.2
141–147	17	0.2	99.4
147–153	29	0.3	99.7
153–159	9	0.1	99.8
>=159	17	0.2	100.0
Total	8914	100.0	

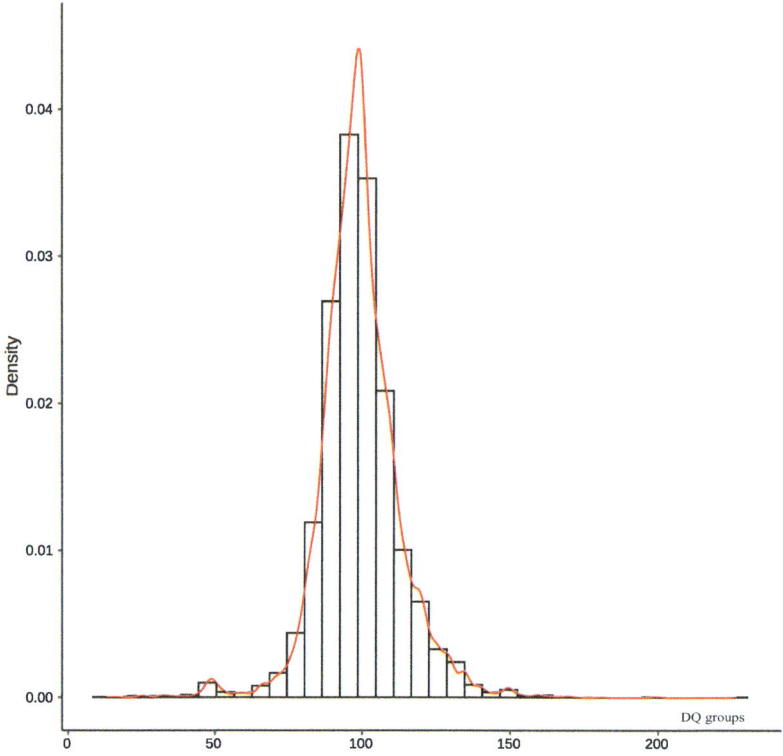

Fig. 7.1 Histogram and probability density curve of overall DQs grouped with an interval of 6 for the sample of 8,914 children

patterns but also by various factors including nutrition, care, and environment. The test items mainly evaluate neuroreflexes and muscle tone, with higher scores indicating normal development in infants and lower scores indicating the presence of pathological brain and nerve damage. The initial or final item data of a scale may be unstable due to limited expansion and lack of adjacent references. After excluding item data at 1 month, the data from 8,612 children aged 2 to 84 months in the sample showed a similar trend to the overall representative sample. The overall and subscale DQs all followed a normal distribution, as shown in Table 7.3. The skewness and kurtosis values were significantly better than

Table 7.3 Descriptive statistics of overall and subscale DQs for the 8,612 children aged 2–84 months

Scales	Median	M ± SD	(95% CI)	Skewness*	Kurtosis**
Overall scale	99	99.2 ± 13.0	98.9–99.5	−0.202	3.543
Subscale					
Gross motor	99	99.0 ± 14.6	98.7–99.3	0.053	1.668
Fine motor	96	95.7 ± 14.8	95.4–96.0	0.197	1.326
Adaptability	99	100.5 ± 16.2	100.1–100.8	0.575	2.418
Language	100	101.2 ± 16.5	100.8–101.5	0.544	2.069
Social behavior	100	100.9 ± 14.7	100.6–101.2	0.697	2.783

*Std. Error of Skewness = 0.026; **Std. Error of Kurtosis = 0.053

those without data exclusion. See Table 7.4 for the frequency distribution of DQs grouped with an interval of 6, and Fig. 7.2 for the according histogram and probability density curve. Furthermore, excluding the item data at 84 months did not result in significant changes in the statistics, so the analysis of this portion of data was retained.

7.1.4 Analysis of Data Distribution Among Children Aged 0–4 Years and 4–6 Years

Based on the developmental characteristics, assessments for children under 4 years primarily focus on developmental progress, milestones, and adaptive maturity levels. As the visual-motor integration skills gradually improve in children aged 4 and above, the according assessments involve more in-depth and broader domains, including perception, discrimination, memory, quantity, vocabulary, analogies, and even tasks that involve executive functions. The 4–6 years period represents a turning point in cognitive growth to some extent. Therefore, data analysis was conducted separately for children aged 0–4 years and 4–6 years.

(1) **Characteristics of data distribution among children aged 0–4 years**

Table 7.4 Frequency distribution of overall DQs grouped with an interval of 6 among the 8,612 children aged 2–84 months

Group for overall DQs	Frequency	Valid Percent	Cumulative Percent
<51	67	0.8	0.8
51–57	16	0.2	1.0
57–63	17	0.2	1.2
63–69	39	0.5	1.6
69–75	70	0.8	2.4
75–81	194	2.3	4.7
81–87	552	6.4	11.1
87–93	1251	14.5	25.6
93–99	1993	23.1	48.8
99–105	1931	22.4	71.2
105–111	1190	13.8	85.0
111–117	596	6.9	91.9
117–123	354	4.1	96.0
123–129	175	2.0	98.1
129–135	81	0.9	99.0
135–141	49	0.6	99.6
141–147	16	0.2	99.8
147–153	10	0.1	99.9
153–159	9	0.1	100.0
>=159	2	0.0	100.0
Total	8612	100.0	

After excluding the item data at 1 month, the skewness and kurtosis values of DQs for children aged 0–4 years exhibited significant improvements. The descriptive statistics of overall and subscale DQs with (2–60 months: $n = 7,356$) and without (1–60 months: $n = 7,658$) the exclusion of item data at 1 month are presented in Tables 7.5 and 7.6, respectively. The histogram and probability density curve of the DQ scores for the 1–60 months age range are shown in Fig. 7.3, following a normal distribution pattern. To avoid redundancy, the frequency distribution and probability density curve for the 2–60 months age range are omitted.

(2) **Characteristics of data distribution among children aged 4–6 years**

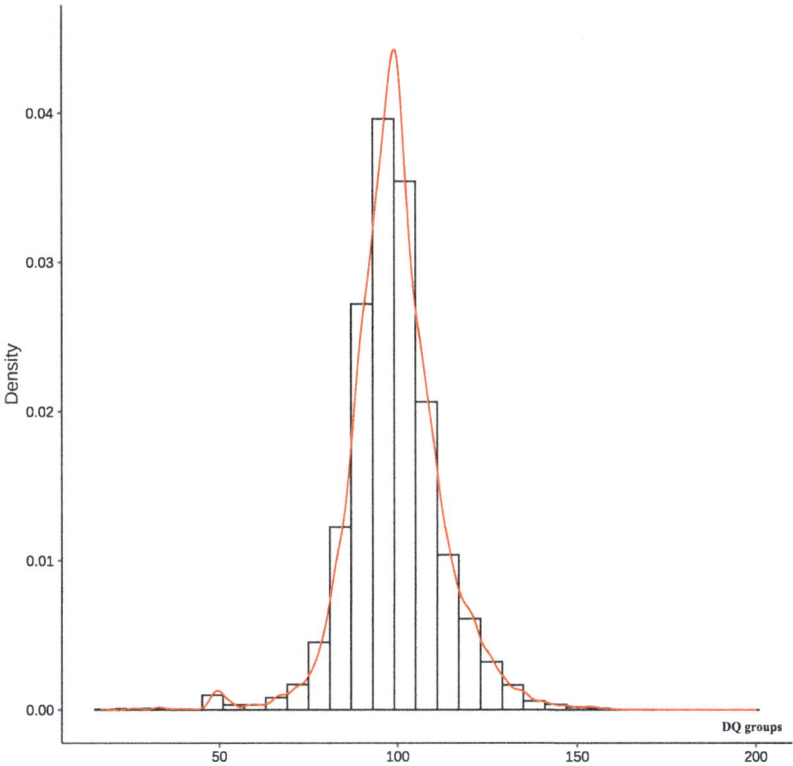

Fig. 7.2 Histogram and probability density curve of overall DQs grouped with an interval of 6 for the 8,612 children aged 2–84 months

Test items for the age range of 4–6 years constitute a complete assessment measure, encompassing main test ages from 36 to 84 months. Table 7.7 presents the medians, means, and 95% confidence intervals of the overall and subscale DQs, as well as the skewness (mostly below 1) and kurtosis (close to 1) values. Figure 7.4 displays the histogram and probability density curve of DQs for the 36–84 months age range, which also followed the normal distribution. From the above tables, we can see that the mean of fine motor DQs in the age ranges of 0–4 years and 4–6 years was about 3 points and 5 points lower than that of the overall DQs, respectively. This finding demonstrates the vital role played by the

Table 7.5 Descriptive statistics of overall and subscale DQs for the 7,658 children aged 1–60 months

Scales	Median	M ± SD	(95% CI)	Skewness*	Kurtosis**
Overall scale	99	100.0 ± 14.6	99.7–100.3	0.127	4.633
Subscale					
Gross motor	100	100.3 ± 18.0	99.9–100.7	0.932	5.867
Fine motor	96	96.9 ± 18.3	96.5–97.3	0.991	6.043
Adaptability	100	101.1 ± 17.9	100.7–101.5	0.853	4.143
Language	100	101.7 ± 19.4	101.2–102.1	0.165	4.440
Social behavior	100	101.8 ± 17.2	101.4–102.2	1.123	5.664

*Std. Error of Skewness = 0.028; **Std. Error of Kurtosis = 0.056

Table 7.6 Descriptive statistics of overall and subscale DQs for the 7,356 children aged 2–60 months

Scales	Median	M ± SD	(95% CI)	Skewness*	Kurtosis**
Overall scale	99	99.4 ± 13.5	99.1–99.7	−0.238	3.258
Subscale					
Gross motor	99	99.3 ± 15.6	98.9–99.6	0.034	1.492
Fine motor	96	95.8 ± 15.4	95.5–96.2	0.191	1.140
Adaptability	100	100.9 ± 16.9	100.5–101.3	0.552	2.111
Language	100	101.6 ± 17.3	101.2–102.0	0.499	1.724
Social behavior	100	101.2 ± 15.3	100.9–101.6	0.687	2.509

*Std. Error of Skewness = −0.029; ** Std. Error of Kurtosis = 0.057

development of fine motor skills in infants and toddlers, as it can have an impact on the cognitive abilities of school-age children.

7.1.5 Frequency Distribution, Histograms, and Probability Density Curves of DQs for the Five Subscales

The DQs for the gross motor, fine motor, adaptability, language, and social behavior subscales were also grouped with an interval of 6 for the 8,612 children aged 2 to 84 months. See Tables 7.8, 7.9, 7.10, 7.11, 7.12 for the frequency distribution of DQs for each subscale, and Figs. 7.5, 7.6,

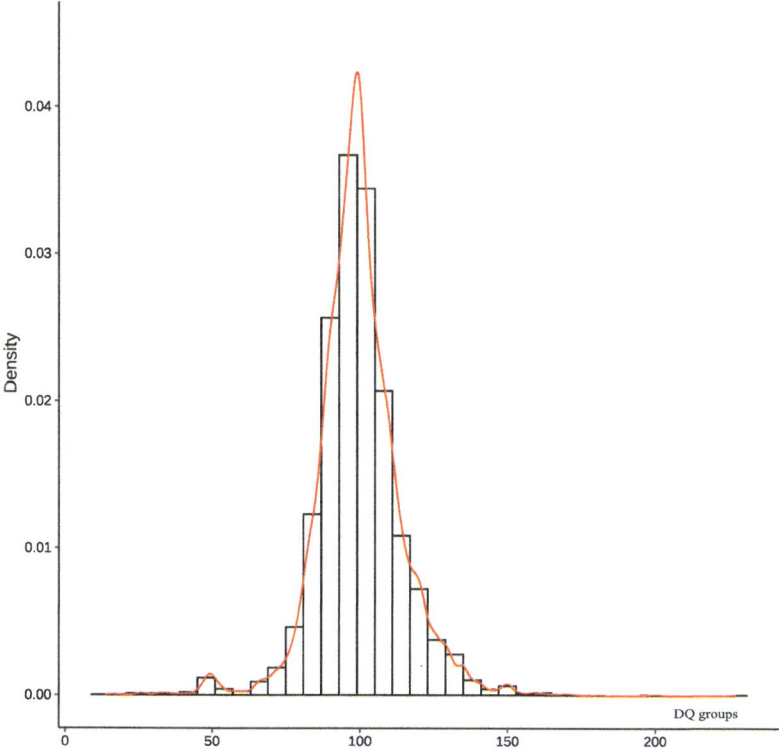

Fig. 7.3 Histogram and probability density curve of DQs grouped with an interval of 6 for the 7,658 children aged 1–60 months

7.7, 7.8, 7.9 for the corresponding histograms and probability density curves.

(1) **Frequency distribution, histogram, and probability density curve of gross motor DQs**

See Fig. 7.5 and Table 7.8.

(2) **Frequency distribution, histogram, and probability density curve of fine motor DQs**

Table 7.7 Descriptive statistics of overall and subscale DQs for the 2,872 children aged 4–6 years (36–84 months)

Scales	Median	M ± SD	(95% CI)	Skewness*	Kurtosis**
Overall scale	101	102.0 ± 12.3	101.6–102.5	0.574	1.649
Subscale					
Gross motor	101	101.3 ± 13.3	100.8–101.8	0.325	1.302
Fine motor	96	96.8 ± 14.6	96.3–97.3	0.512	1.072
Adaptability	102	102.8 ± 15.1	102.2–103.3	0.342	0.771
Language	103	104.8 ± 15.8	104.3–105.4	0.550	1.459
Social behavior	103	104.6 ± 14.5	104.0–105.1	0.471	1.340

*Std. Error of Skewness = 0.046; **Std. Error of Kurtosis = 0.091

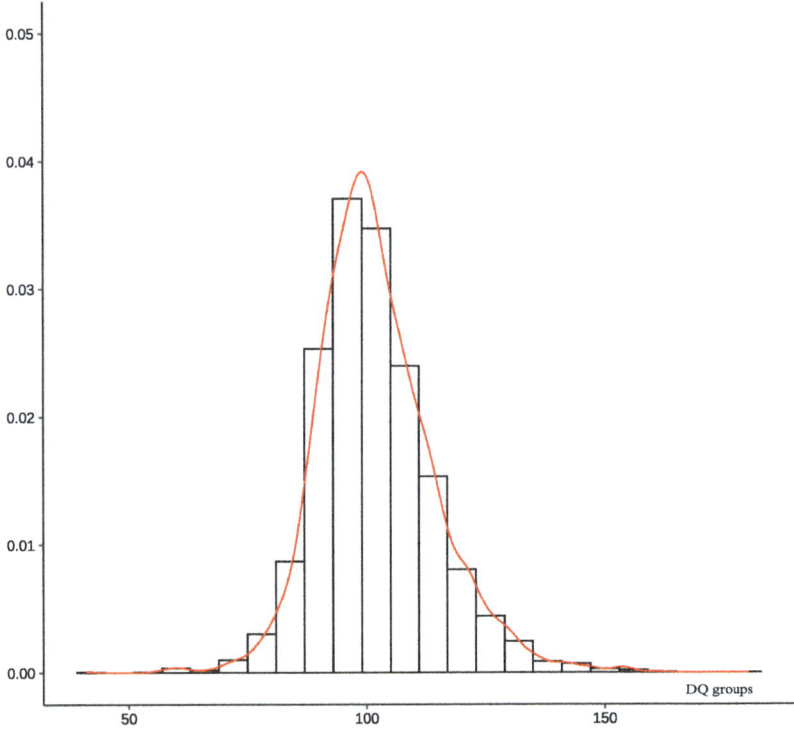

Fig. 7.4 Histogram and probability density curve of overall DQs grouped with an interval of 6 for the 2,872 children aged 4–6 years (36–84 months)

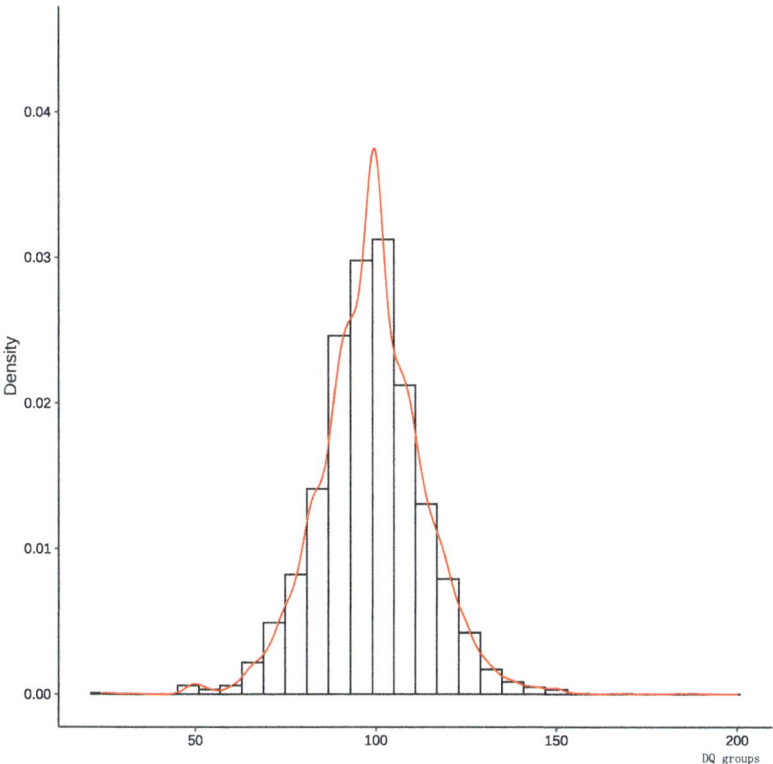

Fig. 7.5 Histogram and probability density curve of gross motor DQs grouped with an interval of 6 for the 8,612 children aged 2–84 months

See Fig. 7.6 and Table 7.9.

(3) **Frequency distribution, histogram, and probability density curve of adaptability DQs**

See Fig. 7.7 and Table 7.10

(4) **Frequency distribution, histogram, and probability density curve of language DQs**

Table 7.8 Frequency distribution of gross motor DQs grouped with an interval of 6 among the 8,612 children aged 2–84 months

Group for gross motor DQs	Frequency	Valid Percent	Cumulative Percent
<51	38	0.4	0.4
51–57	17	0.2	0.6
57–63	22	0.3	0.9
63–69	97	1.1	2.0
69–75	191	2.2	4.2
75–81	407	4.7	9.0
81–87	727	8.4	17.4
87–93	1160	13.5	30.9
93–99	1454	16.9	47.8
99–105	1698	19.7	67.5
105–111	1170	13.6	81.1
111–117	697	8.1	89.2
117–123	499	5.8	94.9
123–129	220	2.6	97.5
129–135	109	1.3	98.8
135–141	50	0.6	99.3
141–147	29	0.3	99.7
147–153	18	0.2	99.9
153–159	3	0.0	99.9
>=159	6	0.1	100.0
Total	8612	100.0	

See Fig. 7.8 and Table 7.11.

(5) **Frequency distribution, histogram, and probability density curve of social behavior DQs**

See Fig. 7.9 and Table 7.12.

7.1.6 DQs Corresponding with the Quartiles for the Sample

The above analysis indicates the stable data of the Erxin Scales and confirms its qualified psychometric properties. As the fine motor DQs were lower than the overall DQs, the distribution of overall and subscale DQs among the representative sample was further examined utilizing quartiles and also including the 5th and 95th percentiles (see Table 7.13).

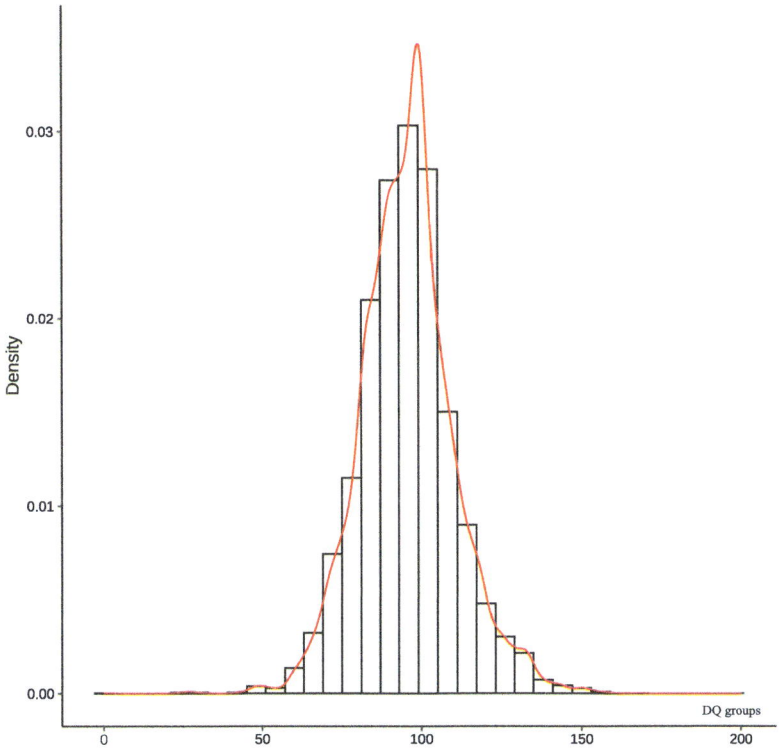

Fig. 7.6 Histogram and probability density curve of fine motor DQs grouped with an interval of 6 for the 8,612 children aged 2–84 months

This analysis allows us to gain insights into the underlying patterns and characteristics of the data. The fine motor DQs at the 5th, 25th, 50th, and 75th percentiles were 9, 5, 3, and 2 points lower, respectively, than the corresponding overall DQs. They were also lower the DQs for other subscales, indicating a relative lag in this domain. While brain neurodevelopment is influenced by genetic predisposition, the combined effects of genetic and environmental factors cannot be overlooked. The development of fine motor skills requires even more environmental stimuli.

Table 7.9 Frequency distribution of fine motor DQs grouped with an interval of 6 among the 8,612 children aged 2–84 months

Group for fine motor DQs	Frequency	Valid Percent	Cumulative Percent
<51	29	0.3	0.3
51–57	14	0.2	0.5
57–63	54	0.6	1.1
63–69	152	1.8	2.9
69–75	330	3.8	6.7
75–81	542	6.3	13.0
81–87	1069	12.4	25.4
87–93	1353	15.7	41.1
93–99	1501	17.4	58.6
99–105	1540	17.9	76.5
105–111	896	10.4	86.9
111–117	451	5.2	92.1
117–123	309	3.6	95.7
123–129	148	1.7	97.4
129–135	132	1.5	98.9
135–141	44	0.5	99.4
141–147	26	0.3	99.7
147–153	13	0.2	99.9
153–159	7	0.1	100.0
>=159	2	0.0	100.0
Total	8612	100.0	

7.1.7 Means and Medians of DQs for Children at Different Main Test Ages

The means of the overall and subscale DQs were analyzed across different test ages and were found to be stabilized within 90–110 except for that at the test age of 1 month (see Table 7.14). We could see that the fine motor DQs were comparatively lower at 18–27 months of age. A closer look at the fine motor skills for these test ages revealed that the original scale items remained unchanged, with the addition of one new item at test ages of 21 months and 27 months. The pass rate for the item "Imitate pulling the zipper" added at 21 months was 67.5%, while that for the item "Insert the zipper slider into the bottom stop" at 27 months was only 13.4%, lower than what was achieved during the item testing phase. Nonetheless, the pass rate for the item "Insert the zipper slider into the bottom stop" at 30, 33, 36, and 42 months of age was 31.7%, 45.2%, 76.1%, and

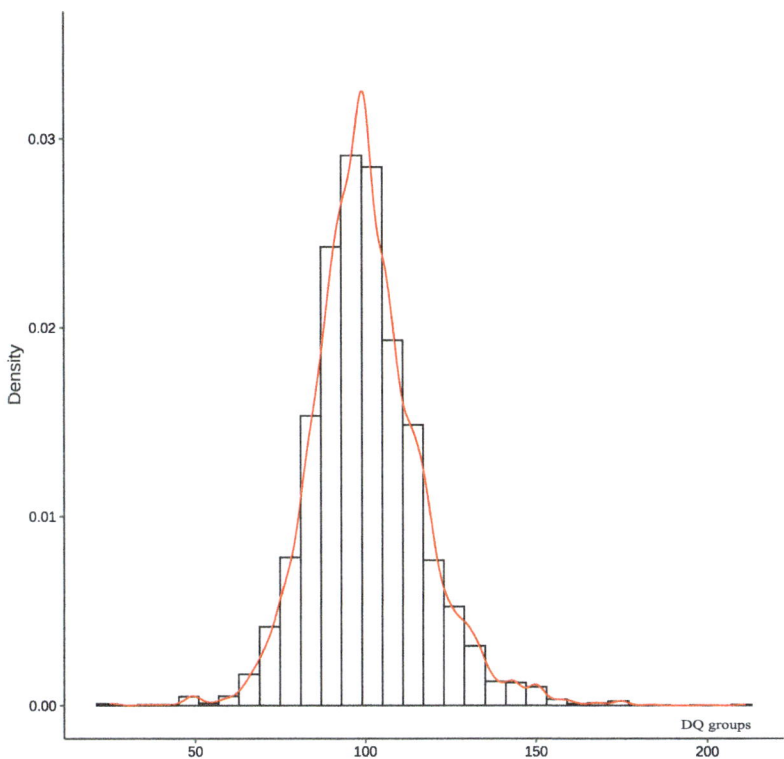

Fig. 7.7 Histogram and probability density curve of adaptability DQs grouped with an interval of 6 for the 8,612 children aged 2–84 months

90.9%, respectively; its gradual increase with age reveals the progressive development of visual-motor integration skills. The pass rate (36.6%) for the retained item "Imitate drawing vertical lines" at 27 months was also not high. Two insights could be gained from this. Firstly, children aged 18–27 months are in a critical development period of hand-eye coordination. It is thus necessary for the maternal and child health care system to enhance popularization of knowledge in this regard, thereby promoting the development of fine motor skills in infants and young children and improving their cognitive abilities. Secondly, the pass rates for items in the same domain should be considered together instead of separately during scale revision, so as to ensure their difficulty levels for the same test age are

Table 7.10 Frequency distribution of adaptability DQs grouped with an interval of 6 among the 8,612 children aged 2–84 months

Group for adaptability DQs	Frequency	Valid Percent	Cumulative Percent
<51	35	0.4	0.4
51–57	5	0.1	0.5
57–63	21	0.2	0.7
63–69	72	0.8	1.5
69–75	168	2.0	3.5
75–81	376	4.4	7.9
81–87	761	8.8	16.7
87–93	1159	13.5	30.2
93–99	1495	17.4	47.5
99–105	1474	17.1	64.6
105–111	1115	12.9	77.6
111–117	697	8.1	85.7
117–123	538	6.2	91.9
123–129	243	2.8	94.7
129–135	217	2.5	97.3
135–141	69	0.8	98.1
141–147	66	0.8	98.8
147–153	52	0.6	99.4
153–159	17	0.2	99.6
>=159	32	0.4	100.0
Total	8612	100.0	

within a reasonable range. Additionally, the fine motor DQs at 24 months were the lowest (mean: 89.9, median: 87). The domain consists of only one item ("Thread through the buttonhole"), which was deemed stable and aligned with the age level by the panel of experts during revision. However, further research is needed in the administration of the test item to investigate its operation details and optimize the testing tools.

7.2 Number of Items and Age Range for the Erxin Scales

7.2.1 Number of Items in the Revised Erxin Scales

The 0- to 4-year section of the Erxin Scales include 221 items, and an additional 40 items were added for the extended age range up to 6 years. Therefore, the gross motor, fine motor, adaptability, language, and social behavior subscales consist of 50 items, 52 items, 55 items, 52 items, and 52 items, respectively. In addition, a newly developed Communication

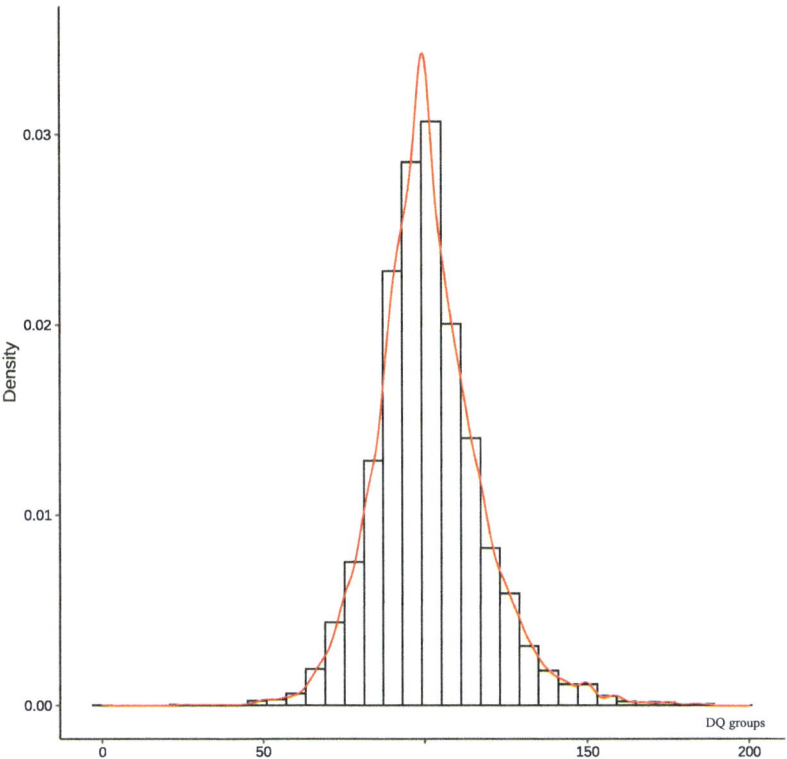

Fig. 7.8 Histogram and probability density curve of language DQs grouped with an interval of 6 for the 8,612 children aged 2–84 months

Warning Behavior Subscale was added, which includes 33 items. As a result, the Erxin Scales after revision comprise a total of 294 items.

7.2.2 Age Range for the Scales

The revised version of the Erxin Scales is suitable for assessing children from 1 month to 6 years of age, with a minimum age for assessment of 27 days and a maximum of 72 months. Although the most appropriate age range for the scale is from 2 to 72 months, it could be extended up to 8 or 9 years for children with intellectual disabilities, depending on their developmental level.

Table 7.11 Frequency distribution of language DQs grouped with an interval of 6 among the 8,612 children aged 2–84 months

Group for language DQs	Frequency	Valid Percent	Cumulative Percent
<51	21	0.2	0.2
51–57	16	0.2	0.4
57–63	25	0.3	0.7
63–69	87	1.0	1.7
69–75	174	2.0	3.7
75–81	372	4.3	8.1
81–87	630	7.3	15.4
87–93	1082	12.6	27.9
93–99	1437	16.7	44.6
99–105	1619	18.8	63.4
105–111	1122	13.0	76.5
111–117	714	8.3	84.8
117–123	530	6.2	90.9
123–129	297	3.4	94.4
129–135	200	2.3	96.7
135–141	97	1.1	97.8
141–147	63	0.7	98.5
147–153	60	0.7	99.2
153–159	24	0.3	99.5
>=159	42	0.5	100.0
Total	8612	100.0	

7.3 Classification Criteria for DQs of the Erxin Scales

7.3.1 Classification Criteria of Well-known Developmental or Intelligence Scales

Different intelligence scales or ability tests may have slightly different criteria for intelligence classification due to variations in research methods and target populations. For example, WPPSI adopts the concept of deviation IQ with a standard deviation of 15, while SB5 uses a standard deviation of 16 [3]. As shown in Table 7.15, WPPSI and BS5 have different classification criteria for intelligence [4], but they generally agree on the classification of average and lower intelligence levels. BSID uses percentile rankings based on developmental indices [5, 6], and its classification for average and lower intelligence levels is consistent with WPPSI and BS5, with a cut-off value of 70 for defining delayed development. GDS draws on adaptive behavior development as the basis for evaluation,

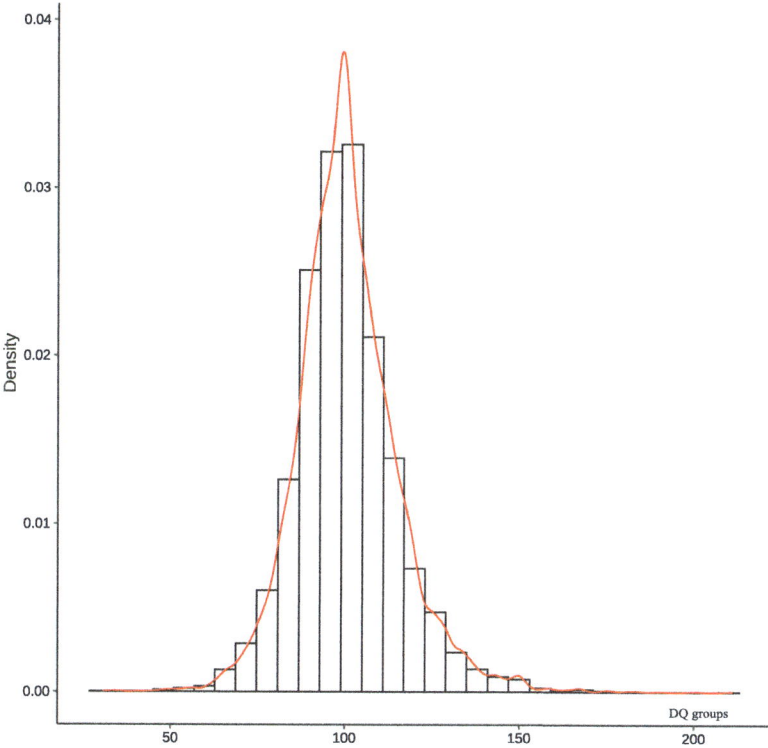

Fig. 7.9 Histogram and probability density curve of social behavior DQs grouped with an interval of 6 for the 8,612 children aged 2–84 months

classifying scores below 75 as delayed development and scores below 85 as suggestive of organic impairment [3, 5, 6]. The original Erxin Scales used the same cut-off value for delayed development as BSID [5].

7.3.2 DQ Classification and Evaluation of the Erxin Scales

Standardization is an important step in the development of psychological measures and is an essential component of all assessment tools. It involves establishing normative values that accurately evaluate the psychological development of children, providing a reference range or standard for assessing child development. In psychometrics, such reference range or standard is referred to as a norm. Standardization, along with other essential psychometric tests such as reliability and validity, is imperative prior to the utilization of any psychological scales.

Table 7.12 Frequency distribution of social behavior DQs grouped with an interval of 6 among the 8,612 children aged 2–84 months

Group for social behavior DQs	Frequency	Valid Percent	Cumulative Percent
<51	10	0.1	0.1
51–57	11	0.1	0.2
57–63	15	0.2	0.4
63–69	57	0.7	1.1
69–75	123	1.4	2.5
75–81	274	3.2	5.7
81–87	615	7.1	12.8
87–93	1155	13.4	26.2
93–99	1632	19.0	45.2
99–105	1750	20.3	65.5
105–111	1167	13.6	79.1
111–117	748	8.7	87.7
117–123	464	5.4	93.1
123–129	226	2.6	95.8
129–135	159	1.8	97.6
135–141	76	0.9	98.5
141–147	49	0.6	99.1
147–153	45	0.5	99.6
153–159	12	0.1	99.7
>=159	24	0.3	100.0
Total	8612	100.0	

Table 7.13 Overall and subscale DQs at the quartiles and the 5th and 95th percentiles for the sample of 8,914 children

	Percentiles				
	5%	25%	50%	75%	95%
Overall scale	81	92	99	106	123
Subscale Gross motor	75	90	99	108	125
Fine motor	72	87	96	104	125
Adaptability	77	91	100	109	130
Language	76	91	100	110	132
Social behavior	79	92	100	109	129

Table 7.14 Means, standard deviations, and medians of DQs for the 8,914 children at different main test ages

Main test age	Number of cases	Overall DQs	Gross motor DQs	Fine motor DQs	Adaptability DQs	Language DQs	Social behavior DQs
1	302	113.9 ± 28.6 111	125.3 ± 43.8 136	122.7 ± 44.8 111	106.5 ± 33.6 100	103.10 ± 46.7 100	115.4 ± 40.2 100
2	303	94.1 ± 27.2 100	96.7 ± 27.9 95	99.3 ± 22.8 100	107.0 ± 34.5 100	106.0 ± 28.7 100	106.6 ± 27.7 100
3	337	97.6 ± 19.3 100	96.7 ± 20.9 100	99.2 ± 20.5 100	111.8 ± 18.3 117	107.5 ± 18.5 103	108.6 ± 16.9 103
4	318	99.3 ± 15.7 100	97.6 ± 18.2 98	97.3 ± 15.7 98	100.4 ± 12.4 100	106.0 ± 18.4 103	100.8 ± 13.7 100
5	308	103.5 ± 11.8 103	104.2 ± 13.2 106	100.3 ± 13.9 100	101.6 ± 15.3 100	106.2 ± 15.1 104	104.4 ± 13.1 104
6	390	101.6 ± 9.1 102	100.0 ± 10.7 100	100.2 ± 11.7 100	103.5 ± 13.1 103	101.1 ± 13.6 100	102.0 ± 11.7 102
7	319	100.5 ± 9.8 100	98.7 ± 11.0 97	97.9 ± 10.8 99	100.2 ± 11.5 101	99.2 ± 12.8 100	101.5 ± 12.2 100
8	315	99.4 ± 7.8 99	99.0 ± 11.4 99	95.9 ± 8.8 96	98.4 ± 9.1 99	98.6 ± 13.1 98	100.3 ± 9.1 100
9	318	97.4 ± 8.2 97	96.8 ± 11.8 98	93.5 ± 9.1 94	95.4 ± 9.5 95	97.3 ± 11.0 97	98.8 ± 9.3 100
10	321	95.6 ± 7.9 96	96.2 ± 10.2 97	92.6 ± 10.4 93	93.2 ± 9.3 93	97.0 ± 10.5 95	97.5 ± 8.3 94
11	301	95.2 ± 7.9 95	96.6 ± 10.2 97	93.3 ± 10.9 93	92.2 ± 10.5 91	96.6 ± 9.2 97	96.6 ± 8.3 96
12	366	96.0 ± 10.7 96	96.0 ± 12.6 95.5	96.0 ± 12.7 96	94.2 ± 12.9 96	95.8 ± 11.1 95	95.4 ± 10.3 94
15	316	98.2 ± 12.1	101.3 ± 15.4	95.5 ± 12.3	97.0 ± 13.3	92.0 ± 13.8	90.9 ± 12.1

(continued)

Table 7.14 (continued)

Main test age	Number of cases	Overall DQs	Gross motor DQs	Fine motor DQs	Adaptability DQs	Language DQs	Social behavior DQs
18	333	98 96.9 ± 10.4 96	100 98.2 ± 13.4 90	97 92.0 ± 13.5 91	98.5 95.7 ± 13.7 97	90 91.4 ± 14.4 91	90 90.9 ± 13.1 91
21	298	95.2 ± 9.1 95	96.7 ± 12.7 98	90.3 ± 15.3 91	96.6 ± 14.8 95	94.2 ± 15.9 93.5	94.5 ± 13.7 94
24	304	95.5 ± 11.9 95	94.1 ± 14.5 93	89.9 ± 17.0 87	97.7 ± 17.7 95.5	97.4 ± 19.3 98	97.0 ± 14.3 97.5
27	296	95.7 ± 11.1 95	95.4 ± 15.0 98	89.5 ± 15.8 90	98.3 ± 16.6 96	98.4 ± 16.8 99	97.4 ± 11.8 96.5
30	296	97.3 ± 12.1 98	97.3 ± 15.0 98	92.7 ± 17.3 92	102.3 ± 18.3 100	101.9 ± 16.8 103	100.2 ± 14.0 98
33	301	100.3 ± 14.0 99	99.4 ± 16.1 99	94.4 ± 15.6 95	101.8 ± 18.4 100	102.2 ± 17.7 101	99.5 ± 15.3 97
36	326	103.9 ± 14.9 103	104.6 ± 16.3 105	97.6 ± 17.9 96	105.3 ± 20.1 104	107.1 ± 20.9 105	107.1 ± 18.4 107
42	309	103.7 ± 14.6 103	103.0 ± 14.2 104	96.4 ± 17.7 95	105.8 ± 19.7 106	110.4 ± 20.5 111	109.5 ± 17.7 109
48	318	108.6 ± 15.4 106.5	105.5 ± 16.0 104	100.2 ± 19.1 97	109.6 ± 18.0 110	113.1 ± 19.0 113	112.1 ± 16.5 112
54	329	105.3 ± 12.5 104	104.7 ± 13.7 104	97.8 ± 16.0 96	106.4 ± 14.4 107	109.0 ± 14.8 108	109.2 ± 14.5 109
60	334	104.4 ± 10.4 104	104.2 ± 12.2 104	99.7 ± 13.5 99	104.8 ± 12.3 106	108.5 ± 12.3 108	106.8 ± 11.8 107
66	317	102.4 ± 9.7 103	101.1 ± 10.9 102	97.8 ± 11.4 98	102.2 ± 12.0 103	103.7 ± 11.1 104	103.8 ± 11.1 106

Main test age	Number of cases	Overall DQs	Gross motor DQs	Fine motor DQs	Adaptability DQs	Language DQs	Social behavior DQs
72	322	99.1 ± 9.0 99	99.3 ± 10.2 100	96.3 ± 11.5 97	99.5 ± 10.7 101	100.4 ± 10.03 102	100.8 ± 10.0 102
78	316	97.1 ± 7.2 98	95.9 ± 9.3 97	94.5 ± 9.2 95	97.5 ± 8.5 99	97.2 ± 7.9 98	97.5 ± 7.9 99
84	301	93.3 ± 5.0 93	92.5 ± 7.0 93	90.4 ± 7.6 91	93.2 ± 6.6 94	93.12 ± 6.3 94	93.4 ± 5.6 94

Table 7.15 Intelligence/ IQ/DQ classification by different scales

WPPSI IP	SB5 IQ	BSID DQ	GDS*	Erxin Scales (1985–2005 applied version) DQ	
Very superior: $\geq$ 130	Very gifted or highly advanced: $\geq$ 140	Very superior: >130	Possible to be organically impaired: 75–85		
Superior: 120–129	Superior or gifted: 120–140	Superior: 120–129			
High average: 110–119	High average: 110–120	High average: 110–119		Superior: > 130	Excellent
Average: 90–109	Average: 90–110	Average: 90–109		High average: 115–129	Smart
Low average: 80–89	Low average: 80–90	Low average: 80–89		Average: 85–114	Normal
Borderline: 70–79	Borderline impaired or delayed: 70–80	Borderline: 70–79		Low average: 70–84	Below normal
Extremely low: <70	Impaired or delayed: <70	Delayed: <70	Delayed: <75	Delayed: $\leq$ 69	Low

*Adaptability DQ and evaluation

Assessing intelligence in infants and toddlers can be challenging due to their incomplete neuropsychological development, particularly when there are suspected pathological factors affecting brain function. Early assessments conducted before the age of 2 may yield inconsistent or weak correlations with later assessments. This is caused by the maturation process in infants and toddlers and is not a flaw of the assessment itself. One inherent feature of brain development lies in its high sensitivity to environmental influences [7]. In certain domains, such as motor skills and language, individual differences and environmental and educational factors can influence the measured abilities. These abilities may not be fully expressed at the time of measurement or may not have developed sufficiently for effective assessment. Therefore, caution must be exercised when evaluating infants and toddlers with exceptional intellectual abilities (giftedness) or intellectual disabilities (intellectual impairment), and detailed gradation in classification should be avoided. Referring to the IQ evaluation of WPPSI and SB5, developmental indices of BSID, and DQ classification of the original Erxin Scales, the revised Erxin Scales provide six levels of developmental assessment: superior, high average, average, low average, borderline, and delayed. This classification system adheres to cultural norms in China and features appropriate evaluation descriptions.

Admittedly, a further classification of DQs below 70 based on the severity of developmental delay was not made because of the limited number of individuals with such low DQ levels in the sample. Another reason lies in the absence of concurrent clinical assessment or comparative studies with other diagnostic scales, as well as the lack of subsequent clinical follow-ups.

7.4 Normative Reference Values for the Erxin Scales

7.4.1 Formation of Normative Reference Values

Based on the descriptive statistics of DQs (including means, 95% confidence intervals, medians, quartiles, and normal distribution data) derived from the representative sample, and referring to the norm classification of well-known scales, the revised Erxin Scales' DQ scores are categorized into six norm levels: superior, high average, average, low average, borderline, and delayed. The sample size and composition ratio of the overall and subscale DQs at each norm level are shown in Table 7.16.

7.4.2 Classification and Evaluation of DQ Norm Levels

The Erxin Scales provide a set of reference standards, i.e., norms, for assessing DQs. The composition ratio ranges for overall and subscale DQs at different norm levels in the representative sample are presented in Table 7.17. The distribution of the norm levels is as follows: Superior level accounts for 2.7–5.9%, high average level accounts for 12.6–20.3%, average level accounts for 51.7–64.5%, low average level accounts for 12.8–20.5%, borderline level accounts for 2.3–8.0%, and delayed level accounts for 1.8–3.5%. The table also indicates the levels of DQs within the representative sample, providing medical suggestions and guidance for children with lower DQs.

Table 7.16 Sample sizes and composition ratios of the overall and subscale DQs at different norm levels

DQ norm level	Overall scale Number of cases (%)	Gross motor subscale Number of cases (%)	Fine motor subscale Number of cases (%)	Adaptability subscale Number of cases (%)	Language subscale Number of cases (%)	Social behavior subscale Number of cases (%)
<70	159 (1.8)	226 (2.5)	308 (3.5)	181 (2.0)	217 (2.4)	138 (1.5)
70–80	209 (2.3)	491 (5.5)	712 (8.0)	458 (5.1)	448 (5.0)	336 (3.8)
80–90	1137 (12.8)	1299 (14.6)	1826 (20.5)	1329 (14.9)	1184 (13.3)	1162 (13.0)
90–110	5751 (64.5)	4897 (54.9)	4607 (51.7)	4772 (53.5)	4732 (53.1)	5127 (57.5)
110–130	1414 (15.9)	1662 (18.6)	1119 (12.6)	1723 (19.3)	1811 (20.3)	1719 (19.3)
≥130	244 (2.7)	339 (3.8)	342 (3.8)	451 (5.1)	522 (5.9)	432 (4.8)

Table 7.17 Classification and evaluation of DQ norm levels for the Erxin Scales

Overall and subscale DQ level	Composition ratio (%)	DQ level within the representative sample	Evaluation	Suggestion	Guidance
130≤DQ	2.7–5.9	Superior	Excellent	Regular follow-up	
110≤DQ<130	12.6–20.3	High average	Good		
90≤ DQ<110	51.7–64.5	Average	Normal		
80≤DQ<90	12.8–20.5	Low average	Below normal	Increase in evaluation frequency	Family intervention
70≤DQ<80	2.3–8.0	Borderline	Low	Relevant medical assessment	Rehabilitation training
DQ<70	1.8–3.5	Delayed	Very low	Specialized medical assessment	Rehabilitation training

7.4.3 Percentiles for DQs at Main Test Ages

To understand the growth patterns of children, provide a basis for comparative studies, and better interpret the assessment results, this English edition also includes the reference percentiles for overall and subscale DQs at different main test ages, which are urgently needed for clinical and research purposes. In doing so, comparative measurement information is offered, equipping evaluators with scientifically accurate reference for comparing cognitive progress made by children during continuous monitoring of developmental trajectories or longitudinal follow-up studies. It also helps parents understand their child's development level compared to same-age peers and appreciate the importance of assessment and monitoring. Please refer to Tables 1–6 in Appendix A for specific information, where Table 1 presents relevant data on overall DQs, while Tables 2–6 provide data on DQs for the gross motor, fine motor, adaptability, language, and social behavior subscales, respectively. The reference ranges of DQs from the 3rd to 97th percentiles at the main test ages for children from 1 to 84 months of age are also provided.

7.5 Risk Index Classification of the Communication Warning Behavior Subscale

The risk index classification for the added Communication Warning Behavior Subscale is as follows: A score below 7 is considered normal, a score between 7 and 12 requires follow-up observation, a score between 12 and 30 indicates a risk of developmental deviation and communication difficulties, a score above 30 suggests a suspicion of ASD, and a score exceeding 50 indicates a high likelihood of ASD. To facilitate clinical interpretation and evaluation and to reflect the screening function of the scale, the percentage composition of the healthy control group ($n = 1,596$) from the sampled region is presented in Table 7.18. After administering the assessment, the assessor should consider the overall and subscale DQs and refer to the norm cut-offs to provide detailed interpretation and recommendations regarding the risk index.

7.6 Stepwise Age Correction for Preterm Infants

The revised Erxin Scales fully consider the applicability of its testing tools for preterm infants, reflected such as in the adjustments made to the handle thickness and weight of the bell stick. Unique considerations have also been given to the age correction for preterm infants, which

Table 7.18 Risk index classification and evaluation of the communication warning behavior subscale

Risk index classification	Composition ratio of risk index in healthy children (%)	Risk index classification and evaluation	Suggestion	Guidance
Index<7	78.7	Normal	Follow-up according to regular physical examinations	
7≤index<12	9.6	Risk of developmental deviations or unfavorable behaviors	Increase in follow-up frequency; reassessment within 1–3 months	Close observation to avoid missed diagnosis
12≤index<30	9.8	Risk of communication disorders	Differential diagnosis based on developmental level or reassessment using other methods	Timely intervention, regular assessment, and follow-up
30≤index<50	1.8	Suspicion of ASD	Professional reassessment based on developmental level	Involvement of institutions and families in rehabilitation training; regular assessment
50≤index	0.1	High likelihood of ASD	Further specialized diagnostic assessment	Involvement of institutions and families in rehabilitation training; regular assessment

involves subtracting the number of weeks they were preterm from their chronological age. When using the original or revised Erxin Scales, it is recommended to input the information based on the actual date of birth during assessment, on the basis of which the assessment result displays the mental age (developmental age) and DQ. Age correction is only taken into account when interpreting the assessment report and decided based on the chronological age, mental age, DQ, and clinical performance.

For preterm infants, especially those with a young chronological age, their developmental age outweighs the DQ. Comparing the developmental age with the corrected age allows us to assess their extent of catch-up growth, and a good match between the two indicates successful catch-up. In other words, a small discrepancy between the two ages suggests ideal catch-up growth, while a large discrepancy indicates poor catch-up or even lagging behind. Furthermore, it is essential for assessors to be familiar with the specific content of assessments for preterm infants. While considering appropriate catch-up growth, attention should also be given to screening for organic or functional impairments in them. For example, it is necessary to investigate potential damage to the retina, optic nerve, or hearing when abnormalities are observed in tasks such as watching black-and-white targets, gazing at faces, or responding to sounds; if there is a delay in gross motor or fine motor development, neurological disorders such as cerebral palsy should be considered. The particularity of preterm infants merits targeted analysis of and solutions to specific issues; longitudinal follow-up and monitoring of communication behaviors and intellectual development are necessary. Recommendations regarding age correction are as follows: For infants aged 0–6 months, compare their developmental age with the corrected age (using whole-month correction); for infants older than 6 months, compare their developmental age with the age corrected half-month (using half-month correction by subtracting half of the weeks they were preterm); for preterm children over two years old, age correction and evaluation are no longer necessary. Examples are provided in Table 7.19 for further clarification.

To prevent parents from losing confidence due to assessments and encourage them to actively engage in interventions, the Erxin Scales adopt a stepwise age correction method, providing parents with evaluation information that is easier to understand and accept. This approach motivates parents to engage in early interventions, aiming to effectively promote the positive development of preterm infants' motor skills, cognition, and other abilities. Although the Erxin Scales have demonstrated good assessment validity for preterm infants in clinical settings, further research on this population is needed. Currently, a relevant work is under preparation.

Table 7.19 Illustrations of the stepwise age correction for preterm infants

Chronological age	Recommended age correction	Illustration
27 days–6 months	Chronological age minus the weeks preterm (whole-month correction)	Take an infant born at 32 weeks with 8 weeks (2 months) preterm as an example. If the chronological age is 5 months, the corrected age would be 3 months (chronological age of 5 months minus 2 months preterm). While interpreting the assessment report, the obtained developmental age would be compared with the corrected age of 3 months
7–24 months	Chronological age minus half of the weeks preterm (half-month correction)	Take an infant born at 32 weeks with 8 weeks (2 months) preterm as an example. If the chronological age is 7 months, the age correction would be 6 months (chronological age of 7 months minus half of the weeks preterm, which is 1 month). While interpreting the assessment report, the obtained developmental age would be compared with the half-month corrected age of 6 months
Over 24 months	No correction	

References

1. Ma, B. R. (2004). *Medical statistics*. People's Medical Publishing House.
2. Piñon, M. F. (2010). *Theoretical background and structure of the Bayley scales of infant and toddler development* (3rd ed.). Bayley–III Clinical Use and Interpretation (pp. 1–28). Academic Press.
3. Liu, X. Y., Lin, C. J., & Xue, Q. B. (1999). *Child health care*. Jiangsu Science and Technology Press.
4. Zhang, J. J., & Gao, Z. M. (1989). *Children intelligence test and training*. Science and Technology Press.
5. Yang, Y. F. (2016). *Rating scales for children's developmental behavior and mental health*. People's Medical Publishing House.
6. Xu, S. S., Huang, H., & Zhang, J. S. (2010). Research and application of diagnostic developmental scales for infants. *Chinese Journal of Child Health Care, 18*(11), 859–861.
7. DeMaster, D., Bick, J., Johnson, U., Montroy, J. J., Landry, S., & Duncan, A. F. (2019). Nurturing the preterm infant brain: Leveraging neuroplasticity to improve neurobehavioral outcomes. *Pediatric Research, 85*(2), 166–175.

CHAPTER 8

Application and Administration of the Scales

Developmental assessment results are influenced by factors such as the attitude of the assessor, the testing atmosphere, and the emotional state and health condition of the test subjects. It should be noted that these results are not fixed and unchanging, and regular monitoring is necessary to understand the developmental trends of children. Test management is a crucial aspect for the administration of the Erxin Scale. This chapter presents important considerations before administrating the Erxin Scale, including qualifications certification of the examiner and assessor, assessor's competence, testing environment, testing timing, preparation and organization of testing tools, special instructions for administering the Erxin Scale, scoring information, and management of test records.

8.1 Management

8.1.1 Management of Examiners and Assessors

1) **Examiner qualifications**

The training program for instructors and assisting teachers (examiners) sets the following requirements: The training for Erxin Scales instructors is conducted by members who participated in the development and revision of the scales or those who have undergone rigorous foundational training. They should possess theoretical and practical knowledge of the

© The Author(s), under exclusive license to Springer Nature Singapore Pte Ltd. 2024
C. Jin et al., *Erxin Scales: Child Developmental Scale of China*,
https://doi.org/10.1007/978-981-99-9997-2_8

development and revision of the Erxin Scales, as well as the necessary skills to perform standardized operations. Individuals who have passed the assessment conducted by the main members of the scale revision team are eligible to serve as examiners in the training program. The training materials center around the Chinese edition of *Children Neuropsychological and Behavior Scale-Revision 2016* published by Beijing Publishing House or this English edition of "Erxin Scales: Child Development Scale of China." The training adheres to professional ethics, considering the specificity, professionalism, standardization, and consistency required in psychological testing.

2) **Assessor training and certification**

Institutions intending to conduct assessments must participate in the specialized training program launched by the Erxin Scales revision team. Participants in formal Erxin Scales training should include physicians and therapists from various levels of maternal and child health hospitals, children's hospitals, pediatric departments of general hospitals, preventive healthcare departments, community health service organizations, and medical rehabilitation institutions. They should also include practitioners in early childhood education, special education professionals, managers of childcare institutions, managers of non-profit social rehabilitation institutions, and other professionals engaged in child growth and development-related fields.

Participants should first acquire knowledge of the theoretical foundations of developmental scales, the development and revision process of the Erxin Scales, data collection procedures for representative samples, and the formation in psychometrics. Subsequently, they are supposed to study the instruction manual for the Erxin Scales, including the operation details and scoring criteria for the items, as well as other matters meriting attention during test administration. In addition, they should observe practical demonstrations, followed by hands-on training. Upon successful completion of theoretical and practical assessments, participants will be awarded a certification endorsed by Chunhua Jin, the person in charge of the Erxin Scales revision work and its dedicated promotor.

8.1.2 Specific Testing Requirements

1) **Testing environment**

The testing should ideally take place in a clean, tidy, quiet, and comfortable room free from distractions. There should be no noise or other individuals present during testing. The lighting in the room should come from overhead sources, avoiding curiosity-inducing stimuli for infants and young children. The walls of the room should have a warm, solid color tone, with minimal unnecessary decorations. The furniture, including the table and chairs, should be suitable for both the assessors, the children, and their parents.

2) **Test subjects and duration**

The Erxin Scales are designed for individuals aged 27 days to 6 years. In cases of significant developmental delay, the age range can be extended up to 8 or 9 years. Generally, the testing duration is approximately 30–50 minutes, with around 30–40 minutes for children under 2 years old and 40–50 minutes for children aged 2–6 years.

3) **Testing preparation**

   a) Testing toolkit: The testing tools in the toolkit should be organized appropriately. Before and after each assessment, the assessor should check if all the required tools are present. If any tools are missing, they should be promptly replenished.
   b) Test forms: To facilitate the assessment process and minimize waste, specially designed test record forms specific to the Erxin Scales should be used. The selection of the form should be based on the age of the child being assessed. The front side of the form contains basic information about the subjects, including their name, gender, and other important demographic information. The inner side of the form includes the test items and their sequential number, categorized according to the main test ages, covering domains such as gross motor skills, fine motor skills, adaptive abilities, language, social behavior, and communication warning behaviors.
   c) Other objects: Prior to the assessment, it is necessary to prepare pens, a stopwatch, and clean drinking water.

8.1.3 Requirements for the State of the Child Being Assessed

The assessment should be conducted when infants and young children are naturally awake and in good physical health. If the child is crying, hungry, in a poor state, or drowsy, it is advisable to postpone or reschedule the assessment to avoid influencing the results.

8.2 Specific Requirements for the Assessor

8.2.1 Kind Reminders

Before starting the assessment, it is important to provide parents with kind reminders: The child is not expected to finish all the test items; some items may be achievable, while others may not. It is common for children to refuse to perform certain tasks during the assessment, even if they can do them at home; parents should not feel anxious about this. Moreover, parents should not provide unsolicited prompts or use nonverbal cues such as gestures or eye contact to suggest specific responses, as this may affect the reliability of the assessment results.

8.2.2 Establishing a Friendly Relationship

During the assessment, typically only one parent accompanies the child. The assessor should build a relaxed and appropriate rapport with the parent, showing care and liking for the child. It is also important to establish and maintain positive and effective communication with the child being assessed. The assessor should always show a warm and friendly attitude, using gentle language and a kind demeanor when interacting with the child. The assessment should commence once the child is familiar with the environment. It is particularly important to establish an emotional connection with slightly older children before initiating the assessment procedures. Throughout the assessment, the assessor should pay attention to the child's reactions and behaviors in order to make accurate judgments and provide timely responses. It is crucial to avoid entering the assessment process without mutual communication, using simplistic and rigid approaches. When a child completes a test item, the assessor can express appreciation through smiling, nodding, or using neutral and encouraging language such as "Well done," "Take your time," "Give it a try," or "You can do it." These expressions help to stimulate the child's interest in the assessment and generate positive responses. It is not permissible to place the testing toolkit on the table.

8 APPLICATION AND ADMINISTRATION OF THE SCALES   183

8.2.3 Following an Ascending Order of Difficulty

During the assessment, it is advisable to start with easier items and then progress to more difficult ones. Generally, it is recommended to group together items that require maintaining the same posture or position to avoid frequent changes. Items involving question-and-answer tasks and hands-on activities should be arranged appropriately, and assessments of gross motor items should be scheduled based on specific circumstances (e.g., the child's emotions and persistence). An item can be temporarily skipped if the child shows no interest in it, and an alternative item that the child enjoys, such as that involves colored blocks or spot-the-difference games, can be introduced. Questions or tasks requiring the child to follow instructions should be administered when the child is relatively at ease, and the questioning should strictly adhere to the specified instructions without arbitrary modifications.

8.2.4 Recording the Scores

The symbol "O" should be used to indicate passes, rather than symbols like "$\sqrt{}$" or " × ," to avoid placing unnecessary psychological pressure on the child. If it is not possible to complete all the test items in one session, a separate time should be scheduled to start from the beginning, thus re-administering the assessment.

8.2.5 Data Input and Report Output

The previously manual processes of age calculation, scoring, score conversion, and DQ calculation involved in the Erxin Scales are all automated now, reducing the possibility of human calculation errors. After the assessment is completed, both the passed and failed items are entered into a computer system and saved. The electronic version of the assessment report can be shared with parents and can also be printed if needed. Finally, the assessor provides relevant interpretations based on the obtained scores and comparison with the normative data. The report includes the child's average developmental age (mental age), overall DQ, developmental ages and quotients of specific domains (gross motor, fine motor, adaptability, language, and social behavior), as well as the index obtained from the Communication Warning Behavior Subscale, which helps identify ASD risk. It also provides guidance to parents on how to promote their child's development based on the DQ scores. This serves as a bridge for the communication between the assessor and the parents, facilitating the interpretation of the test results.

8.3 BE PROFICIENT IN THE ASSESSMENT PROCEDURE OF THE ERXIN SCALES

8.3.1 Familiarizing Yourself with the Instructions

To administrate the Erxin Scales, a copy of the Chinese edition of *Children Neuropsychological and Behavior Scale-Revision 2016* or the instruction manual for the English edition of "Erxin Scales: Child Development Scale of China" should be referred to. The instructions for each test item should be memorized, and standardized instructions be followed during the assessment.

8.3.2 Memorizing the Specific Assessment Procedure

Firstly, a main test age should be selected based on the chronological age (selecting the younger main test age corresponding to the chronological age). After finishing the testing for the main test age, two age segments earlier (in the direction of ages younger than the main test age) should be tested. If the child passes the items in a domain for two consecutive age segments, passes would be assumed for all previous items in that domain; otherwise, testing continues backwards until the child passes the items in a domain for two consecutive age segments. Then, testing proceeds in the opposite direction (ages older than the main test age), and in each domain, testing continues until the child fails the items in a domain for two consecutive age segments. The Communication Warning Behavior Subscale adopts a cumulative scoring rule: All items before the main test age need to be observed; if a behavior is not observed or its presence is not clear, the parent should be asked to assist in confirming the behavior's existence rather than its occasional appearance. If a positive answer occur after the main test age, observation and inquiry about subsequent items should be continued; the assessment regarding the domain could be stopped if two consecutive items receive negative responses.

CHAPTER 9

Instruction Manual for the Erxin Scales

9.1 OPERATIONS AND PASSING/SCORING CRITERIA FOR ITEMS OF ERXIN SCALES

1 month old

Domain	No.	Item	Operation/measure	Passing/scoring criterion
Gross motor	1	Head upright for 2 seconds when sitting up with shoulders supported	Place the infant in a supine position. The assessor stands facing the infant, smiles and talks to the infant until they look at the assessor's face. At this point, the assessor gently grasps the infant's shoulders and lifts the infant up to a sitting position to observe the infant's ability to control their head	The head of the infant who is in a sitting position can stay upright for 2 seconds or more

(continued)

The original version of the chapter has been revised: Figures and Tables have been updated. A correction to this chapter can be found at https://doi.org/10.1007/978-981-99-9997-2_11

© The Author(s), under exclusive license to Springer Nature Singapore Pte Ltd. 2024, corrected publication 2025
C. Jin et al., *Erxin Scales: Child Developmental Scale of China*, https://doi.org/10.1007/978-981-99-9997-2_9

(continued)

1 month old

Domain	No.	Item	Operation/measure	Passing/scoring criterion
	2	Tilt and raise the head when lying prone	**Warning/reminder:** Place four fingers together on the outside of the scapula, ensuring that the index finger does not touch the infant's neck. Maintain a moderate speed (neither too fast nor too slow) when lifting the infant up by grasping the shoulders Note: For full-term infants, Item #12 ("Head upright for about 5 seconds when sitting up by pulled the wrist") should be assessed before this item Let the infant lie prone, with forearms bent as if supporting themselves. Use a toy to coax the infant to lift the head. Observe the head movement	Pass if the infant lifts the head upwards, turns it, or momentarily raises the head
Fine motor	3	Clench a fist when the palm is touched	Place the infant in a supine position. The assessor places the index finger or thumb from the ulnar side into the infant's palm and lifts the hand upwards	The infant can tightly clench the fist, and when the assessor raises their hand upwards, they can still feel the infant tightly clenching the fist to maintain the body from sinking
	4	Natural state of hands	**Warning/reminder:** When the thumb or index finger is placed in the infant's palm, it can be pressed against the palm center The assessor observes the natural state of the infant's hands when they are awake	Pass if the hands are generally in a fist-like position, with the thumbs not reaching the palm center or tightly gripping though tucked inwards

(continued)

9 INSTRUCTION MANUAL FOR THE ERXIN SCALES   187

(continued)

1 month old

Domain	No.	Item	Operation/measure	Passing/scoring criterion
			Warning/reminder: 1. Fail if the hands are completely relaxed and in an open state 2. Fail if, for infants under 4 months old, the thumbs are tucked inwards tightly and reach the palm center, or if the hands are completely relaxed and in an open state 3. Fail if, for infants over 4 months old, the thumbs are still tucked inwards	
Adaptability	5	Eyes cross the midline following the red ball	Place the infant in a supine position. The assessor holds a red ball and gently shakes it about 20 cm above the infant's face to attract their attention. The assessor then moves the red ball in an arc-shaped trajectory towards one side of the infant's head, then reverses and moves along the arc through the midline to the other side of the head. Observe the movements of the infant's head and eyes	Pass if when the assessor moves the red ball towards the midline, the infant tracks the red ball with the eyes and looks beyond the midline, with or without turning the head
			Warning/reminder: At least one successful attempt out of three is required	
	6	Watch black-and-white target	Place the infant in a supine position. The assessor holds a black-and-white target and slowly moves it about 20 cm above the infant's face to attract their attention	The infant's eyes clearly fixate on the black-and-white target

(continued)

(continued)

1 month old

Domain	No.	Item	Operation/measure	Passing/scoring criterion
Language	7	Make small guttural sound	**Warning/reminder:** The "red ball" item should be tested before the "black-and-white target" item Observe the infant making sounds or vocalizations when they are awake	Pass if it is observed or informed that the infant in the awake state can make small guttural sound
			Warning/reminder: *R (means need to require to child's parents) The assessor can properly tease the infant but should avoid touching their body	
	8	Respond to sound	Place the infant in a supine position. The assessor gently shakes a brass bell about 10–15 cm above the infant's ear on one side and observes their response. Then repeat the operation on the other side	Pass if the infant exhibits one or more responses (e.g., reduced or increased movement, cessation of activity, staring, widening of the eyes, frowning)
			Warning/reminder: Both sides are required to be tested, but passing on one side is sufficient. Please make a note if any side fails	
Social behavior	9	Stare at the speaker	The assessor faces the infant's face, smiles, and speaks	Pass if the infant can stare at the assessor
			Warning/reminder: The assessor should avoid touching the infant's face or body during the test	

(continued)

9 INSTRUCTION MANUAL FOR THE ERXIN SCALES 189

(continued)

1 month old

Domain	No.	Item	Operation/measure	Passing/scoring criterion
	10	Eyes track people who move around	Place the infant horizontally on a bed or reclining in the parent's arms. Talk and engage with the infant to gain their attention. The assessor then walks back and forth, observing whether the infant's eyes follow them **Warning/reminder:** The assessor should maintain an upright position while teasing the infant, avoiding bending over or touching the infant's body	Pass if the infant's eyes track the assessor
Communication warning behavior	11	Have sleep disorders after birth	Inquire about the infant's sleeping patterns **Warning/reminder:** R Sleep disorder is operationalized as significantly affecting the mother and the entire family's life	Points are scored if there are sleep disorders, lack of regularity, and restlessness

2 months old

Domain	No.	Item	Operation	Passing/scoring criterion
Gross motor	12	Head upright for about 5 seconds when sitting up by pulled the wrist	Place the infant in a supine position. The assessor places their thumb in the infant's palm, with the remaining four fingers holding the infant's wrist, and gently pulls the infant into a sitting position. Observe the infant's ability to control their head **Warning/reminder**: Maintain a moderate speed when pulling the infant's wrist to sit them up	The head of the infant pulled to a sitting position can stay upright for 5 seconds or more
	13	Head lifted off the bed when lying prone	Let the infant lie prone, with forearms bent as if supporting themselves. Use a toy to coax the infant to lift their head. Observe the infant's response	The infant can independently lift the head off the bed surface for 2 seconds or more
Fine motor	14	Hold the bell stick for a moment	Place the infant in a supine position. Place a bell stick in the infant's hand	The infant holds the bell stick for 2 seconds or more
	15	Thumb separates when the hand is tapped lightly	The assessor gently taps the back of the infant's hands separately when they are awake. Observe the natural relaxation state of the infant's thumbs **Warning/reminder**: Fail if the thumb is clearly tucked inwards and reaches the center of the palm	Pass if lightly tapping the back of the infant's hand can make the previously tightly clenched fist open
Adaptability	16	Watch the big toy immediately	Place the infant in a supine position. Shake a doll about 20 cm above the infant's face. Observe the infant's response	The infant can notice the doll immediately

(continued)

(continued)

2 months old

Domain	No.	Item	Operation	Passing/scoring criterion
	17	Eyes turn up and down following the red ball	**Warning/reminder:** Item #27 (Watch toy on the front of the chest immediately) should be tested before this item. At least one successful attempt out of three is required. Place the infant in a supine position. The assessor lifts a red ball and gently shakes it about 20 cm above the infant's face to attract their attention. First, slowly move it upward beyond the head, and then move it downward towards the chin **Warning/reminder:** Item #28 ("Eyes and head turn 180° following the red ball") should be tested before this item	Pass if the infant's eyes turn up and down following the red ball, with or without moving the head
Language	18	Pronounce "a," "o," "e" or other vowels	Inquire whether the infant can pronounce consonants or tease the infant to make sounds **Warning/reminder:** R The assessor can properly tease the infant but should avoid touching their body	The infant can pronounce "a," "o," "e" or other vowels in the awake state
	19	Make complex reactions to sounds	Place the infant in a supine position. Gently shake a brass bell about 10–15 cm above the infant's ear on one side, and observe the infant's response. Repeat the operation on the other side	The infant shows facial expressions (frowning, staring, smiling, etc.) and changes in body movements (increased or decreased activity) when hearing sounds

(continued)

(continued)

2 months old

Domain	No.	Item	Operation	Passing/scoring criterion
Social behavior	20	Smile spontaneously	**Warning/reminder:** Pass is considered when the infant shows both facial expressions and changes in body movements. Passing on one side is sufficient, but please make a note if any side fails. Observe or inquire if the infant spontaneously smiles without external stimuli **Warning/reminder:** R Smiling during sleep does not count	The infant can smile spontaneously, either with or without sound
	21	Respond when teased	Place the infant in a supine position. The assessor bends over and teases the infant by nodding, smiling, or talking. Observe the infant's response **Warning/reminder:** Do not touch the infant while trying to elicit a response. Blank stares or daydreaming do not count	Pass if the infant exhibits one or several of such expressions as smiling, making sounds, and moving limbs
Communication warning behavior	22	Easily agitated and difficult to soothe	Under normal circumstances, infants after birth have a basic sleep routine. Apart from a few hungry cries before feeding, most of the time is spent in peaceful sleep **Warning/reminder:** R Being easily agitated and difficult to soothe is operationalized as causing exhaustion for the entire family	Points are scored if the infant is easily agitated, cries frequently, and is difficult to soothe

3 months old

Domain	No.	Item	Operation	Passing/scoring criterion
Gross motor	23	Head upright when held straight	Hold the infant upright and observe their ability to control the head and neck **Warning/reminder**: Fail if the infant shows a tilted neck or habitual tilted neck	The infant can raise the head upright and maintain stable for 10 seconds or more
	24	Head raised 45° when lying prone	Let the infant lie prone, with forearms bent and the head in a midline position. Use a toy to engage the infant to raise the head. Observe the infant's response	The infant can raise the head off the bed by themselves, with the face at a 45° angle to the bed, for at least 5 seconds
Fine motor	25	Hold the bell stick for 30 seconds	Let the infant lie down or hold them in a sitting position. Place the bell stick in the infant's hand **Warning/reminder**: Fail if using the bed for support	The infant can hold the bell stick for 30 seconds without using the bed for support
	26	Put hands together	Place the infant in a supine position. Observe whether the infant can put the hands together spontaneously or with the assessor's assistance **Warning/reminder**: Fail if the hands are only put together for less than 3 seconds Assistance is allowed once	The infant puts the hands together for 3–4 seconds

(continued)

(continued)

3 months old

Domain	No.	Item	Operation	Passing/scoring criterion
Adaptability	27	Watch the toy on the front of the chest immediately	Place the infant in a supine position. The assessor moves a doll about 20 cm above the infant along the midline from below to until reaching the area between the infant's nipples and the chin. Observe the infant's response **Warning/reminder:** Do not shake the toy At least one successful attempt out of three is required	Pass if the infant notices the doll immediately when it is moved to the area between the nipples and the chin
	28	Eyes and head turn 180° following the red ball	Place the infant in a supine position. The assessor holds a red ball and gently shakes it about 20 cm above the infant's face to attract their attention. Then the assessor slowly moves the red ball along an arc-shaped trajectory from one side of the head, crossing the midline, and returning to the other side of the head. Observe the movements of the infant's head and eyes **Warning/reminder:** At least one successful attempt out of three is required	The infant's eyes and head turn 180° following the red ball

(continued)

9 INSTRUCTION MANUAL FOR THE ERXIN SCALES 195

(continued)

3 months old

Domain	No.	Item	Operation	Passing/scoring criterion
Language	29	Laugh out loud	Tease the infant to laugh without physical contact **Warning/reminder**: R	The infant giggles
Social behavior	30	Laugh when seeing people	Observe the infant's facial expressions when they are not teased by anyone **Warning/reminder**: The assessor should not engage in proximity-based touching or social behaviors Fail if the infant shows blank stares	The infant smiles when seeing people
	31	Actively observe the surrounding environment	Observe the infant's reactions to people and the environment when they are not teased	The infant shows signs of observing the surrounding environment, with their eyes looking around
Communication warning behavior	32	Rarely look at the mother's face	Inquire of the mother about the infant's behavior during feeding or when awake and playing **Warning/reminder**: R Observe the infant's initial communication with the mother	Points are scored if the infant rarely looks at the mother's face during feeding or when awake

4 months old

Domain	No.	Item	Operation	Passing/scoring criterion
Gross motor	33	Stand for a while when the armpits are held	The assessor supports the infant under the armpits with both hands and relax their hands after the infant is placed in an upright position. Observe the infant's response **Warning/reminder**: During the observation, the hands supporting the infant's armpits should be relaxed slightly to ensure safety No weight-bearing on the lower limbs needs to be noted	The infant can maintain a standing position with their legs for 2 seconds or more
	34	Head raised 90° when lying prone	Let the infant lie prone, with forearms bent and the head in a midline position. Use a toy to engage the infant to raise their head. Observe the infant's response	The infant can raise the head off the bed by themselves, with the face at a 90° angle to the bed, for at least 5 seconds
Fine motor	35	Watch and shake the bell stick	Hold the infant in a sitting position and place a bell stick in the infant's hand, encouraging the infant to shake it	The infant can focus on the bell stick and shake it a few times
	36	Try to grab something	Shake the bell stick in front of the infant and observe the infant's hand movements **Warning/reminder**: The infant can be in a supine or sitting position. Touching the infant's hand is allowed to attract their attention	Pass if the infant shows excitement and attempts to lift the arms or make grabbing movements

(continued)

9 INSTRUCTION MANUAL FOR THE ERXIN SCALES 197

(continued)

4 months old

Domain	No.	Item	Operation	Passing/scoring criterion
Adaptability	37	Make eye contact	The assessor or the mother speaks to the infant. Observe whether the infant makes eye contact with people **Warning/reminder**: Do not touch the infant's body	The infant can make eye contact with an adult and maintain it for at least 5 seconds
	38	Yell loudly	Observe or inquire whether the infant makes loud noises when happy or displeased **Warning/reminder**: R Fail if the loud noises are high-pitched and lack tone variations	Pass if the loud noises vary in tone
Language	39	Babble in quiet time	Observe or inquire about the sounds the infant makes when they are quiet **Warning/reminder**: R The observation should be made when the infant is awake, and check whether the sounds they make are louder than "a," "o," "e" or other vowels pronounced at the age of 2 months	The infant can produce nonsyllabic, meaningless sounds, similar to babbling
	40	Find the sound source	Hold the infant in a sitting position. The assessor gently shakes a brass bell about 15–20 cm above the infant's ear from behind. Observe the infant's response	The infant can turn the head towards the sound source; passing on one side is sufficient

(continued)

(continued)

4 months old

Domain	No.	Item	Operation	Passing/scoring criterion
			Warning/reminder: Both sides should be tested, and if only one side passes, it should be noted	
Social behavior	41	Watch the figure in the mirror	Place an unframed mirror horizontally about 20 cm in front of the infant. The assessor or the mother teases the infant via the mirror. Observe the infant's response	Pass if the infant watches the figure in the mirror either spontaneously or when teased, or if the infant shows changes in facial expressions or body movements in response to the figure
			Warning/reminder: Item #51 ("React to the figure in the mirror") should be tested before this item. The duration of attention should be at least 5 seconds	
	42	Happy when seeing the mother or other relatives	Observe the infant's facial expressions when seeing the mother or other relatives, or hearing their voices	The infant becomes happy when seeing the mother or other relatives
			Warning/reminder: R	
Communication warning behavior	43	Make no response to others' smiling faces	Observe whether the infant responds with a smiling face when the assessor or others smile at the infant	Points are scored if the infant does not respond with a smiling face to others' social smile
			Warning/reminder: R Points should be scored if the infant shows a dull facial expression, no changes in expression while awake, or a consistently cold and unsmiling expression	

5 months old

Domain	No.	Item	Operation	Passing/scoring criterion
Gross motor	44	Sit up by pulled the wrist lightly	Place the infant in a supine position. The assessor holds the infant's wrist (placing the thumb from the ulnar or radial side into the infant's hand while the other four fingers hold the infant's wrist) and gently pulls the infant into a sitting position **Warning/reminder**: Fail if the infant cannot actively cooperate and exert effort to sit up, fails to maintain an alignment between their head and trunk during the process of sitting up, or stands up directly without going through the sitting position	Pass if the infant can actively sit up with effort, and maintain a nearly straight alignment between their head and trunk without any backward delay in the head movement
	45	Sit up by oneself with the head tilted forward	Place the infant in a sitting position on the bed **Warning/reminder**: Fail if the infant's body leans forward at an angle, even if the infant is capable of lifting the head and supporting themselves with the hands on the bed	Pass if the infant sits up by themselves for 5 seconds or more, and leans forward with a curved back forming a C-shaped sitting posture, with or without support from hands on the bed

(continued)

(continued)

5 months old

Domain	No.	Item	Operation	Passing/scoring criterion
Fine motor	46	Grab the toy nearby	Hold the infant in a sitting position, with their hands on the table. Place a toy (e.g., a bell stick) about 2.5 cm away from the infant's palm and encourage the infant to reach for it **Warning/reminder**: To pass, the infant should be able to hold onto the toy and lift it off the tabletop; otherwise, it would be considered a failure	Pass if the infant can grab the toy with one or both hands and take it away from the tabletop
	47	Play hands spontaneously	Observe whether the infant can put their hands together and play with them **Warning/reminder**: Assistance is allowed once It is acceptable to either place the infant in a supine position or hold them in a sitting position	The infant spontaneously brings the two hands together to play
Adaptability	48	Notice the small pellet	Place a pellet on the table and point to the pellet or move it around to attract the infant's attention. During the operation, the assessor uses their finger to push the pellet and quickly moves their hand away to observe the infant's reaction to the pellet	The infant clearly notices the pellet

(continued)

9 INSTRUCTION MANUAL FOR THE ERXIN SCALES 201

(continued)

5 months old

Domain	No.	Item	Operation	Passing/scoring criterion
	49	Hold a building block and look at another	**Warning/reminder**: 1. When using a finger to stop the rolling pellet, the hand should be quickly moved away to prevent the infant from focusing on the assessor's finger instead of the pellet itself 2. The surface of the testing table should be dark in color (preferably in dark green) Hold the infant in a sitting position. Place one building block in the infant's hand, then place another block on the table within the infant's reach, and appropriately tease the infant. Observe the infant's response to the second building block **Warning/reminder**: Fail if the first block is not retained in the hand while the infant is looking at the second block	Pass if the infant holds the first block in their hand, and when the second block approaches, their gaze immediately follows, clearly fixating on the second block
Language	50	Produce sounds when seeing familiar people or toys	Observe or inquire about the sounds the infant makes when they see familiar people or toys **Warning/reminder**: R Pass if the infant becomes excited in response to visual sensory stimulation and spontaneously emits vocalizations with tone variations resembling speech	The infant can produce babbling sounds resembling speech, with consonant-vowel combinations such as "ma," "pa," "ba," etc.

(continued)

(continued)

5 months old

Domain	No.	Item	Operation	Passing/scoring criterion
Social behavior	51	React to the figure in the mirror	Place an unframed mirror vertically about 20 cm in front of the infant and observe the infant's response	The infant shows facial expression changes (e.g., smiling, surprise, contemplation) or accompanying body movements (e.g., patting, kissing, hugging, biting) in response to their own figure in the mirror
			Warning/reminder: The assessor and the parent should not appear in the mirror	
	52	Excited to see food	Observe or inquire about the infant's response when seeing food (e.g., milk bottles, cookies, water)	The infant displays an excited expression when seeing a milk bottle or the mother's breast, fixating their gaze on it, and showing signs of happiness and a desire to eat
			Warning/reminder: R Observe the infant's reaction before food touches their lips	

(continued)

(continued)

5 months old

Domain	No.	Item	Operation	Passing/scoring criterion
Communication warning behavior	53	Overly quiet	The infant is excessively quiet and shows limited social interaction behaviors, leading the parents to feel that "the infant requires minimal care or supervision." **Warning/reminder:** R For a normal 5-month-old or older infant in the awake state, the quiet period should not be too long (approximately around 5 minutes). When it is silent, the infant often initiates vocalizations (e.g., "ah," "oh," "uh") or produces long sounds with tone variations to explore or perceive the presence of people around and attract attention. If there is no response after several vocalizations, the infant will start to cry loudly or fuss Points should be scored if the infant, in the awake state, does not initiate interactions or vocalizations for an extended period to perceive the presence of people around	Points are scored if the infant in the awake state remains quiet for an extended period in the room without actively producing sounds or showing behaviors like crying or fussing to seek attention

6 months old

Domain	No.	Item	Operation	Passing/scoring criterion
Gross motor	54	Turn over from supine to prone position	Place the infant in a supine position. Use a toy to encourage the infant to roll over	The infant can independently turn from supine to prone position and free the hand pressed underneath If the infant can only turn over on one side and free the hand, it could be considered a pass
			Warning/reminder: R Proficiency in turning over is emphasized Fail if the infant cannot free the hand pressed underneath, or if the infant is not proficient in turning over and has the awareness but cannot complete the action, with merely occasional successful attempts or half-completed attempts that require multiple tries	
	55	Strike the table	Hold the infant in a sitting position. The assessor demonstrates striking the table. Encourage the infant to do the same	The infant strikes or hits the table to produce sounds, either spontaneously or following the demonstration
			Warning/reminder: Fail if the infant merely touches the table occasionally	
Fine motor	56	Tear and crumple paper	Use a piece of pink soft paper from the testing toolkit and place it in the infant's hand, allowing the infant to grasp the paper. Observe the infant's response	The infant can crumple the paper with both hands two or more times, or tear the paper
			Warning/reminder: It is required to use the uniformly standardized pink soft paper provided in the testing toolkit. The assessor should not give demonstration	

(continued)

(continued)

6 months old

Domain	No.	Item	Operation	Passing/scoring criterion
	57	Rake the fingers to get the building block on the table	Hold the infant in a sitting position and place a building block on the table within the infant's easy reach. Observe the infant's response **Warning/reminder**: It is required to lift the building block off the table	Pass if the infant extends the hand to touch, grip, and pick up the building block
Adaptability	58	Grasp one building block in each hand	Hold the infant in a sitting position and sequentially hand two building blocks to the infant. Observe the infant's response **Warning/reminder**: The blocks can be reached for by the infant or be placed in the infant's hands by the assessor. Pass is considered as long as the blocks are held by the infant for 10 seconds or more	The infant holds one building block in each hand for 10 seconds or more
	59	Look for fallen toys	The assessor holds a red ball at the same horizontal level as the infant's eyes to attract the infant's attention. When the infant notices the red ball, the assessor immediately releases it but keeps the hand in the original position. Observe the infant's response **Warning/reminder**: The infant makes searching movements but may not necessarily find the ball After the infant notices the red ball, the assessor must not make any sound, and their hand should not move downward with the falling ball	The infant immediately lowers the head and searches for the red ball after it falls to the ground

(continued)

(continued)

6 months old

Domain	No.	Item	Operation	Passing/scoring criterion
Language	60	Turn around and look for who called the name	The assessor or the parent calls the infant's name from behind. Observe the infant's response **Warning/reminder**: The caller should stand upright and be at least 50 cm away from the infant's body, avoiding getting too close to the infant's ears to prevent a reaction caused by airflow impact	The infant turns their head to search for the person calling them
	61	Understand the gesture to hug	The assessor extends the hand as if to pick up the infant (without making any sound cues). Observe the infant's response **Warning/reminder**: It is allowed that the assessor holds the infant while the mother or caregiver extends their hand to indicate they want to hold the infant. At least one successful attempt out of two is required Fail if the infant only bends down without extending the hand	The infant understands and extends the hand towards the assessor or the mother (caregiver)
Social behavior	62	Feed oneself food	Observe or inquire whether the infant can bring a cookie or other food to their mouth and chew when they have it in their hand **Warning/reminder**: R Fail if the infant only sucks the food, without showing a biting motion	The infant can put cookies or other food into their mouth and chew

(continued)

(continued)

6 months old

Domain	No.	Item	Operation	Passing/scoring criterion
	63	Play hide and seek	The assessor hides their face behind an A4 paper with a small hole in the center (approximately 0.5 cm in diameter). Then, the assessor calls the infant's name, and slowly reveals their face on one side (left or right) of the paper and makes a sound like "meow" when the infant looks towards the sound. Repeat the above operation on the same side twice. On the third time, the assessor calls the infant's name from behind the paper and observes the infant's actions and facial expressions through the hole **Warning/reminder**: Each time, the infant's name should be called from behind the paper, and then the assessor's face should appear on the same side of the paper (if the first time is on the right, the second time must also be on the right, and vice versa). On the third time, the infant should be observed from behind the paper through the hole. The assessor is not allowed to move the paper or reveal their face from above or below the paper It is considered an incorrect operation for the assessor to keep their head still while moving the paper back and forth	The infant actively participates in the game, actively gazes at the area where the assessor's face is visible, and smiles happily. On the third call, the infant's gaze returns to the direction where the assessor's face was last seen, or their body and head tilt towards the direction where the assessor's head emerged, waiting for the assessor to appear again

(continued)

(continued)

6 months old

Domain	No.	Item	Operation	Passing/scoring criterion
Communication warning behavior	64	Sensitive to advertisement jingles	Inquire whether the infant shows no response or ignores their name being called, but is sensitive to music, advertisement jingles, or specific sounds **Warning/reminder:** R This item requires positive identification of abnormal sensitivity behavior in infants	Points are scored if the infant makes no response or pays no attention when their name is called, but shows a particularly sensitive reaction to certain music or advertisement jingles (e.g., being highly responsive to the sound of an ambulance, even at a very low volume)

7 months old

Domain	No.	Item	Operation	Passing/scoring criterion
Gross motor	65	Prop oneself up on the ground with feet when the armpits are held	Support the infant under the armpits, allowing them to be suspended with their feet approximately 20–30 cm above the bed, and then quickly lower them from the upright position. Observe the posture of the feet when they touch the bed surface	Pass if the infant can place the entire soles of their feet on the bed or immediately transition from tiptoeing to full-foot contact

(continued)

(continued)

7 months old

Domain	No.	Item	Operation	Passing/scoring criterion
	66	Sit upright by oneself	**Warning/reminder:** Fail if the lower limbs cannot bear weight or the infant remains on tiptoes without being able to transition to full-foot contact. If one foot has high muscle tension and exhibits tiptoeing while both feet are in contact with the bed, it would also be considered a failure. Place the infant in a sitting position on the bed	The infant sits upright by themselves without needing support from hands on the bed for at least 1 minute
Fine motor	67	Rake the fingers to get the pellet	**Warning/reminder:** Minor body sway is allowed. Hold the infant in a sitting position. Place a pellet on the table, and encourage the infant to get it	Pass if the infant successfully performs raking or scratching actions with all fingers and uses the entire palm to get the pellet
	68	Grasp another building block with the other hand after grabbing a block with one hand	**Warning/reminder:** This item requires the tabletop to be dark in color (preferably in dark green). Hold the infant in a sitting position and present one building block to the infant. Once the infant grabs it, present another block. Observe the infant's response	The infant voluntarily reaches out to grab the building blocks on the table, using the other hand to successfully grab the second block after grasping the first block and retaining it in one hand

(continued)

(continued)

7 months old

Domain	No.	Item	Operation	Passing/scoring criterion
Adaptability	69	Pass the first building block to the other hand, and then go on to get the second building block	**Warning/reminder:** To pass, the infant should be able to hold the blocks in both hands Hold the infant in a sitting position and present one building block to the infant. Once the infant holds it, present another block towards the hand holding the first block. Observe the infant's response **Warning/reminder:** The first building block should be passed directly to the other hand. If there are actions such as placing the first block on the table or putting it in the mouth during the process, it is considered a failure	After passing the first block to the other hand, the infant goes on to pick up the second block. Actively initiating a change of hands is also considered a pass
	70	Reach for toys in the distance	Hold the infant in a sitting position and place a toy on the table that is out of the infant's reach. Observe the infant's response	The infant stoops down and gets the toy successfully
Language	71	Produce bilabial sounds such as "da-da" and "ma-ma" without specific reference	Observe or inquire about the infant's vocalizations when they are awake **Warning/reminder:** R Pass if the infant can produce sounds such as "da-da" and "ma-ma" that resemble calling for someone (though without specific reference to the father or the mother)	The infant produces bilabial sounds such as "da-da" and "ma-ma," though without specific reference

(continued)

(continued)

7 months old

Domain	No.	Item	Operation	Passing/scoring criterion
Social behavior	72	Hold feet to play or suck	Place the infant in a supine position. Observe the infant's performance when they hold their feet spontaneously or with the assessor's assistance **Warning/reminder**: Assistance is allowed once	The infant can hold their feet to play or exhibit behaviors such as sucking or nibbling their toes
	73	Show resisted reaction to strangers	Observe or inquire about the infant's response to strangers **Warning/reminder**: R Pass if the infant shows a sense of unfamiliarity when seeing strangers	Pass if the infant shows behaviors such as resisting being held, crying, being unhappy, or being surprised, when seeing strangers

(continued)

(continued)

7 months old

Domain	No.	Item	Operation	Passing/scoring criterion
Communication warning behavior	74	Do not engage in "conversations" with others	Inquire if the infant exhibits the following behavior: When the room is quiet and there are no sounds, the infant makes sounds like "goo goo" or "yah yah," similar to trying to communicate or engage with someone, to check if someone is present. If there is a response, the infant continues to play or "converse" with the person; by comparison, if there is no response, the infant becomes uneasy and may cry or fuss to seek attention. The infant stops crying when hearing someone making a sound or comforting them **Warning/reminder**: R	Points are scored if the infant does not engage in "conversations" with others

9 INSTRUCTION MANUAL FOR THE ERXIN SCALES 213

8 months old

Domain	No.	Item	Operation	Passing/scoring criterion
Gross motor	75	Hold onto objects with both hands to stand up	Place the infant on the bed. Assist the infant in grasping the railing with both hands to assume a standing posture, without their chest leaning against the railing. Observe **Warning/reminder**: The chest should not be leaned against the railing, and the body should maintain a balance and would not fall even if there is a slight sway	The infant supports the entire body weight by holding onto the railing and maintains a standing posture for 5 seconds or more
	76	Sit by oneself and rotate freely to reach for objects	Entice the infant siting on the bed with a toy, and observe whether the infant can freely rotate the upper body to reach for the toy Or, gently push the infant's shoulder to one side to observe their side balance, and look for infant's efforts to return to an upright position and resistance to falling **Warning/reminder**: The ability to maintain front and side balance is expected at this age, but not necessarily posterior balance When performing operations involving front, side, and especially posterior balance, special care should be taken to protect the infant	The infant sitting by themselves does not require hand support, allowing free upper body movement to reach for objects. Or, the infant can maintain balance without falling when pushed from one side or demonstrates efforts to regain balance

(continued)

(continued)

8 months old

Domain	No.	Item	Operation	Passing/scoring criterion
Fine motor	77	Pinch a pellet with thumb and other fingers	Hold the infant in a sitting position. Place a pellet on the table, and encourage the infant to pick it up	The infant can pinch the pellet using the thumb and other fingers
	78	Try to take the third building block after grabbing two building blocks	Continuously present two building blocks for the infant to successfully grab them, and then present a third block to encourage the infant to take it **Warning/reminder**: Pass is considered only when the infant attempts to pick up the third block (although it may not be successful) and the previously held blocks do not fall	The infant shows an intention to pick up the third block, (but may not necessarily succeed), with the first two blocks still in hand
Adaptability	79	Consciously imitate shaking the bell	The assessor demonstrates shaking the bell (using the bell stick provided in the testing toolkit) and encourage the infant to do the same **Warning/reminder**: The assessor should not say the word "shake" during the demonstration If the infant does a smashing motion instead of shaking the bell, it is considered a failure If no demonstration is given, the infant voluntarily shaking the bell is considered a pass This item does not require the infant to gaze at the bell stick while shaking it	The infant can consciously shake the bell

(continued)

(continued)

8 months old

Domain	No.	Item	Operation	Passing/scoring criterion
	80	Try to grasp constantly moved toys with hands	Use a toy to entice the infant to reach for it. When the infant is about to reach it, move the toy slightly further away and observe the infant's response **Warning/reminder**: The infant's movements should be coherent and include a stooping motion with reaching hands	The infant consistently pursues the toy, making efforts to reach it, but may not necessarily obtain it
Language	81	Imitate the sounds of coughing or tongue movements	Produce the sounds of coughing or tongue movements in front of the infant and observe their response. Or, inquire whether the infant can imitate the sounds of coughing or tongue movements **Warning/reminder**: R Observe whether the infant can imitate the sounds of coughing or tongue movements Inquire whether the infant can imitate the sounds of coughing or tongue movements, or produce onomatopoeic words (such as imitating sounds made by living beings like dogs ("woof woof") or cats ("meow meow"), or imitating sounds made by inanimate objects like a hammer hitting the ground ("clang clang") or an electric drill ("squeak squeak")	The infant can imitate the sounds of coughing or tongue movements, or produce onomatopoeic words such as imitating animal noises (e.g., "woof woof," "meow meow," "plop plop") or snoring. One successful imitation is sufficient

(continued)

(continued)

8 months old

Domain	No.	Item	Operation	Passing/scoring criterion
	82	Express needs with gestures	The assessor inquires of the parent about the following questions: (1) Whether the infant frequently reaches out the hands to express the desire to be held; (2) Whether the infant spreads out the hands to indicate "no"; (3) Whether the infant smacks the lips or uses gestures to express that something tastes good **Warning/reminder:** R Apart from the examples mentioned above, other actions, such as when the parent asks, "Are you full?" and the infant pats their belly to indicate being full, can also be considered for a pass	Pass if the infant demonstrates two or more of these behaviors
Social behavior	83	Understand adult facial expressions	The assessor or the parent scolds or praises the infant. Observe the infant's response	Pass if the infant demonstrates signs of distress or excitement
Communication warning behavior	84	Lack active cooperation when picked up	Inquire about the infant's feeling and behavior when they are picked up by someone	Points are scored if the infant, when picked up by someone, does not cling to the person or arch their back, or feels limp and heavy, making it difficult to hold them

(continued)

(continued)

8 months old

Domain	No.	Item	Operation	Passing/scoring criterion
			Warning/reminder: R When picking up an infant, one should feel the infant actively cooperating and clinging. Otherwise, points should be scored	

9 months old

Domain	No.	Item	Operation	Passing/scoring criterion
Gross motor	85	Walk forward with both hands held by someone	The assessor holds the hands of the infant who is in a standing position, applying proper force, and encourages the infant to walk forward	The infant makes the effort to move their legs in a coordinated manner, taking three or more steps forward. Minor body sway is allowed
	86	Crawl on hands and knees	Place the infant in a prone position. Use a toy to entice the infant to crawl	The infant can lift their chest and abdomen off the bed, supporting themselves on all fours and crawling forward
			Warning/reminder: The infant should crawl on hands and knees The infant should support themselves on all fours, lifting the chest and abdomen off the bed, and crawling proficiently No specific requirement for the crawling posture Fail if the infant moves forward by crawling on their stomach or moves their legs while retreating (with the abdomen barely leaving the bed)	

(continued)

(continued)

9 months old

Domain	No.	Item	Operation	Passing/scoring criterion
Fine motor	87	Pinch a pellet with thumb and index finger	Hold the infant in a sitting position. Place a pellet on the table, and encourage the infant to pick it up	The infant can pick up the pellet using the thumb and index finger
	88	Take out the building blocks from the cup	The assessor, with the infant's gaze, puts one or two building blocks into a cup and encourages the infant to take them out (such as by saying, "Can you give the blocks to Auntie or Mommy?") **Warning/reminder:** Pouring out does not count During the operation, the use of pronouns such as "me" or "him/her" or saying "take" or "get" is not allowed The number of blocks in the cup should not exceed two	The infant can take out the building blocks on their own
Adaptability	89	Beat two building blocks against each other	The assessor presents two building blocks and demonstrates beating them against each other. Then, let the infant hold one block in each hand, and encourage the infant to do the same (such as by saying, "Baby, give it a try")	The infant can bring their hands together at the midline and intentionally beat the blocks against each other. Accuracy is not required during beating

(continued)

(continued)

9 months old

Domain	No.	Item	Operation	Passing/scoring criterion
	90	Fiddle with or pinch the tongue of the bell	**Warning/reminder**: Fail if there is merely occasional contact between the blocks. The assessor should not use the word "beat." The assessor gently shakes a brass bell to attract the infant's attention, and then hand the bell to the infant to observe their response **Warning/reminder**: When the assessor hands the bell to the infant, the tongue of the bell should be presented facing down; the assessor can shake the bell while handing it to the infant, and observes if the infant searches for and fiddles with or pinches the tongue of the bell with their fingers	Pass if the infant consciously looks for and fiddles with or pinches the tongue of the bell
Language	91	Make welcoming gestures	The assessor only says "Welcome" without demonstrating any gestures. Encourage the infant to express welcome using gestures **Warning/reminder**: R The assessor does not demonstrate any gestures Pass if the infant claps their hands upon hearing "Welcome." Fail if the infant hears the assessor say "Welcome" but does not make any movements, and instead claps their hands only when they see the parent saying "Welcome" and clapping their hands	The infant can make welcoming gestures

(continued)

(continued)

9 months old

Domain	No.	Item	Operation	Passing/scoring criterion
	92	Make goodbye gestures	The assessor only says "Goodbye" without demonstrating any gestures. Encourage the infant to express goodbye using gestures **Warning/reminder**: R The assessor says "goodbye" without demonstrating the waving gesture Pass if the infant waves upon hearing "Goodbye." Fail if the infant hears the assessor say "Goodbye" but does not wave, and instead waves only when they see the parent saying "Goodbye" and waving their hand	The infant can make goodbye gestures
Social behavior	93	Shake head or push away something uninterested	Observe or inquire about the infant's response to objects uninterested **Warning/reminder**: R When infants are uninterested in or do not want a given object, they usually shake their head, push the object away, or turn their body to avoid the object If the infant does not express a lack of interest in the given object but instead takes it and throws it away or tosses it, it would be considered a failure as the infant has not clearly expressed a rejection	Pass if the infant clearly shakes their head or pushes away unwanted objects

(continued)

9 INSTRUCTION MANUAL FOR THE ERXIN SCALES

(continued)

9 months old

Domain	No.	Item	Operation	Passing/scoring criterion
Communication warning behavior	94	Exhibit no stranger anxiety towards unfamiliar individuals, nor show attachment to family	From 7 to 12 months old, infants experience a peak period of stranger anxiety. They may show surprise, alertness, or even fear when encountering unfamiliar people. While a minority of infants may not exhibit stranger anxiety, they usually show a clear attachment to their family **Warning/reminder**: R Points are scored when the infant shows no reaction towards either family members or strangers In cases where the infant does not exhibit stranger anxiety towards anyone, the assessor observes the infant's reaction when seeing family members. If the infant displays a gaze of attachment to their family/caregiver, it indicates a sense of closeness. If this behavior is not observed, points should be scored	Points are scored if the infant displays no surprise or alertness towards strangers, nor exhibits attachment to their family

10 months old

Domain	No.	Item	Operation	Passing/scoring criterion
Gross motor	95	Make protective action	The assessor stands at the edge of the bed or table and supports the infant from behind. Lift the infant with both hands extended from the infant's back under the armpits to the front of their chest (supporting the infant's torso, with the head lower than the level of the hips, or making the infant's body form an angle of about 30° with the horizontal, with the head lowered). Then, quickly perform a plunging motion and observe the infant's response **Warning/reminder**: During the operation, the plunging motion should be fast, as slow speed cannot elicit the infant's protective action of extending the forearms and opening the hands	Infant extends both arms forward with open hands, displaying a protective gesture
	96	Sit up by oneself	Place the infant in a prone position. Entice the infant with a toy, and observe if the infant can sit up	The infant can sit up in a relatively coordinated manner from a prone position without assistance and maintain a stable sitting posture

(continued)

(continued)

10 months old

Domain	No.	Item	Operation	Passing/scoring criterion
			Warning/reminder: Either "lying prone → lying on one's side → sitting up" or "lying prone → kneeling → sitting up" is acceptable	
Fine motor	97	Coordinate the fingertips of the thumb and index finger skillfully	Hold the infant in a sitting position. Place a pellet on the table, and encourage the infant to pick it up	The infant can pinch the pellet via coordinating the fingertips of the thumb and index finger skillfully and quickly
Adaptability	98	Initiatively remove the cup and play with the building blocks hidden inside	Place building blocks on the table, and with the infant's gaze, cover the blocks with a cup (with the cup handle facing the infant). Encourage the infant to take the blocks (the assessor can ask, "Where are the blocks?") **Warning/reminder:** Fail if the infant only removes the cup without taking away the building blocks	The infant can initiatively remove the cup and take away the building blocks hidden inside it
	99	Look for something hidden in the box	Shake a box containing a coin in front of the infant. Then, avoiding the infant's gaze, take out the coin and give the infant an empty box. Observe the infant's response	The infant can actively search for the coin inside the box

(continued)

(continued)

10 months old					
Domain	No.	Item	Operation		Passing/scoring criterion
Language	100	Imitate "mama," "papa," "nana" or other sounds resembling language	**Warning/reminder:** The assessor should refrain from speaking, such as saying "shake" or "open." Make sounds or vocalizations resembling language, such as "mama," "papa," "nana" and "da," in front of the infant. Observe if the infant can imitate these sounds **Warning/reminder:** R Observe or inquire if the infant can imitate sounds resembling language Pass if the infant can imitate sounds like "papa," "mama," and "nana," but this does not guarantee a pass for Item #81 ("Imitate the sounds of coughing or tongue movements")		Pass if the infant can imitate any of these sounds
Social behavior	101	Know the names of common objects and the address terms of people	The assessor asks the infant, "Where is Mommy?" "Where is the lamp?" "Where is Auntie?" or other questions about the address terms of people or object names. Observe the infant's response		The infant can use eye gaze to indicate or point out two or more people or objects

(continued)

(continued)

10 months old

Domain	No.	Item	Operation	Passing/scoring criterion
	102	Get something as instructed	Place a doll, a ball, and a cup side by side on a table within the infant's reach. Encourage the infant to pick one of them according to the instructions **Warning/reminder**: Each object should be asked twice. Questions should be asked alternately instead of continuously	The infant can comprehend the instructions and successfully get one or more specific objects
Communication warning behavior	103	Often shout loudly or make strange sounds	Inquire if the infant frequently shouts or makes strange noises without any apparent reason **Warning/reminder**: R Points are scored for frequent and unexplained loud shouting, but not for occasional or infrequent loud shouting with valid reasons	Points are scored if the infant often shouts loudly or makes strange sounds

11 months old

Domain	No.	Item	Operation	Passing/scoring criterion
Gross motor	104	Stand by oneself for a while	Place the infant in an upright position. The assessor releases the hands once the infant stands steadily. Observe the infant's standing ability	The infant can stand alone for 2 seconds or more

(continued)

(continued)

11 months old

Domain	No.	Item	Operation	Passing/scoring criterion
	105	Hold onto the railing to squat down and pick something up	**Warning/reminder**: Minor body sway is allowed Let the infant stand while holding onto the railing without leaning. Place a toy near the infant's feet and encourage the infant to squat down and get it **Warning/reminder**: Minor body sway is acceptable as long as the infant does not fall Fail if the infant can squat to get the object but fails to stand up	The infant can squat down with one hand holding onto the railing, pick up the toy with the other hand, and then stand up
Fine motor	106	Put building blocks into a cup	The assessor demonstrates putting building blocks into a cup. Encourage the infant to do the same **Warning/reminder**: The assessor should not say "put them in."	The infant can consciously put the building blocks into the cup and release them from their hand
Adaptability	107	Open the towel and look for the building block wrapped inside	With the infant's gaze, wrap a building block in a towel, then unwrap it and wrap it again. Encourage the infant to find the block	The infant consciously opens the towel and looks for the building block wrapped inside it, and successfully picks the block up

(continued)

(continued)

11 months old					
Domain	No.	Item		Operation	Passing/scoring criterion
				Warning/reminder: This item emphasizes the entire process of the infant opening the towel to search for the building block. If the infant shakes the scarf directly to uncover the block, the item should be retested. If the infant only opens one or two corners of the scarf and pulls or shakes the other corners, but successfully picks up the building block after making searching motions, it is considered a pass	
	108	Imitate patting the doll		The assessor demonstrates patting a doll and encourages the infant to do the same, such as by saying, "Let's put the little sister to sleep."	The infant imitates the adult's action by lightly patting the doll
				Warning/reminder: The assessor should not say "pat."	
Language	109	Pronounce single-syllable sounds consciously		Observe or inquire about the infant's conscious vocalization	The infant consciously and correctly produces single-syllable sounds such as "ba," "ma," "na," etc., regardless of pronunciation accuracy
				Warning/reminder: R Pass if the infant frequently produces sounds such as "ba," "ma," "na," "zou," "yi," "nai," "woof," etc.	

(continued)

(continued)

11 months old				
Domain	No.	Item	Operation	Passing/scoring criterion
	110	Know the meaning of "no" / "don't"	When the infant is trying to pick up a toy and play with it, the assessor says, "Don't move it" or "Don't take it." Observe or inquire about the infant's response **Warning/reminder**: R The assessor should not make any gestures	The infant stops the action of picking up the toy
Social behavior	111	Drink water from a cup	Observe or inquire if the infant can drink water from a cup held by an adult **Warning/reminder**: R	The infant can drink water from a cup, with a small amount of spillage allowed
	112	Take off a hat	The assessor puts a hat on the infant's head and observes if the infant can take off the hat **Warning/reminder**: The action of taking off the hat should not be a forceful grabbing motion	The infant can take off the hat using one or both hands
Communication warning behavior	113	Avoid eye contact	Observe the infant's eye contact with others, including their ability to engage in eye communication	Points are scored if the infant makes no eye contact, avoids eye contact, or their gaze tends to drift and be unstable when looking at others

(continued)

(continued)

11 months old

Domain	No.	Item	Operation	Passing/scoring criterion
			Warning/reminder: R For example, points should be scored if the infant quickly looks away or exhibits a blank expression with drifting and unstable gaze when making eye contact with someone, or if the infant often stares directly at others as if they are fixated on them, but does not engage in eye contact or show an intention to communicate This domain is assessed primarily via observation, so inquiries with the parent is not necessary as long as the behavior is directly observable during assessment	

12 months old

Domain	No.	Item	Operation	Passing/scoring criterion
Gross motor	114	Stand steadily by oneself	Place the child in an upright position. The assessor releases the hands once the infant stands steadily. Observe the infant's standing ability **Warning/reminder:** Minor body sway is allowed	The child can stand alone for 10 seconds or more

(continued)

(continued)

12 months old

Domain	No.	Item	Operation	Passing/scoring criterion
	115	Walk forward with one hand held by someone	The assessor holds one of the child's hands and walks with them without exerting force. Observe the child's walking ability. **Warning/reminder**: Fail if the child leans forward or relies on the support of an adult's arm to walk	The child can independently take steps and, when holding someone's hand, can coordinate the movement of both legs, taking at least three or more steps forward
Fine motor	116	Hold a pen in whole palm to draw lines	The assessor demonstrates drawing lines on paper with a pen and encourages the child to imitate. **Warning/reminder**: Demonstrate in the same direction. There must be visible lines drawn on the paper; drawing random dots with the pen tip does not count	The child can hold the pen and draw lines on the paper
	117	Try to put the pellet into the vial	Present a pellet and a transparent vial. The assessor takes the vial, demonstrates and instructs in putting the pellet into the vial (such as by saying, "Come, look at Auntie"). Encourage the child to do the same	The child pinches the pellet and attempts to put it into the vial, but success is not necessary

(continued)

(continued)

12 months old

Domain	No.	Item	Operation	Passing/scoring criterion
Adaptability	118	Cap the bottle	**Warning/reminder:** The assessor should not say "put it in." Fail if the child of this age does not use the thumb and index finger to pinch the pellet and make an attempt to put it into the vial Place a bottle cap upside down on the table. The assessor demonstrates covering the bottle with the cap and encourages the child to do the same	The child can flip the bottle cap and put it back on the bottle, though not necessarily in a stable manner, and it may fall off. Pass as long as the child flips the bottle cap and puts it back on the bottle
Language	119	Consciously call people	**Warning/reminder:** The assessor can say, "Let's see how Auntie does it, give it a try," but should not say "cap" or "cover." Observe or inquire if the child actively and consciously and accurately calls out when they see their mother, father, or other people **Warning/reminder:** R If the child can clearly use other terms of address such as "grandpa," "grandma," "aunt," etc., it could also be considered a pass	The child can actively and correctly address their father, mother, or other people. Fail if the child calls everyone "mom."

(continued)

(continued)

12 months old

Domain	No.	Item	Operation	Passing/scoring criterion
	120	Handing something over when asked	Give the child a toy and then the assessor or the parent says, "Give this to Auntie or Mommy," without reaching out their hand. Observe the child's response **Warning/reminder**: During the operation, the assessor should only speak without making reaching gestures, and should not say "give it to me."	The child can hand the toy to the assessor or the parent and voluntarily release it to them
Social behavior	121	Actively cooperate to wear clothes	Observe or inquire about the child's cooperation when getting dressed by an adult **Warning/reminder**: R	The child cooperates and exhibits actions such as extending their hand or leg when getting dressed, but not necessarily puts on the clothing successfully
	122	Engage in joint attention	Observe or inquire if the child can pay attention to a certain scene or event pointed out by the parents and observe it together with them? **Warning/reminder**: R Pass if, for example, you point with your finger and say, "Look, there's a little dog," and the child follows the direction you are pointing in	The child engages in joint attention

(continued)

9 INSTRUCTION MANUAL FOR THE ERXIN SCALES 233

(continued)

12 months old

Domain	No.	Item	Operation	Passing/scoring criterion
Communication warning behavior	123	Fail to look in the direction pointed by others	Talk about topics that can engage the child in joint attention, such as pointing to a lamp and saying, "Where is the lamp?" or pointing in a certain direction and saying, "Look, there's a cat." Observe the child's response **Warning/reminder**: R Observe the child's joint attention behavior, and when speaking, use finger pointing gestures with exaggerated tone and facial expressions	Points are scored if the child does not look in the direction pointed by others

15 months old

Domain	No.	Item	Operation	Passing/scoring criterion
Gross motor	124	Walk freely by oneself	Observe the child's walking ability **Warning/reminder**: The child is allowed to extend both arms for balance Fail if the child is unable to control the pace and still runs forward even after adjusting their rhythm	The child walks freely without swaying, controls the pace, and avoids inertia-driven forward movements

(continued)

(continued)

15 months old

Domain	No.	Item	Operation	Passing/scoring criterion
Fine motor	125	Spontaneously draw	The assessor presents paper and a pen, encouraging the child to draw **Warning/reminder**: The drawn lines should have curves Demonstration is not allowed for this item	The child can freely draw random lines on the paper with a pen
	126	Take or pour the pellets out of the vial	Present a transparent vial with pellets inside and hand it to the child, saying, "What should Auntie do if she wants the little beans (pellets)?" or "Give the little beans (pellets) to Mommy." Encourage the child to take out the pellets **Warning/reminder**: When encouraging the child to take out the pellets, the phrase "pour out" should not be used	The child can take out or pour out the pellets
Adaptability	127	Turn the pages of a book twice	The assessor demonstrates turning the pages of a book and encourages the child to do the same **Warning/reminder**: When demonstrating, turn one page at a time	Pass if the child turns the pages of the book twice or more

(continued)

(continued)

15 months old

Domain	No.	Item	Operation	Passing/scoring criterion
	128	Cover the round box	The assessor takes out a round box, demonstrates covering the box, and encourages the child to do the same (while demonstrating, the assessor can say, "Baby, look at Auntie.") **Warning/reminder:** The assessor should not say "cover it." The demonstration should include the action of flipping the lid of the box	The child can cover the round box and close it tightly
Language	129	Point out the eyes, ears, mouth, nose, and hands	The assessor asks the child, "Where are your eyes?" "Where are your ears?" "Where is your nose?" etc. Observes the child's response **Warning/reminder:** Before operating the item, the parent should be reminded not to speak or physically assist the child. If the child points to a body part of the parent, such as the ear, with their hand, the parent should not move their head towards the child. If this happens, ask about other body parts	The child can correctly identify three or more body parts
	130	Speak 3–5 words	Observe or inquire about the child's conscious speech	The child consciously says 3–5 words other than "mom" and "dad."

(continued)

(continued)

15 months old

Domain	No.	Item	Operation	Passing/scoring criterion
			Warning/reminder: R The words spoken should be recorded. For example: 1 grandpa, 2 grandma, 3 eat, 4 water, 5 want, 6 walk, 7 don't have, 8 don't want, 9 big, 10 take, 11 bye, 12 aunt, 13 outside, 14 thank you, 15 brother, 16 no	
Social behavior	131	Take off socks correctly	Observe or inquire about the child's method of taking off socks	The child can consciously and correctly remove socks without pulling or tugging them from the toes
			Warning/reminder: R	
Communication warning behavior	132	Do not point to objects with hand	Inquire about the child's reaction or behavior when seeing something they like or want	Points are scored if the child does not use pointing to indicate liking or wanting something, but instead pulls others to the object
			Warning/reminder: R The observation/inquiry should focus on whether the child uses their own hand to point to objects. Points should be scored if the child consistently relies on adults and uses the adult's hand, instead of their own, to point	

9 INSTRUCTION MANUAL FOR THE ERXIN SCALES

18 months old

Domain	No.	Item	Operation	Passing/scoring criterion
Gross motor	133	Throw a ball with no specific direction	The assessor demonstrates throwing a ball over the shoulder and encourages the child to do the same **Warning/reminder:** Demonstrate throwing the ball over the shoulder (avoid reminding the child during their operation)	The child raises their hand above their shoulder and throws the ball with or without specific direction, but the distance should be greater than their arm length
Fine motor	134	Imitate drawing lines	The assessor demonstrates drawing random lines with a crayon and encourages the child to imitate **Warning/reminder:** Demonstrate in the same direction There are no requirements for the pose when holding the crayon	The child can draw lines freely with a smooth start and stop, with no specific direction
Adaptability	135	Stack four building blocks	Demonstrate stacking two building blocks and knock them down. Then, present the blocks one by one and encourage the child to stack them up **Warning/reminder:** At least one successful attempt out of three is required	The child stacks four or more building blocks

(continued)

(continued)

18 months old

Domain	No.	Item	Operation	Passing/scoring criterion
	136	Put the round building block into the template correctly	Place a round building block under the hole of the template, with the hole close to the child's body. The assessor says to the child, "This is the home for a little friend (pointing to the template surface, not the hole). Please help this little friend (pointing to the round block) find its own home." Do not demonstrate	The child can correctly place the round block into the hole in one attempt
Language	137	Correctly deliver three building blocks as requested	Ask the child to pass two building blocks to Mommy and Auntie, and place another one on the table, respectively **Warning/reminder:** The assessor should not reach out their hand	The child can correctly deliver the building blocks as requested
	138	Consciously say 10 words or phrases	Observe or inquire about the child's conscious speech and record	The child consciously says 10 or more words or phrases other than "mom" and "dad."

(continued)

9 INSTRUCTION MANUAL FOR THE ERXIN SCALES

(continued)

18 months old

Domain	No.	Item	Operation	Passing/scoring criterion
			Warning/reminder: R The words or phrases spoken should be recorded. Commonly spoken words include: 1 grandpa, 2 grandma, 3 eat, 4 water, 5 want, 6 walk, 7 don't have, 8 no, 9 big, 10 take, 11 bye, 12 aunt, 13 outside, 14 thank you, 15 brother, 16 don't want, 17 push, 18 this, 19 that, 20 kitchen, 21 stinky, 22 pee, etc.	
Social behavior	139	Have control of urination during the daytime	Observe or inquire about the child's urine control, or if they wet their pants during the day	Pass if the child indicates the need to urinate voluntarily or when prompted, with minimal daytime accidents
			Warning/reminder: R	
	140	Eat with a spoon	Observe or inquire if the child can use a spoon by themselves	The child can eat with a spoon on their own, with minimal spills allowed
			Warning/reminder: R	
Communication warning behavior	141	Do not request to be held	Inquire if the child requests to be held	Points are scored if the child does not exhibit behaviors such as reaching out, tiptoeing, or leaning forward to express an expectation or request to be held
			Warning/reminder: R	

21 months old

Domain	No.	Item	Operation	Passing/scoring criterion
Gross motor	142	Walk on tiptoes	The assessor demonstrates walking on tiptoes and encourages the child to do the same **Warning/reminder:** R Fail if the heels touch the ground during walking	The child can take three or more consecutive steps by walking on tiptoes, with the heels not touching the ground
	143	Hold onto the handrail and walk up the stairs	Place a toy on the stairs. Encourage the child to go upstairs and get it	The child can hold onto the handrail and proficiently climb three or more steps
Fine motor	144	Thread the crystal thread through the buttonhole	The assessor demonstrates threading a crystal thread through a buttonhole. Encourage the child to do the same	The child can thread the crystal thread through the buttonhole for at least 0.5 cm, without needing to pull the thread
	145	Imitate pulling the zipper	Demonstrate pulling the zipper up and down once each **Warning/reminder:** The assessor should secure the ends of the zipper while encouraging the child to pull it	The child moves the zipper slider back and forth via coordinating both hands. Pass if the child pulls half of the zipper

(continued)

(continued)

21 months old

Domain	No.	Item	Operation	Passing/scoring criterion
Adaptability	146	Stack 7–8 building blocks	Demonstrate stacking two building blocks and knock them down. Then, present the blocks one by one, and encourage the child to stack them up **Warning/reminder**: At least one successful attempt out of three is required	The child can stack 7–8 building blocks
	147	Identify the color red	Present the four-color picture (red, yellow, blue, and green). Ask the child, "Which one is red?" **Warning/reminder**: At least one successful attempt out of three is required	The child can correctly identify the color red in the picture
Language	148	Answer simple questions	The assessor asks, "What is this (a ball)?" "Who is that (the person with the child)?" "What is Daddy doing (going to work)?"	The child can answer all the questions correctly
	149	Say sentences consisting of 3–5 words	Observe or inquire about the child's conscious speech **Warning/reminder**: R	The child can consciously speak sentences consisting of 3–5 words with a subject-predicate or subject-object structure

(continued)

(continued)

21 months old

Domain	No.	Item	Operation	Passing/scoring criterion
Social behavior	150	Freely express personal needs	Observe or inquire if the child can clearly express their needs **Warning/reminder**: R Pass if, for example, the child wants to eat meat during a meal and they point and say "meat." Fail if the child only uses gestures (a verbal expression of personal needs is required)	The child can express three or more needs, such as "eating, drinking, playing with cars, going out." Incomplete language expression and accompanying gestures are allowed
	151	Play imaginative plays-	Observe or inquire if the child plays imaginative plays, such as pretending to feed dolls or stuffed animals, tucking them in, giving them injections, etc. **Warning/reminder**: R	Pass if the child plays imaginative plays
Communication warning behavior	152	Lack imagination	Inquire if the child engages in pretend play activities such as playing doctor, pretending to fly an airplane while sitting on a chair, using a cardboard tube as a microphone, etc. **Warning/reminder**: R	Points are scored if there is no this kind of behaviors

24 months old

Domain	No.	Item	Operation	Passing/scoring criterion
Gross motor	153	Jump off the ground with both feet	The assessor demonstrates jumping off the ground with both feet simultaneously. Encourage the child to do the same. **Warning/reminder:** The child can jump with the feet either together or apart	The child can jump off the ground with both feet simultaneously and also land with both feet, repeating this action two or more times
Fine motor	154	Thread the crystal thread through the buttonhole and pull the thread out	The assessor demonstrates threading a crystal thread through a buttonhole and pulling it out. Encourage the child to do the same	The child can thread the crystal thread through the buttonhole and pull the thread out
Adaptability	155	Turn the book page by page	The assessor demonstrates turning the pages of a book one by one. Encourage the child to do the same	The child can turn the pages of a book by pinching one at a time, and continuously turn three or more pages

(continued)

(continued)

24 months old

Domain	No.	Item	Operation	Passing/scoring criterion
	156	Put the round building block into the inverted template correctly	On the basis of the child being able to put the round building block into the template correctly, flip the template 180°, with the round block remaining in its original position. The assessor says to the child, "This is the home for a little friend (pointing to the template). Please help this little friend (pointing to the round block) find its own home." Do not demonstrate	After the template is inverted, the child can correctly place the round block into the hole in one attempt
Language	157	Say two or more sentences of poems or nursery rhymes	Encourage the child to recite Tang poetry, Song lyrics, nursery rhymes, etc. **Warning/reminder**: Prompted parts do not count. To pass, the child must independently produce two or more sentences	The child can spontaneously or with slight prompting, complete two or more sentences of Tang poetry or nursery rhymes after an opening is given
	158	Speak out the use of common objects	The assessor asks the child about the uses of a bowl, pen, stool, and ball **Warning/reminder**: The four objects (bowl, pen, stool, and ball) could not be substituted by others	The child can state the use of three or more objects

(continued)

(continued)

24 months old

Domain	No.	Item	Operation	Passing/scoring criterion
Social behavior	159	Say hello or goodbye to someone	Encourage the child to greet someone, with or without demonstration	The child can spontaneously or imitatively say phrases like "hello" and "goodbye."
	160	Ask "What is this?"	Observe or inquire if the child spontaneously asks, "What is this?" when they see something **Warning/reminder**: R	The child spontaneously asks "What is this?"
Communication warning behavior	161	Exhibit no sharing or showing off behaviors	Inquire if the child exhibits sharing or showing off behaviors. For example, if they extend their hand to show you candy or a toy but retract their hand when you try to take it **Warning/reminder**: R Most children at this age are unwilling to share their favorite toys or objects with others. When persuaded by their mother or other family members, although the child may appear reluctant, they can show or let others play with the toys, which should be considered normal sharing behavior	Points are scored if there is no sharing or showing off, or no behaviors indicating preference for specific objects

(continued)

(continued)

24 months old

Domain	No.	Item	Operation	Passing/scoring criterion
	162	Enjoy circling or rotating own body	Inquire about the characteristics of the child's activities In typically developing children, spinning in circles is done with an intention to perform to interact with others, entertain or seek attention, and require encouragement and approval from others **Warning/reminder:** R Points are scored if, for example, the child rotates their body when picking up any object or circles themselves when self-excited	Points are scored if the child engages in repetitive activities such as running back and forth or going up and down stairs, frequently spins or twists their body, or enjoys circling (here, circling is a self-stimulatory behavior not requiring attention or interaction from others)

27 months old

Domain	No.	Item	Operation	Passing/scoring criterion
Gross motor	163	Go upstairs by oneself	Encourage the child to go upstairs without holding onto the handrail	The child ascends the stairs without holding onto the handrail, steadily climbing three or more steps. Placing both feet on the same step is allowed

(continued)

(continued)

27 months old

Domain	No.	Item	Operation	Passing/scoring criterion
	164	Go downstairs by oneself	**Warning/reminder**: Demonstration is allowed, but when demonstrating ascending the stairs, the assessor must alternate feet, one on each step. See Appendix B, 2. Staircase for Testing for the staircase specifications. Encourage the child to go downstairs without holding onto the handrail	The child descends the stairs without holding onto the handrail, steadily going down three or more steps. Placing both feet on the same step is allowed
Fine motor	165	Imitate drawing vertical lines	**Warning/reminder**: Demonstration is allowed, but when demonstrating descending the stairs, the assessor must alternate feet, one on each step. See Appendix B, 2. Staircase for Testing for the staircase specifications. The assessor demonstrates drawing a vertical line, ensuring that the testing paper is placed upright. Encourage the child to imitate. **Warning/reminder**: Demonstrate in the same direction	The child can draw a vertical line with a length of ≥ 2.5 cm, and the angle between the drawn line and the vertical line should be $<30°$

(continued)

(continued)

27 months old

Domain	No.	Item	Operation	Passing/scoring criterion
	166	Insert the zipper slider into the bottom stop	Present an opened zipper, and demonstrate insert the slider into the bottom stop. Encourage the child to do the same **Warning/reminder**: Demonstrate in the same direction It is not required for the zipper slider to be fully inserted into the bottom stop during assessment	Pass if the child can insert the zipper slider into the bottom stop
Adaptability	167	Know the difference between big and small	The assessor shows the child a big circle and a small circle, and asks the child to give the big one to Mommy or Auntie **Warning/reminder**: At least two successful attempts out of three is required The assessor should use the circles contained in the testing toolkit, preferably placing them on the table. If lifting them is necessary, both hands should be on the same horizontal plane (consistency in both height and position) and maintain stable to avoid any potential discrepancies that could mislead the child or disrupt the assessment	The child can correctly give the big circle to Mommy or Auntie

(continued)

(continued)

27 months old

Domain	No.	Item	Operation	Passing/scoring criterion
	168	Correctly put the building blocks of different shapes into the corresponding holes	Place circular, square, and triangular building blocks next to their corresponding holes on the template. The assessor says to the child, "These are the homes for the little friends (pointing to the template). Please help these little friends (pointing to the three blocks) find their own homes." **Warning/reminder**: Demonstration is not allowed. The triangular block should be placed in the same orientation as the template	The child can place the blocks into the corresponding holes in one attempt. Prompts could only be provided for the isosceles triangle, such as by suggesting a change in direction
Language	169	Say a sentence consisting of 7–10 words	The assessor says the sentence "On Sunday, Mommy took me to the park." One repetition is allowed. Encourage the child to repeat it **Warning/reminder**: Maintain a moderate speech rate	The child can repeat seven or more words without affecting the meaning of the sentence
	170	Understand and act on the instructions	The assessor says to the child, "Please raise your hand" and "Please lift your foot." One repetition but no demonstration is allowed. Observe the child's response	The child can raise the hand or lift the foot according to the instructions

(continued)

(continued)

27 months old

Domain	No.	Item	Operation	Passing/scoring criterion
Social behavior	171	Take off clothes or pants without help	**Warning/reminder:** The assessor should avoid any suggestive actions, including eye gestures Observe or inquire if the child can take off clothes or pants by themselves **Warning/reminder:** R Taking off clothes does not include unbuttoning	The child can take off clothes or pants without help
	172	Have the concept of right and wrong	The assessor asks the child, "Is it right to hit people?" Observes the child's reaction or response	Pass if the child shakes their head or says "no."
Communication warning behavior	173	Have a preference for circular objects	Inquire about the child's favorite toys **Warning/reminder:** R Points should be scored if the child has a preference for a limited number of toys, tends to enjoy playing with circular objects, or shows a strong focus on specific objects	Points are scored if, for example, the child prefers to play with wheels or wheel-like objects rather than a toy car

(continued)

9 INSTRUCTION MANUAL FOR THE ERXIN SCALES   251

(continued)

27 months old

Domain	No.	Item	Operation	Passing/scoring criterion
	174	Engage in monotonous play with toys	Engage in monotonous play with toys: Inquire if the child's play with toys is limited to only 1–2 types, or if use unconventional ways to play toys, or if the child frequently engages in playing one particular play without getting tired of it **Warning/reminder**: R	Points are scored if the child often arranges the toys in a straight line and even in an organized manner

30 months old

Domain	No.	Item	Operation	Passing/scoring criterion
Gross motor	175	Stand on one foot for 2 seconds	The assessor demonstrates standing on one foot. Encourage the child to do the same **Warning/reminder**: Minor body sway or extending the arms to maintain balance is allowed	The child can stand on one foot without holding onto any object for 2 seconds or more
Fine motor	176	Thread through 3–5 buttons	The assessor demonstrates threading a crystal thread through a buttonhole and pulling it out. Encourage the child to do the same	The child can proficiently thread through 3–5 buttons

(continued)

(continued)

30 months old

Domain	No.	Item	Operation	Passing/scoring criterion
	177	Imitate building a bridge with building blocks	The assessor demonstrates using two blocks at the bottom and one block on top to build a bridge with a hole. Keep the model intact, and encourage the child to do the same **Warning/reminder**: The assessor must not prompt the presence of the hole in the bridge	The child can build a bridge with a hole according to the model
Adaptability	178	Know the difference between one and many	The assessor places one block and several blocks respectively on two sides, and asks the child to identify which side has more. If the child identifies the side with more blocks, the assessor then points to the other side and asks, "How many are there?" **Warning/reminder**: Fail if the child only gives one correct response	The child first correctly identifies the side with more blocks, and then answers "One."

(continued)

9 INSTRUCTION MANUAL FOR THE ERXIN SCALES 253

(continued)

30 months old

Domain	No.	Item	Operation	Passing/scoring criterion
	179	Correctly put the building blocks of different shapes into the inverted template	On the basis of the child being able to place three blocks into the template correctly, flip the template 180° while keeping the three blocks in their original positions. The assessor says to the child, "These are the homes for the little friends (pointing to the template). Please help these little friends (pointing to the three blocks) find their own homes." No demonstration is given	The child can correctly place the blocks into the corresponding holes on the inverted template in one attempt. Prompts could only be provided for the isosceles triangle, such as by suggesting a change in direction
Language	180	Tell the names of 10 pictures	Present the pictures (24 in total). Point to each picture and encourage the child to say its name **Warning/reminder**: Note for the first picture: A correct answer would be "polar bear" or "white bear." If the child only says "bear," the assessor should follow up with the question: "What kind of bear?" If the child cannot provide "polar bear" or "white bear" as the answer, their response is considered incorrect	The child can correctly tell the names of 10 or more pictures
	181	Speak out one's own name	The assessor asks the child, "What is your name?"	The child can correctly state their full name when asked

(continued)

(continued)

30 months old

Domain	No.	Item	Operation	Passing/scoring criterion
Social behavior	182	Pour water back and forth from two cups without spilling	Pour 1/3 cup of water into a cup without handles. The assessor demonstrates pouring the water back and forth into another cup and encourages the child to do the same	The child pours the water back and forth between two cups (one cup filled with 1/3 water, the other cup empty) twice without spilling water
	183	Correctly answer or point out where the peel should be thrown	Present the picture. The assessor says to the child, "It is wrong to litter. Where do you think this child should throw the fruit peel?" Encourage the child to answer	The child can correctly answer or indicate that the peel should be thrown in the trash bin
Communication warning behavior	184	Play alone and exhibit unsociable behavior	Inquire if the child can play with peers of the same age **Warning/reminder:** R Points are scored if the child often engages in solitary play when playing with other children, and does not actively participate in games or activities with other children even when accompanied by adults	Points are scored if the child has no desire to play with peers and exhibits unsociable behavior
	185	Show a lack of interest in people around	Inquire about the child's behavior when someone comes to their house **Warning/reminder:** R	Points are scored if the child displays indifference and does not pay attention in most cases when someone visits their home

33 months old

Domain	No.	Item	Operation	Passing/scoring criterion
Gross motor	186	Perform standing long jump	The assessor demonstrates jumping with the feet together over a sheet of 16K white paper (20 cm wide), or over the A4 paper placed horizontally in front of their feet. Encourage the child to do the same **Warning/reminder**: The child can jump with the feet either together or apart Fail if the child performs a stepping motion instead of jumping	The child jumps with both feet off the ground over the paper without stepping on it
Fine motor	187	Imitate drawing a circle	The assessor demonstrates drawing a circle and encourages the child to imitate **Warning/reminder**: Demonstrate in the same direction The assessor should draw a closed circle while demonstrating	Pass if the child draws a closed circle where both ends meet, and the circle has no obvious angles
	188	Insert all the zipper slider into the bottom stop and try to zip it up	Present an opened zipper, and demonstrate inserting the zipper slider into the bottom stop and zipping it up. Encourage the child to do the same **Warning/reminder**: Showing the attempt to zip it up is sufficient Demonstrate in the same direction	The child can fully insert the zipper slider into the bottom stop and try to zip it up

(continued)

(continued)

33 months old

Domain	No.	Item	Operation	Passing/scoring criterion
Adaptability	189	Stack 10 building blocks	Demonstrate stacking two building blocks and knock them down. Then, present the blocks one by one, and encourage the child to stack them up **Warning/reminder**: At least one successful attempt out of three is required	The child can stack 10 building blocks
	190	Execute three commands consecutively	The assessor takes out a small towel and a brass bell and instructs the child to do three things: wipe the table, shake the bell, and open the door. The assessor may repeat the instructions once (the order of the three tasks must remain consistent and cannot be changed; no requirement for which task to do first) After the child starts, no further reminders or prompts are given **Warning/reminder**: The assessor is allowed to provide slight body language assistance when giving instructions, but should not demonstrate the entire operation. Body language assistance is not allowed while repeating the instructions	The child can perform all the tasks without forgetting any one, but the order of tasks can be reversed

(continued)

(continued)

33 months old

Domain	No.	Item	Operation	Passing/scoring criterion
Language	191	Tell one's own sex	The assessor asks the child about their gender. If the child is a girl, the assessor asks, "Are you a girl or a boy?" If the child is a boy, the assessor asks, "Are you a boy or a girl?"	The child can correctly state their own gender
	192	Understand the meaning of "inside" and "outside"	The assessor puts a pellet into a transparent vial and asks, "Is the pellet inside or outside the vial?" Then, the assessor takes the pellet out of the vial and asks, "Is the pellet outside or inside the vial?" **Warning/reminder**: The assessor must ask the questions according to the provided instructions and should not change the sentences arbitrarily	Pass if the child can correctly state whether the pellet is inside or outside
Social behavior	193	Put on shoes	The assessor takes off the child's shoes, holds them with the toes facing the child, and encourages the child to put them on	The child can successfully put on the shoes; distinguishing left from right is not required The child can unbutton a specific button on their own, instead of pulling or tearing it

(continued)

(continued)

33 months old

Domain	No.	Item	Operation	Passing/scoring criterion
	194	Can unbutton	Present a doll and encourage the child to unbutton the doll's clothes. The assessor should assist in fastening the doll's clothes **Warning/reminder**: The assessor should observe the child's unbuttoning process. Pass if the button is unbuttoned instead of pulled apart	
Communication warning behavior	195	Laugh spontaneously without apparent reason	Inquire if the child laughs spontaneously without any apparent reason **Warning/reminder**: R	Points are scored if the child often laughs spontaneously without any apparent reason
	196	Talk to oneself using language others cannot understand	Inquire about the child's speech condition **Warning/reminder**: R	Points are scored if the child talks to themselves without emotional exchange partners, using self-created, strange language that others cannot understand

9 INSTRUCTION MANUAL FOR THE ERXIN SCALES 259

36 months old

Domain	No.	Item	Operation	Passing/scoring criterion
Gross motor	197	Jump with alternating feet	The assessor demonstrates jumping in place with alternating feet and knees raised up. Encourage the child to do the same **Warning/reminder**: Movement within the range of one foot is allowed while alternating feet	The child can jump with alternating feet in a coordinated manner, with both feet leaving the ground by 5 cm
Fine motor	198	Imitate drawing intersecting lines	The assessor demonstrates drawing intersecting lines. Encourage the child to imitate **Warning/reminder**: Demonstrate in the same direction	The child can draw two intersecting straight lines with relatively continuous strokes
	199	Tighten the screw	The assessor shows a screw and a nut and instructs the child to screw them together. If the child does not know how, the assessor can demonstrate **Warning/reminder**: Demonstrate in the same direction	The child can use both hands to assemble the screw and nut
Adaptability	200	Know the meaning of "3"	The assessor shows three building blocks and asks the child, "How many blocks are these?"	The child can correctly state "three blocks."

(continued)

(continued)

36 months old

Domain	No.	Item	Operation	Passing/scoring criterion
	201	Identify two colors	Present the four-color picture (red, yellow, blue, and green). Ask the child to identify the corresponding colors, starting with a non-red color to avoid the child's possible recitation of the sequence	The child answers correctly for two or more colors
Language	202	Tell the names of 14 pictures	Showing pictures (24 in total), the assessor points to each picture and encourages the child to say the name of the picture	The child can correctly tell the names of 14 or more pictures
	203	Pronounce clearly	Observe the child's pronunciation while speaking	Most of the child's speech is clear, and even if there are occasional unclear pronunciations, it does not hinder communication
Social behavior	204	Know the meanings of "hungry," "cold," and "tired"	The assessor asks the child, one by one, "What do you do when you're hungry?" "What do you do when you're cold?" "What do you do when you're tired?"	The child can correctly answer two or more of the questions: Eating, dressing, resting, etc.

(continued)

(continued)

36 months old

Domain	No.	Item	Operation	Passing/scoring criterion
	205	Can button	Present a doll and encourage the child to button the doll's clothes. The assessor should assist in fastening the doll's clothes	The child can button up a specific button on their own
Communication warning behavior	206	Constantly repeat a sentence or question	Inquire about the child's language communication situation: Does the child engage in repetitive questioning, such as repeating a particular sentence or a specific question? (e.g., constantly saying "want car, want car, want car...") **Warning/reminder:** R Points are scored if the child talks incessantly to the point where family members feel overwhelmed or get the impression that the child is relentless in pursuing their goals	Points are scored if the child keeps talking incessantly, constantly repeating a particular sentence, or endlessly asking the same question

(continued)

(continued)

36 months old

Domain	No.	Item	Operation	Passing/scoring criterion
	207	Exhibit persistent, repetitive actions	Inquire if the child exhibits repetitive actions that are generally difficult to be stopped	Points are scored if, for example, the child persistently repeats the action of turning the lights on and off, or engages in other repetitive behaviors. For instance, repeatedly using the elevator: If someone else presses the elevator button while the child is inside, they will refuse to go home, and will only return home when they wait for the elevator to reach the ground floor again, then press the button themselves to take the elevator to the floor where their home is located
			Warning/reminder: R Repetitive actions are extremely difficult to redirect or transfer Points should be scored, for example, when going out, the child insists that everyone in the house must go out, and if even one person is left behind, they may cry or shout until everyone is out. Points should not be scored if such behavior only occurs once	

42 months old

Domain	No.	Item	Operation	Passing/scoring criterion
Gross motor	208	Go upstairs with alternating feet	The assessor demonstrates going upstairs with alternating feet, without holding onto the handrail. Encourage the child to do the same **Warning/reminder:** See Appendix B, 2. Staircase for Testing for the staircase specifications	The child climbs at least three steps of the stairs, one foot per step
	209	Jump down the last step of the stairs with the feet together	The assessor demonstrates standing on the last step of the staircase, with the feet together, and jumping to the ground. Encourage the child to do the same **Warning/reminder:** Slight body sway upon landing is allowed Fail if the distance between two feet exceeds 10 cm upon landing	Pass if the child jumps down and lands on the ground steadily, keeping the feet close together Pass if the child jumps with the feet together, and lands on the ground with the feet less than 10 cm apart (equivalent to the length of the A4 paper folded along the shorter side)

(continued)

(continued)

42 months old

Domain	No.	Item	Operation	Passing/scoring criterion
Fine motor	210	Assemble a circle and a square using plastic boards	The assessor asks the child to make a circle using four plastic boards and make a square using two equilateral triangle boards, with a time limit of 2 minutes **Warning/reminder:** Fail if exceeding the time limit	Pass if the child succeeds in assembling both the circle and the square, and the assembled square should form an angle of less than 30° with the horizontal line (judging the angle relative to the horizontal line while facing the child)
	211	Can use scissors	The assessor demonstrates cutting a straight line on a sheet of paper with scissors. Encourage the child to do the same **Warning/reminder:** Demonstrate in the same direction	Pass if the child can cut a straight line with a length of ≥ 10 cm and a deviation angle of $<15°$ from the primary cutting direction
Adaptability	212	Know the meaning of "5"	The assessor shows five building blocks and asks the child, "How many blocks are these?"	The child can correctly state "five blocks."

(continued)

(continued)

42 months old

Domain	No.	Item	Operation	Passing/scoring criterion
	213	Identify four colors	The assessor presents the four-color picture (red, yellow, blue, and green), and asks the child to identify the corresponding colors, starting with a non-red color to avoid the child's possible recitation of the sequence	The child answers correctly for all four colors
Language	214	Use antonyms	The assessor asks the following questions respectively: (1) Fire is hot, what about ice? (2) An elephant's trunk is long, what about a rabbit's tail? (3) Hair is black, what about teeth? (4) Wood is hard, what about cotton? **Warning/reminder**: Correct answers: (1) Ice is cold; (2) A rabbit's tail is short; (3) Teeth are white; (4) Cotton is soft Answering "ice is ice" is incorrect	The child answers correctly for two or more of the questions
	215	Tell the shape of the figures (△ ○ □)	The assessor shows the triangle (△), circle (○), and square (□) blocks one by one, and asks the child, "What shape is this?" **Warning/reminder**: To pass, all three shapes must be correctly identified	The child can correctly name the three given shapes

(continued)

(continued)

42 months old

Domain	No.	Item	Operation	Passing/scoring criterion
Social behavior	216	Put on a coat by oneself	Observe whether the child can put on a coat by themselves **Warning/reminder**: R	The child can put on the coat and button or zip it by themselves
	217	Know the reason to wash hands before eating	The assessor asks the child, "Why do we need to wash our hands before eating?" **Warning/reminder**: Fail if the answer is "will have a stomachache" or "need to eat."	Pass if the child can answer correctly, such as "hands are dirty," "there are bugs," "there are bacteria," or "to avoid getting sick."
Communication warning behavior	218	Lack empathy	Inquire whether the child uses facial expressions or gestures to show concern for a family member who is feeling unwell or unhappy **Warning/reminder**: R	Points are scored if the child seems to lack empathy. For example, if their hand accidentally touches a hot cup, they do not show a painful expression or reach out for comfort. Similarly, if their mother's hand is burned by a hot cup, they do not exhibit caring actions or behaviors

48 *months old*

Domain	No.	Item	Operation	Passing/scoring criterion
Gross motor	219	Stand on one foot for 5 seconds	The assessor demonstrates standing on one foot and encourages the child to do the same **Warning/reminder**: Fail if the child can only stand for less than 5 seconds Pass if the child can stand steadily for 5 seconds or more at the second attempt	The child can stand on one foot for at least 5 seconds, with stable balance and minimal sway
	220	Jump down the last step of the stairs with the feet together and land steadily	The assessor demonstrates standing on the last step of the staircase, with the feet together, and jumping to the ground. Encourage the child to do the same	Pass if the child jumps with the feet together, and lands on the ground steadily with the feet less than 5 cm apart
Fine motor	221	Imitate drawing a square	The assessor demonstrates drawing a square and encourages the child to imitate **Warning/reminder**: Demonstrate in the same direction	The child can imitatively draw a square. Slight tilting of the drawn square is allowed, with one angle <45°

(continued)

(continued)

48 months old				
Domain	No.	Item	Operation	Passing/scoring criterion
	222	Assemble screws as shown in picture	The assessor shows the picture of an assembled screw for 5 seconds, then takes it away and gives the child the separate screw, washer, and nut, asking the child to assemble them from memory. If any part is dropped, the assessor can prompt by saying, "What else is there?"	Pass if the child can independently assemble the screw, washer, and nut in the correct order without or with minimal prompting
Adaptability	223	Find out three differences	The assessor presents a set of spot-the-difference pictures, and asks the child to identify the differences between the two pictures. Use a teddy bear for demonstration and instruction, with a time limit of 2 minutes	Pass if the child can find out at least three differences, including the demonstrated one
	224	Identify the missing parts in pictures (3/6)	The assessor presents a set of incomplete pictures, and asks the child what is missing in each picture. Use the first picture for demonstration and instruction **Warning/reminder**: Correct answers are as shown in the corresponding missing parts	To pass, the child must correctly respond to three or more of the given pictures, including the demonstrated one

(continued)

9 INSTRUCTION MANUAL FOR THE ERXIN SCALES

(continued)

48 months old

Domain	No.	Item	Operation	Passing/scoring criterion
Language	225	Imitate saying a compound sentence	The assessor says the sentence "Mom told me not to fight with other children." One repetition is allowed. Encourage the child to repeat it **Warning/reminder:** Maintain a moderate speech rate while demonstrating. The child's repetition should not change the meaning of the sentence	The child can repeat the sentence in a relatively complete manner, with occasional omissions or misspellings, but maintaining the basic structure of a compound sentence
	226	Know the use of pot, mobile phone, and eyes	The assessor asks the following questions respectively: (1) What is a pot used for? (2) What is a mobile phone used for? (3) What are eyes used for? **Warning/reminder:** When asked the use of a mobile phone, the child is required to state its main function: A mobile phone is used as a communication tool or for making phone calls Fail if the child only mentions playing games or watching animations, or says things like sending WeChat messages, chatting, shopping, or even watching videos or TikTok	Pass if the child answers all three questions correctly Correct answers: (1) Used for cooking; (2) A communication tool/used for making phone calls; (3) Eyes can see things, people, or objects, etc.

(continued)

(continued)

48 months old

Domain	No.	Item	Operation	Passing/scoring criterion
Social behavior	227	Play group plays	Inquire whether the child can participate in group plays **Warning/reminder**: R	The child can actively participate in group plays and follow the plays rules
	228	Distinguish between male and female toilets	Present a picture showing male and female toilet signs, and ask the child which toilet they should use and then ask, "Why?" **Warning/reminder**: To pass, both questions should be answered correctly	The child can identify the correct toilet sign and verbally express the meaning of gender
Communication warning behavior	229	Cannot observe or perceive verbal and non-verbal cues	Inquire whether the child observes others' expressions and changes their own behavior according to others' moods	Points are scored if the child does not observe or perceive verbal and non-verbal cues and shows no response to others' emotions such as happiness, anger, or sadness Points are scored if the child fails to notice or realize when their own actions or behaviors are inappropriate for the given situation, and they do not self-regulate or stop themselves unless when forced or loudly scolded by a parent

(continued)

(continued)

48 months old

Domain	No.	Item	Operation	Passing/scoring criterion
			Warning/reminder: R For example, a child initially wanted their mother to give them yogurt but notices her displeasure, thus temporarily abandoning the idea of having yogurt or using language or actions to comfort the mother. If the child does not exhibit such behavior or performance, points should be scored	

54 months old

Domain	No.	Item	Operation	Passing/scoring criterion
Gross motor	230	Stand on one foot for 10 seconds	The assessor demonstrates standing on one foot. Encourage the child to do the same	Pass if the child can stand on one foot for at least 10 seconds, with stable balance and minimal sway
	231	Walk forward 2 meters heel to toe	The assessor demonstrates walking heel to toe in a straight line. Encourage the child to do the same	The child can walk forward 2 meters (six steps) heel to toe; slight body sway is allowed
Fine motor	232	Fold paper with neat edges	The assessor demonstrates folding the rectangular paper in half horizontally and vertically, once each. Encourage the child to do the same **Warning/reminder:** The paper used is of uniform size	The child can fold the paper into a nearly rectangle shape, with a difference in opposite edges less than 1 cm and angle between paper edges less than 15°

(continued)

(continued)

54 months old

Domain	No.	Item	Operation	Passing/scoring criterion
	233	Pick up peanuts with chopsticks	The assessor encourages the child to use chopsticks to pick up a peanut from the table and put it in a box, and repeat the action twice **Warning/reminder:** Three consecutive successful attempts are required Demonstration is not allowed No specific requirements for chopsticks holding gesture	The child can proficiently pick up the peanut at least three times without dropping it in the process
Adaptability	234	Categorization	The assessor gives the child a round button and then shows the first set of templates (including shapes such as circle, square, and triangle). The assessor asks, "Which ones are similar to the object in your hand? Why?" After that, the templates are put away. Then, show the second set of templates (including a square button, triangle, and square), and ask the same question **Warning/reminder:** Correct answers: (1) Select the circle template; they are all circular/round. (2) Select the square button; they are all buttons, with buttonholes and eyelets	The child correctly answers both questions

(continued)

(continued)

54 months old

Domain	No.	Item	Operation	Passing/scoring criterion
	235	Identify the missing parts in pictures (4/6)	The assessor presents a set of incomplete pictures, and asks the child what is missing in each picture. Use the first picture for demonstration and instruction	To pass, the child must correctly respond to four or more of the given pictures, including the demonstrated one
Language	236	Rinse one's own mouth	Observe whether the child knows how to rinse their mouth **Warning/reminder:** The action of rinsing mouth from left to right is required. Demonstration is allowed	The child can rinse mouth fluidly from left to right and spit out water without spraying
	237	Know numbers	The assessor shows pictures and randomly points out numbers within 10, asking the child to identify them	The child correctly identifies all the numbers
Social behavior	238	Know morning and afternoon	If the assessment is conducted in the morning, the assessor asks: (1) Is it morning or afternoon now? (2) Does the sun set in the afternoon or morning? If the assessment is conducted in the afternoon, the assessor asks: (1) Is it afternoon or morning now? (2) Does the sun rise in the morning or afternoon?	The child correctly answers both questions

(continued)

(continued)

54 months old

Domain	No.	Item	Operation	Passing/scoring criterion
	239	Count fingers	**Warning/reminder**: Fail if the child's response does not include the words "morning" or "afternoon." The assessor asks the child how many fingers are on one hand. If answered correctly, the assessor then asks how many fingers there are on two hands	The child can mentally count and say that there are 10 fingers on two hands
Communication warning behavior	240	Cannot express agreement or approval verbally	**Warning/reminder**: Fail if the child counts fingers one by one using hand gestures Inquire whether the child can use words like "yes," "good," "great," etc., to express agreement or approval of others' opinions **Warning/reminder**: R	Points are scored if the child fails to respond with words like "yes," "good," "great," etc., to express agreement or approval

60 months old

Domain	No.	Item	Operation	Passing/scoring criterion
Gross motor	241	Hop on one foot	The assessor demonstrates hopping on one foot in place. Encourage the child to do the same	The child can consecutively hop on one foot three times or more; extending both arms for balance is allowed

(continued)

(continued)

60 months old

Domain	No.	Item	Operation	Passing/scoring criterion
	242	Pedal	**Warning/reminder:** Hoping within the range of one foot is allowed The assessor demonstrates going up and down a single step, starting with the same foot. Encourage the child to do the same **Warning/reminder:** Brief pauses are allowed, but the duration should be within 2 seconds	The child, starting with the same foot, can smoothly and fairly proficiently complete three sets
Fine motor	243	Assemble an oval according to the picture	Place a pre-drawn oval-shaped picture in front of the child, and ask the child to place six plastic boards into it according to the picture without any reminders, with a time limit of 2 minutes **Warning/reminder:** The child should complete the task within 2 minutes Fail if exceeding the time limit	The child places all plastic boards correctly
	244	Try to cut out a circle	The assessor gives the child a half A4-sized paper with a pre-drawn circle (7.5 cm in diameter) on it. Encourage the child to cut out the circle **Warning/reminder:** Show the child a A5 paper (half of A4 paper size) drawn with a standard circle (7.5 cm in diameter), and ask the child to cut it out	The child can cut out the circle roughly, with slight angles allowed

(continued)

(continued)

60 months old

Domain	No.	Item	Operation	Passing/scoring criterion
Adaptability	245	Find out five differences	The assessor presents a set of spot-the-difference pictures, and asks the child to identify the differences between the two pictures. Use a teddy bear for demonstration and instruction, with a time limit of 2 minutes	Pass if the child can find out at least five differences, including the demonstrated one Record the time
	246	Identify the missing parts in pictures (5/6)	The assessor presents a set of incomplete pictures, and asks the child what is missing in each picture. Use the first picture for demonstration and instruction **Warning/reminder**: Correct answers are as shown in the corresponding missing parts	To pass, the child must correctly respond to five or more of the given pictures, including the demonstrated one
Language	247	What is your last name?	The assessor asks the child, "What is your last name?" **Warning/reminder**: Fail if the child's response also includes their first name	The child can correctly state their last name
	248	Name two types of circular objects	The assessor asks the child to name two types of circular objects **Warning/reminder**: If objects like a water cup, which is cylindrical, are mentioned, the child must specifically state that the cup mouth is circular; otherwise, it would be considered a failure	The child can name two or more types of circular objects

(continued)

(continued)

60 months old

Domain	No.	Item	Operation	Passing/scoring criterion
Social behavior	249	Where do you live?	The assessor asks the child, "Where do you live?" and may follow up with "Can you tell me more specifically? How can I take you home?" **Warning/reminder**: Record: Village name/door number, building number, residential area, street, district	Pass if the child's provided address enables others to locate it relatively easily
Communication warning behavior	250	Prefer TV commercials to cartoons	Inquire whether the child likes TV commercials or advertising music more than cartoons **Warning/reminder**: R	Points are scored if the child is more interested in TV commercials or advertising music

66 months old

Domain	No.	Item	Operation	Passing/scoring criterion
Gross motor	251	Catch the ball	The assessor demonstrates catching a ball with both hands instead of the front chest, and then stands 1 meter away from the child and throws the ball to the child, encouraging them to catch it with their hands	The child catches the ball with their hands; one successful catch out of three attempts is sufficient

(continued)

(continued)

66 months old

Domain	No.	Item	Operation	Passing/scoring criterion
			Warning/reminder: Catching it with both arms or using the front chest does not count. A standard-sized tennis ball is used	
	252	Walk backward 2 meters heel to toe	The assessor demonstrates walking backward heel to toe in a straight line. Encourage the child to do the same	The child can walk backward 2 meters (six steps) heel to toe; slight body sway is allowed
Fine motor	253	Can write one's own name	The assessor asks the child to write their own name **Warning/reminder:** It must be the full name rather than a nickname	The child can write their own name correctly
	254	Cut out a smooth circle	The assessor gives the child a half A4-sized paper with a pre-drawn circle (7.5 cm in diameter) on it. Encourage the child to cut out the circle **Warning/reminder:** Show the child a A5 paper (half of A4 paper size) drawn with a standard circle (7.5 cm in diameter) Fail if the cut-out circle has obvious angles or excessive jagged edges	The child can cut out the circle smoothly, without angles or jagged edges
Adaptability	255	Stand between trees	The assessor asks the child, "If one person stands between two trees, then how many people can stand between three trees in a row?"	The child answers, "Two people."

(continued)

(continued)

66 months old

Domain	No.	Item	Operation	Passing/scoring criterion
	256	Cut an apple crosswise	The assessor asks the child, "If you cut an apple crosswise, how many slices will there be?" If the child does not understand, the assessor can use gestures to assist with the cutting motion	Pass if, without prompting or with only prompting gestures from the assessor, the child answers "four slices."
Language	257	Know one's own zodiac sign	The assessor asks the child, "What is your zodiac sign?"	The child can correctly state their own zodiac sign
	258	Count backwards	The assessor first asks, "Can you count backwards?" and then demonstrates and says, "1, 2, 3 backward is... 3, 2, 1. Now, please count backwards starting from 17: 17, 16, 15, 14..." Encourage the child to complete the countdown **Warning/reminder**: The assessor can start counting together with the child from 17, saying "17, 16, 15, 14" and then stop, allowing the child to continue counting on their own	The child can fluently and correctly count backwards from 13 to 1
Social behavior	259	Why takes the crosswalk?	The assessor asks the child, "Why should we use crosswalks, overhead bridges, or underground passages when crossing the road?"	The child can provide a correct response, indicating that it is for safety reasons, such as to avoid being hit by a car, etc.

(continued)

(continued)

66 months old

Domain	No.	Item	Operation	Passing/scoring criterion
	260	Chickens swim in water	The assessor presents a picture of chickens swimming in water and asks the child if the drawing is correct. If the child answers "no," the assessor asks why it is incorrect **Warning/reminder**: The standard answer is that chickens cannot swim or walk in water For the picture presented, if the child answers "incorrect" or says "chickens walk on the road," the assessor should then ask, "What about this?" (pointing to the picture). The correct response at this point is "It's in the water;" if the child cannot give such response, it would be considered a failure	The child answers, "Chickens cannot swim in water."
Communication warning behavior	261	Lack skills in interacting with peers	Inquire about the child's social interactions with their peers **Warning/reminder**: R When engaging in hugging actions, the child often lacks awareness of the concept of "gentleness" or controlling the "intensity." As a result, their actions tend to be heavy, leading to uncomfortable interactions and displeasure among their peers	Points are scored if the child generally does not use language but often resorts to actions such as pushing, pulling, and hugging when attempting to interact with peers

9 INSTRUCTION MANUAL FOR THE ERXIN SCALES 281

72 months old

Domain	No.	Item	Operation	Passing/scoring criterion
Gross motor	262	Hop on one foot continuously with crossed arms	The assessor demonstrates hopping on one foot in place with crossed arms. Encourage the child to do the same **Warning/reminder**: Hoping within the range of one foot is allowed	The child can consecutively hop on one foot in place with crossed arms three times or more
	263	Bounce a ball twice	The assessor demonstrates bouncing a ball. Encourage the child to do the same **Warning/reminder**: The first bounce upon hitting the ground after throwing downwards does not count. At least one successful attempt out of three is required. A standard-sized ball is used	The child consecutively bounces the ball two or more times
Fine motor	264	Assemble a rectangle	The assessor asks the child to use two (right-angled) non-isosceles triangle plastic boards to make a rectangle **Warning/reminder**: When presenting the two triangle boards, their shorter sides should be positioned opposite to each other. The child should complete the task within 2 minutes. Fail if exceeding the time limit	Pass if the child correctly assembles the rectangle
	265	Copy a composite shape	The assessor shows a combination of a square and a circle as a composite shape. Encourage the child to copy it	The child can draw the composite shape without rotation or displacement

(continued)

(continued)

72 months old

Domain	No.	Item	Operation	Passing/scoring criterion
Adaptability			**Warning/reminder**: Specific passing criteria: The distance between the circle and the square should be within 2 millimeters; the circle and the square should be proportionally enlarged or reduced; the ratio of the longer diagonal to the shorter diagonal of the circle or the square should be less than 1.5:1	
	266	Find out seven differences	The assessor presents a set of spot-the-difference pictures, and asks the child to identify the differences between the two pictures. Use a teddy bear for demonstration and instruction, with a time limit of 2 minutes	Pass if the child can find out at least seven differences, including the demonstrated one
	267	Know left and right	The assessor asks the child to touch their right ear with their left hand, their left ear with their right hand, and their right leg with their right hand	Pass if the child performs all the actions correctly
			Warning/reminder: The assessor should avoid any suggestive actions, including eye gestures	

(continued)

(continued)

72 months old

Domain	No.	Item	Operation	Passing/scoring criterion
Language	268	Describe the picture contents	The assessor shows a comic strip containing three pictures and says to the child, "These three pictures tell a story. Can you tell me what the story is about? Why is the little monkey crying?" If the child does not answer the second question after answering the first, the assessor can ask again, "Why is the little monkey crying?"	Pass if the child can describe the basic contents of each picture individually
	269	Work, window, apple and banana (2/3)	The assessor asks: (1) Why do people go to work? (2) Why do houses have windows? (3) What do apples and bananas have in common?	A minimum of two correct answers is required (1) To earn money or make contribution to the country (2) Used for light transmission or ventilation. (3) Fruits

(continued)

(continued)

72 months old

Domain	No.	Item	Operation	Passing/scoring criterion
			Warning/reminder: Here are some examples of evaluating answers: **Work**: Earning money, buying things, supporting oneself, supporting children (✓); studying, grown up (×) **Window**: Pass if the answers are related to light and ventilation, such as seeing things, light transmission, no darkness (✓); air circulation, ventilation (follow-up question about window opening) (✓); keeping warm (follow-up question about how to keep warm; pass if the answer indicates "sunlight for warmth;" fail if the explanation is unreasonable); coldness, wind, rain, soil blocking (×) **Apple and banana**: Fruits, having a pull tab, having peel, being nutritious, containing vitamins, being sweet, growing on trees (picked from trees), being edible (✓); being yellow, having the same peels (×)	
Social behavior	270	What are the four seasons in a year?	The assessor asks the child to name the four seasons of the year	The order of the seasons (spring, summer, autumn, winter) can be reversed
	271	Recognize the signs	The assessor presents two pictures showing different signs and asks, "Which sign represents danger? Why?"	The child can identify the sign of danger in the pictures and explain the reasons correctly

(continued)

(continued)

72 months old

Domain	No.	Item	Operation	Passing/scoring criterion
Communication warning behavior	272	Exhibit resistance to changes in daily habits	The assessor inquires about the child's daily life situations **Warning/reminder:** R Points should be scored if the child shows signs of unease or experiences difficulty in falling asleep when there is a change in the positioning of the bed or items on the bed	Points are scored if the child exhibits resistance to changes in daily habits, such as only drinking from a specific milk bottle and refusing to drink or even crying when a different bottle is used

78 months old

Domain	No.	Item	Operation	Passing/scoring criterion
Gross motor	273	Kick a ball with string	The assessor demonstrates lifting a ball with string using their hand, and after the ball comes to a stop, they kick it using the inner ankle and arch of the foot. Encourage the child to do the same **Warning/reminder:** If the child kicks with the outer side of the foot, one demonstration and correction are allowed Fail if the child kicks with the leg, toe, or outer side of the foot	The child continuously kicks the ball with the inner ankle for two or more times; the foot is allowed to remain off the ground while kicking

(continued)

(continued)

78 months old

Domain	No.	Item	Operation	Passing/scoring criterion
	274	Bounce a ball five times	The assessor demonstrates bouncing a ball. Encourage the child to do the same **Warning/reminder**: The first bounce upon hitting the ground after throwing downwards does not count. At least one successful attempt out of three is required. A standard-sized ball is used	The child consecutively bounces the ball five or more times
Fine motor	275	Copy a hexagon	The assessor shows a hexagon shape and encourages the child to copy it **Warning/reminder**: The gap between the lines should be within 2 millimeters	The child can copy the hexagon, with all six angles drawn accurately and the connecting lines being straight
	276	Try to tie a slipknot	The assessor shows a pair of chopsticks and a string, and demonstrates tying the chopsticks together with a slipknot using the string. Encourage the child to do the same **Warning/reminder**: Item #287 (Tie a slipknot, with no demonstration given unless the first attempt fails) should be assessed before this item The assessor should assist in securing the chopsticks while the child ties the knot. The demonstrated tying technique should follow standardized guidelines	After demonstration, the child can tie the chopsticks with a single or double slipknot

(continued)

(continued)

78 months old

Domain	No.	Item	Operation	Passing/scoring criterion
Adaptability	277	Graphic analogy	The assessor presents a set of graphic shapes and asks which of the four pictures below would fit appropriately in the blank space above. Using the first question for demonstration **Warning/reminder**: Correct answers: 2 3 4 2	The child can correctly respond to three or more questions, including the demonstrated one
	278	Know the use of flour	The assessor asks the child, "What can you make with flour?" **Warning/reminder**: Record: steamed buns, twisted rolls, dumplings, buns, pancakes, noodles, bread, hamburgers, cakes, dough figurines, etc.	The child can provide two or more correct answers
Language	279	Summarize the theme of pictures	The assessor shows a comic strip containing three pictures and says to the child, "These three pictures tell a story. Can you tell me what the story is about? Why is the little monkey crying?" If the child does not answer the second question after answering the first, the assessor can ask again, "Why is the little monkey crying?"	Pass if the child can clearly understand the theme of the story

(continued)

(continued)

78 months old

Domain	No.	Item	Operation	Passing/scoring criterion
			Warning/reminder: Correct answers: The little monkey didn't build a house; because the monkey is lazy and has no house to live in	
	280	Read a clock	The assessor asks the child to tell the time shown in the clock pictures	The child can tell the time shown in two or more pictures
			Warning/reminder: Correct answers: (1) 4: 00 (2) 1: 30 (3) 9: 20	
Social behavior	281	Know the day of the week	The assessor first tells the child what day of the week it is and then asks, "Can you tell me what day of the week it will be the day after tomorrow? What day of the week is tomorrow? What day of the week was yesterday?"	The child can correctly state them all
	282	Read in the rain	The assessor shows a picture of someone reading a book in the rain and asks if the drawing is correct. If the child answers "no," the assessor asks why it is incorrect	The child can provide the correct response: It's raining; you can't read in the rain; you'll get wet, get sick; the book will get wet

(continued)

(continued)

78 months old

Domain	No.	Item	Operation	Passing/scoring criterion
Communication warning behavior	283	Rarely initiate conversations with others and cannot sustain a conversation	The assessor inquires about the child's interactions with others For example, the assessor can say, "What cartoons are you watching now?" When the child deviates from the topic, possibly shifting the conversation to food, toys, or other non-cartoon-related topics, points should be scored accordingly. (The assessor can ask about the child's home situation to assist in judging.) **Warning/reminder**: R If the parent says that the child can communicate normally with family members and maintain a topic, observations should be made during the assessment: If the child cannot engage in reciprocal communication with the assessor, points should be scored accordingly. If the child can generally maintain a topic, no score is given	Points are scored if the child rarely initiates conversations with others and cannot engage in reciprocal conversation to maintain a topic

84 months old

Domain	No.	Item	Operation	Passing/scoring criterion
Gross motor	284	Kick a ball with string continuously	The assessor demonstrates lifting a ball with string using their hand, and after the ball comes to a stop, they kick it using the inner ankle and arch of the foot. Encourage the child to do the same **Warning/reminder**: If the child kicks with the outer side of the foot, one demonstration and correction are allowed Fail if the child kicks with the leg, toe, or outer side of the foot	The child continuously kicks the ball with the inner ankle for three or more times, with each kick followed by the foot touching the ground, displaying good coordination
	285	Pedal alternately	The assessor demonstrates stepping up and down on a single step alternating feet for a total of three sets. Encourage the child to do the same. If the child does not know how to alternate feet, the assessor can remind them to "use the other foot." **Warning/reminder**: The assessor should call out slogans (such as "left up, left down; right up, right down") while demonstrating The child is allowed to pause during the movements, but the pause should not exceed 2 seconds. The assessor should not call out slogans while the child is performing Fail if the child fails to alternate steps while going up the stairs or obvious lacks proficiency in alternating steps	The child can perform three or more sets with alternating feet smoothly and fairly proficiently

(continued)

(continued)

84 months old					
Domain	No.	Item	Operation		Passing/scoring criterion
Fine motor	286	Learn to play the Cat's Cradle game	The assessor demonstrates the basic pattern of the Cat's Cradle game with one string. Encourage the child to follow along		The child can follow the assessor step by step or, after the assessor's demonstration, independently perform picking the string with the middle finger
			Warning/reminder: Picking the string can be done using the middle finger, index finger, or ring finger		
	287	Tie a slipknot (tie shoelaces)	The assessor presents a pair of chopsticks and a string, encouraging the child to tie the chopsticks together with a slipknot using the string		Without demonstration, the child can tie the chopsticks with a single or double slipknot
			Warning/reminder: The assessor should assist in securing the chopsticks while the child ties the knot		
Adaptability	288	Digital analogy	The assessor presents a set of graphic shapes and asks which of the four pictures below would fit appropriately in the blank space above. Using the first question for demonstration		The child can correctly respond to three or more questions, including the demonstrated one
			Warning/reminder: Correct answers: 2 2 2 4		

(continued)

(continued)

84 months old

Domain	No.	Item	Operation	Passing/scoring criterion
	289	What animals have no feet?	The assessor asks the child, "What animals have no feet?" (Foot defined as used for walking.) Or, the assessor can say to the child, "Feet are used for walking. So, what animals have no feet?" **Warning/reminder**: This item requires categorization. If the child's answer includes two animals of the same category, such as "shark" and "tropical fish," it will not be considered a pass. In this case, the assessor can continue to ask, "Are there any others?" If the child can provide another category, such as "snail," "snake," or "earthworm," it will be considered a pass Example of correct answers: Record: Fish (shark, tropical fish), octopus, dolphin (whale), seahorse; mud loach, jellyfish, tadpole; snake, earthworm, snail	The child correctly answers two or more categories of animals without feet, such as snakes and fish
Language	290	Why get a vaccination?	The assessor asks the child, "Why do children need to have a vaccination?" If the child does not understand, the question can be rephrased as, "Why do children need to get vaccinated?"	Pass if the child can state that vaccination is a preventive measure for illness/colds or mention that getting vaccinated prevents getting sick
	291	What do sweaters, pants, and shoes have in common?	The assessor asks the child, "What do sweaters, pants, and shoes have in common?"	The child answers that they are all clothes that we put on to stay warm

(continued)

(continued)

84 months old

Domain	No.	Item	Operation	Passing/scoring criterion
Social behavior	292	Emergency phone numbers	**Warning/reminder:** Fail if the answer is something like "they all have buttons or eyelets." The assessor asks the child what are the emergency phone numbers for a fire, the police (for seeking help), and an ambulance **Warning/reminder:** Correct answers: Fire: 119; Police: 110; Ambulance: 120 (999)	The child can correctly answer two or more phone numbers
	293	Owls catch mice	The assessor presents a picture of an owl catching a mouse and asks if the drawing is correct. If the child answers "no," the assessor asks why it is incorrect	The child answers, "Owls sleep during the day and do not come out to catch mice."
Communication warning behavior	294	Have exceptional abilities in some aspect	The assessor inquires about the child's abilities in areas such as numbers, road signs, word recognition, calculations, and color recognition	Points are scored if the child's ability in a specific aspect, such as numbers, road signs, reading, or calculations, is exceptional and significantly better than their abilities in communication, social interaction, or daily living skills

(continued)

(continued)

84 months old				
Domain	No.	Item	Operation	Passing/scoring criterion
			Warning/reminder: R Points are scored if the child's abilities in a specific aspect are exceptional and beyond their age, while their communication skills and other developmental levels are comparatively lower (especially in social interaction), or if the child's developmental age is lower than their chronological age but they have better abilities in reading, memorizing routes, or recognizing license plates	

Chapter 10
Appendices A, B, and C

10.1 Appendix A: Reference Percentiles for Overall and Subscale DQs at Different Main Test Ages for the Representative Sample

See Tables 10.1, 10.2, 10.3, 10.4, 10.5, and 10.6.

Table 10.1 Overall DQs at the 3rd-97th percentiles across the main test ages from 1 to 84 months

Erxin Scales

Distribution of overall DQs at the percentiles across different main test ages

Month age	Number of cases	<3	3	5	10	15	25	50	75	85	90	95	>=97
1	302	45	45	58	91	91	100	111	130	136	150	159	164
2	303	48	48	48	50	50	80	100	110	120	125	135	139
3	337	50	50	65	67	83	86	100	110	113	117	123	126
4	318	65	65	73	83	88	93	100	108	113	116	122	125
5	308	80	80	84	90	94	98	103	110	115	120	125	128
6	390	83	83	87	90	93	97	102	107	110	112	116	119
7	319	81	81	87	90	93	96	100	106	109	111	116	121
8	315	85	85	88	91	93	95	99	103	106	109	113	118
9	318	83	83	86	88	89	92	97	102	106	109	112	116
10	321	80	80	83	85	88	91	96	100	103	105	109	111
11	301	81	81	83	86	88	91	95	100	102	104	107	109
12	366	79	79	81	84	86	89	96	100	103	107	122	124
15	316	78	78	80	84	87	91	98	104	109	113	122	123
18	333	80	80	82	84	87	89	96	104	108	109	115	117
21	298	77	77	80	84	86	90	95	100	103	106	110	113
24	304	74	74	77	81	84	88	95	102	107	111	116	122
27	296	76	76	78	83	85	89	95	102	105	109	113	118
30	296	75	75	77	83	86	90	98	103	109	111	118	120
33	301	76	76	81	84	88	91	99	107	115	120	127	129
36	326	78	78	81	86	89	93	103	114	120	122	129	133
42	309	78	78	80	86	90	94	103	113	117	121	128	133
48	318	83	83	86	90	93	97	107	118	125	128	136	143
54	329	85	85	88	91	93	97	104	113	118	122	130	131
60	334	84	84	87	91	94	97	104	112	116	118	122	124
66	317	83	83	87	91	93	97	103	108	111	114	120	121
72	322	79	79	86	89	91	94	99	104	107	109	112	114
78	316	82	82	84	88	91	93	98	102	105	107	109	109
84	301	84	84	85	87	88	90	93	97	99	100	101	101

Table 10.2 Gross motor DQs at the 3rd-97th percentiles across the main test ages from 1 to 84 months

Gross Motor Subscale

Distribution of DQs at the percentiles across different main test ages

Month age	Number of cases	<3	3–	5–	10	15	25	50	75	85	90	95 >=97
1	302	45	45	50	91	91	91	136	150	167	200	200 200
2	303	48	48	50	71	71	75	95	119	125	132	149 150
3	337	52	52	65	67	81	83	100	113	117	121	133 133
4	318	65	65	71	73	77	85	98	110	115	122	125 138
5	308	77	77	80	88	90	96	106	115	118	120	125 125
6	390	77	77	82	85	90	93	100	107	108	112	117 119
7	319	80	80	83	87	90	92	97	106	109	111	116 120
8	315	79	79	81	83	88	91	99	106	113	115	119 122
9	318	73	73	78	82	84	89	98	106	109	111	114 117
10	321	74	74	78	83	84	90	97	103	106	108	113 115
11	301	77	77	79	83	87	90	97	103	105	106	110 117
12	366	75	75	76	82	85	89	96	100	108	113	123 124
15	316	76	76	78	80	82	91	100	116	120	122	126 130
18	333	72	72	75	82	83	89	99	108	114	115	117 119
21	298	71	71	73	79	85	91	98	102	112	114	118 120
24	304	64	64	68	76	81	86	93	105	111	112	115 122
27	296	67	67	72	77	78	84	98	104	110	112	121 122
30	296	70	70	71	79	84	89	98	102	111	118	123 130
33	301	69	69	73	81	82	90	99	110	117	120	127 129
36	326	80	80	80	84	88	92	105	115	122	126	131 135
42	309	78	78	80	84	87	93	104	112	117	119	126 129
48	318	74	74	83	88	90	95	104	116	122	124	133 141
54	329	79	79	83	88	91	95	104	114	119	122	129 132
60	334	79	79	84	89	92	97	104	112	117	120	123 127
66	317	79	79	85	87	90	94	102	108	112	114	119 120
72	322	79	79	82	86	88	92	100	107	111	112	114 115
78	316	76	76	79	83	86	90	97	103	105	107	109 109
84	301	77	77	78	82	85	89	93	98	99	100	101 101

Table 10.3 Fine motor DQs at the 3rd-97th percentiles across the main test ages from 1 to 84 months

Fine Motor Subscale

Distribution of DQs at the percentiles across different main test ages

Month age	Number of cases	<3	3–	5–	10	15	25	50	75	85	90	95 >=97
1	302	32	32	45	91	91	91	111	150	167	182	200 200
2	303	48	48	71	71	75	95	100	119	125	125	132 142
3	337	65	65	66	67	81	83	100	117	121	133	133 133
4	318	65	65	71	77	83	88	98	107	113	115	119 125
5	308	73	73	77	82	87	90	100	110	115	118	122 125
6	390	73	73	81	85	90	95	100	108	110	115	117 121
7	319	76	76	81	86	88	92	99	104	107	110	114 120
8	315	80	80	82	83	85	89	96	101	105	106	110 113
9	318	74	74	78	82	84	88	94	100	103	104	109 111
10	321	71	71	76	80	83	86	93	99	102	105	109 114
11	301	74	74	77	80	82	86	93	102	105	106	109 112
12	366	72	72	76	81	83	88	96	103	110	112	114 123
15	316	76	76	77	81	83	87	97	101	104	111	118 121
18	333	72	72	73	75	81	82	91	100	107	108	116 122
21	298	64	64	69	71	73	79	91	99	105	113	119 123
24	304	62	62	67	68	73	80	87	101	107	112	122 127
27	296	61	61	62	70	72	77	90	100	104	107	113 121
30	296	64	64	66	70	74	81	92	102	108	113	126 132
33	301	60	60	64	78	81	86	95	104	108	110	119 130
36	326	68	68	72	77	82	85	96	108	116	122	133 134
42	309	69	69	72	77	79	85	95	107	114	120	131 136
48	318	70	70	73	77	80	86	97	112	122	128	137 142
54	329	72	72	74	79	82	87	96	109	116	121	126 128
60	334	75	75	79	83	85	90	99	109	114	118	123 127
66	317	77	77	79	83	86	90	98	105	110	114	116 119
72	322	73	73	78	83	85	90	97	104	107	110	115 115
78	316	76	76	79	82	85	88	95	101	105	106	109 109
84	301	74	74	76	80	82	86	91	96	100	100	101 101

Table 10.4 Adaptability DQs at the 3rd-97th percentiles across the main test ages from 1 to 84 months

Adaptability Subscale

Distribution of DQs at the percentiles across different main test ages

Month age	Number of cases	<3	3–	5–	10	15	25	50	75	85	90	95	>=97
1	302	45	45	50	85	91	91	100	111	136	150	180	200
2	303	48	48	50	71	71	79	100	132	150	150	167	175
3	337	67	67	81	83	97	100	117	121	129	133	133	138
4	318	76	76	81	88	90	95	100	105	113	115	119	122
5	308	78	78	80	82	87	90	100	110	115	120	130	135
6	390	81	81	83	89	90	93	103	113	117	121	125	129
7	319	76	76	81	86	88	94	101	107	111	114	116	118
8	315	76	76	81	88	90	94	99	104	106	109	113	115
9	318	78	78	80	83	87	89	95	100	104	106	111	114
10	321	75	75	78	83	85	88	93	99	102	104	110	113
11	301	74	74	77	80	82	86	91	98	105	107	110	111
12	366	74	74	75	79	82	85	93	101	107	112	117	122
15	316	71	71	75	79	83	88	98	107	110	114	119	121
18	333	73	73	74	79	82	86	97	105	108	114	117	122
21	298	70	70	71	79	84	86	95	106	112	115	121	126
24	304	68	68	73	76	81	87	96	108	113	119	130	138
27	296	71	71	73	78	82	87	96	106	113	119	127	143
30	296	74	74	79	81	85	91	100	112	118	125	135	150
33	301	72	72	77	81	86	90	100	113	121	126	134	143
36	326	72	72	76	83	85	90	104	122	128	130	137	146
42	309	68	68	74	78	85	94	106	119	128	132	138	141
48	318	74	74	79	87	90	96	110	123	129	134	139	141
54	329	79	79	83	88	91	96	107	117	120	124	130	133
60	334	78	78	84	88	92	97	106	113	117	122	124	127
66	317	76	76	81	85	90	96	103	112	115	116	120	122
72	322	71	71	78	86	90	94	101	107	110	111	114	115
78	316	80	80	84	86	88	91	99	105	106	108	109	109
84	301	79	79	81	84	86	89	94	98	100	101	101	101

Table 10.5 Language DQs at the 3rd-97th percentiles across the main test ages from 1 to 84 months

Language Subscale

Distribution of DQs at the percentiles across different main test ages

Month age	Number of cases	<3	3–	5–	10	15	25	50	75	85	90	95 >=97
1	302	0	0	0	45	50	91	100	136	150	150	182	200
2	302	71	71	71	75	75	95	100	119	143	150	158	175
3	337	67	67	81	83	97	100	103	117	129	133	138	145
4	318	73	73	77	85	90	95	103	119	125	128	134	138
5	308	80	80	80	88	95	98	104	112	120	125	132	139
6	390	80	80	81	85	89	92	100	110	115	117	123	129
7	319	77	77	79	83	86	92	100	106	111	114	126	129
8	315	75	75	76	83	87	90	98	106	113	116	125	128
9	318	78	78	82	84	87	89	97	104	110	112	117	119
10	321	76	76	78	83	87	90	98	104	108	110	113	115
11	301	76	76	80	85	88	91	97	103	106	106	109	111
12	366	78	78	79	83	86	89	95	100	108	111	113	120
15	316	71	71	73	76	78	81	90	101	108	110	116	118
18	333	66	66	66	73	76	82	91	100	107	110	116	122
21	298	63	63	66	73	79	85	94	105	110	114	121	126
24	304	59	59	68	74	76	86	98	108	117	120	129	137
27	296	67	67	71	77	82	88	99	108	114	120	126	133
30	296	74	74	76	81	85	91	103	111	115	119	128	133
33	301	72	72	77	82	86	92	101	111	118	125	134	143
36	326	74	74	77	85	88	93	105	118	127	133	144	151
42	309	74	74	79	85	90	96	111	125	132	138	148	151
48	318	77	77	84	89	92	99	113	125	134	138	147	152
54	329	78	78	85	91	95	100	108	119	125	128	133	136
60	334	84	84	87	93	97	101	108	117	121	125	129	132
66	317	81	81	85	91	93	97	104	111	115	117	121	123
72	322	80	80	83	88	91	94	102	108	111	112	114	115
78	316	80	80	82	87	89	92	98	103	105	106	109	109
84	301	79	79	81	84	86	89	94	98	100	100	101	101

Table 10.6 Social behavior DQs at the 3rd-97th percentiles across the main test ages from 1 to 84 months

Social Behavior Subscale

Distribution of DQs at the percentiles across different main test ages

Month age	Number of cases	< 3	3–	5–	10	15	25	50	75	85	90	95 >=97
1	302	45	45	50	66	80	91	100	150	150	159	182	200
2	303	58	58	71	75	80	95	100	119	143	150	158	167
3	337	81	81	83	90	97	100	103	117	129	133	138	145
4	318	78	78	82	85	88	93	100	110	113	118	125	128
5	308	83	83	85	88	90	96	104	112	118	120	126	130
6	390	80	80	83	89	90	95	102	108	113	115	121	126
7	319	81	81	85	88	90	93	100	109	114	118	125	127
8	315	83	83	85	88	90	95	100	106	110	113	115	116
9	318	77	77	83	88	89	92	100	104	108	110	112	117
10	321	81	81	84	88	89	93	98	103	106	108	111	112
11	301	80	80	83	86	89	92	96	102	105	106	109	110
12	366	78	78	82	84	86	89	94	100	103	108	117	122
15	316	72	72	75	77	78	81	90	99	103	106	111	116
18	333	66	66	69	73	76	82	91	99	105	108	113	117
21	298	66	66	71	78	80	85	94	105	110	113	117	120
24	304	63	63	70	81	86	89	98	106	111	112	119	123
27	296	77	77	78	83	85	89	97	105	109	111	116	119
30	296	76	76	81	86	89	92	98	107	111	116	125	133
33	301	76	76	78	85	87	90	97	106	114	119	129	136
36	326	76	76	82	86	89	95	107	119	126	129	136	142
42	309	74	74	79	88	92	99	109	119	126	130	141	149
48	318	86	86	88	93	96	99	112	125	130	134	139	143
54	329	85	85	88	91	94	99	109	118	122	128	135	137
60	334	83	83	86	91	94	100	107	115	118	121	125	131
66	317	79	79	84	89	91	98	106	112	115	116	119	120
72	322	75	75	81	87	91	96	102	108	111	112	113	114
78	316	80	80	81	85	89	93	99	103	105	106	108	108
84	301	82	82	83	85	87	90	94	98	99	100	101	101

10.2 Appendix B: Inventory of Testing Tools Used in the Erxin Scales

10.2.1 Inventory and Photographs of Testing Tools Used in the Erxin Scales

1. Inventory of testing tools

No	Name	Specification	No	Name	Specification
1	Red ball	1	29	Small white bottle (with peanuts)	1 bottle, several peanuts
2	Black-and-white target	1	30	Big circle	1
3	Bell stick	1	31	Small circle	1
4	Brass bell	1	32	Plastic board for assembling a circle	4 (quadrants)
5	Tennis ball with string	1	33	Plastic board for assembling a square	2 (45°–45°–90° triangles)
6	Tennis ball without string	1	34	Plastic board for assembling a rectangle	2 (30°–60°–90° triangles)
7	Water cup with a handle	1	35	Template set for categorization test	1 round button
8	Doll	1			1 square button
9	Hat	1			1 small circle
10	Towel	1			1 small square
11	Crayon	1			1 small triangle
12	Comic strip	1	36	Large picture set-1	1 set (24 pictures in total)
13	Unframed mirror	1	37	Large picture set-2	1 set of spot-the-difference pictures
14	Hide-and-seek paper	1	38	Four-color picture	1
15	Pink paper	1 dozen	39	Picture for assembling an oval	1
16	Paper for circle cutting	1 sheet	40	Six plastic boards	1 set (6 pieces)
17	Transparent vial	1 vial (with several pieces of VitC)	41	Picture of a child throwing fruit peel	1

(continued)

(continued)

No	Name	Specification	No	Name	Specification
18	Zipper	1	42	Picture for identifying the missing parts	1
19	Scissors	1 pair	43	Screw components	1 screw, 1 washer, 1 nut
20	Water cup without handles	2	44	Picture of an assembled screw	1
21	Red square block	10	45	Picture showing male and female toilet signs	1
22	String used for the Cat's Cradle game	2	46	Picture for sign recognition	2
23	Chopsticks (with string)	1 pair of chopsticks, 1 red string	47	Picture of chickens swimming in water	1
24	Crystal thread (with buttons)	1 crystal thread, 5 small buttons	48	Picture of reading in the rain	1
25	Plastic template	1	49	Picture for describing the contents	1
26	Building blocks in the template set	1 triangle, 1 square, 1 circle	50	Picture of an owl catching a mouse	1
27	Round box	1	51	Picture for graphic analogy	4
28	Coin	1	52	Picture for digital analogy	4

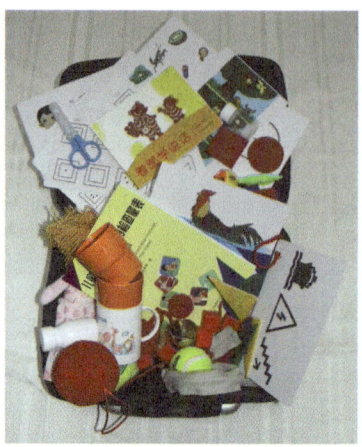

2. Photographs of testing tools

10.2.2 *Staircase for Testing*

The staircase for testing consists of two symmetrical sets of wooden stairs. Each set of stairs is 60 cm long, 25 cm wide, and 16 cm high, with a total of three steps. The balusters are 58 cm high (42 cm high from the step surface to the rake rail, increasing by 16 cm for each additional step). The circumference of the handrail (including the level rail and rake rail) is 8–10 cm. The staircase railing is single-sided. If the railing is made of wood, it can be appropriately thickened to ensure stability. Please refer to the schematic diagram for the dimensions of each component. Place the two set of stairs in alignment, creating a top platform on the step surface that is 60 cm long and 50 cm wide. This allows the child to climb up the stairs from one side, pass through the platform, and then descend the stairs from the other side, completing the stair-climbing action. (Note: When aligning the two sets of stairs, the railing should be on the same side, as shown in the according staircase diagram below.)

If the testing space is not large enough, the two sets of stairs can be used separately. The child being tested can ascend the stairs from one side to reach the third step platform, then turn around and descend the stairs to complete the entire set of actions.

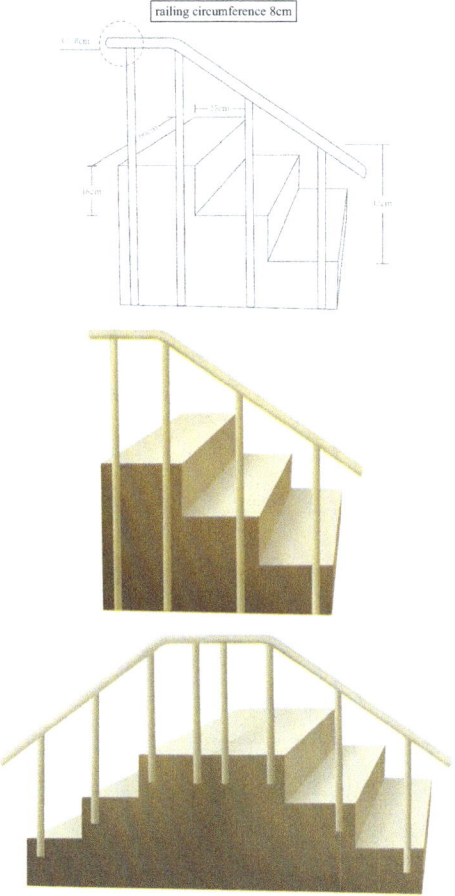

Schematic diagrams of staircase dimensions

10.2.3 Bed for Testing

The testing bed is a stainless-steel pipe bed with guardrails on all four sides. The bed is 140 cm long, 80 cm wide, and 130 cm high. The height of the bed surface from the ground is 70 cm (some test items in the scale require the assessor to be at eye level with the infant, and this height meets the operational requirements). The distance from the bed surface to the upper end of the guardrail is 60 cm. The two short sides of the bed guardrails are fixed, while the two long sides can move up and down along the track and be fixed at the top. The width between the guardrail posts is 12 cm, and the circumference of the guardrail steel pipe is 6–8 cm. Please refer to the schematic diagram for the dimensions of the various parts of the steel pipe bed. The mattress should match the length and width of the bed. If a wooden testing bed is used, stability and safety are important considerations. The dimensions of the various parts can be based on the above specifications, but special attention should be given to ensuring that the spacing between the wooden posts does not exceed 12 cm.

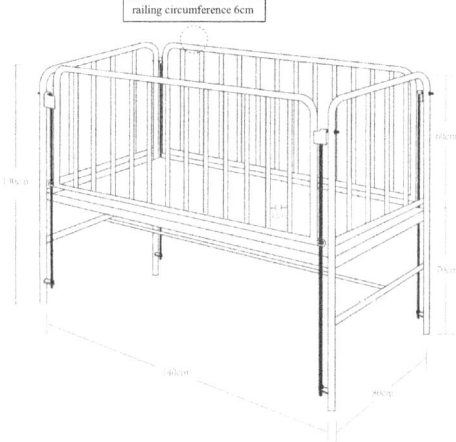

Schematic diagrams of the steel pipe bed

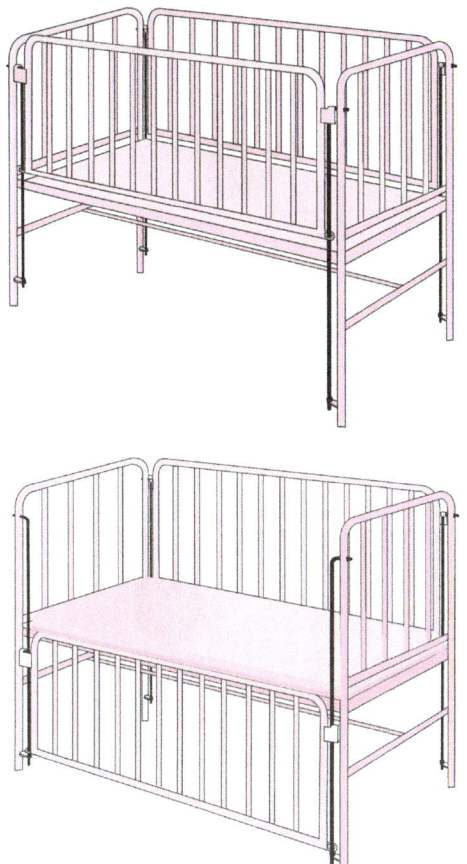

Schematic diagrams of the steel pipe bed

10.3 Appendix C: Pictures of Children Undergoing Assessment for Several Items

The following are selected pictures of an infant at 3 months and 25 days as well as children respectively at 1 year and 16 days, 3 years, 5 years, and 6 years and 4 months undergoing assessment for some items.

Pictures of an infant at 3 months and 25 days undergoing assessment

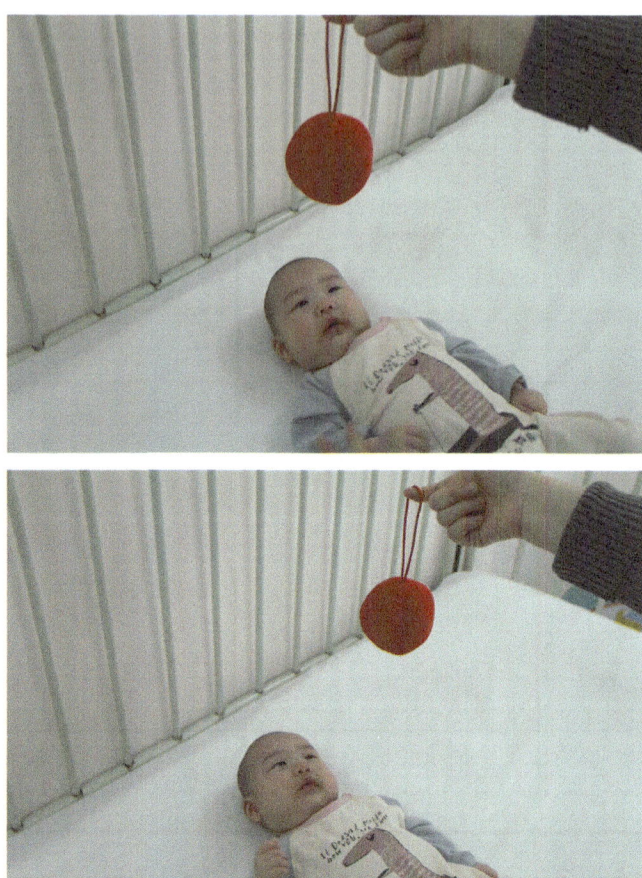

Item #28: Eyes and head turn 180° following the red ball

10 APPENDICES A, B, AND C 309

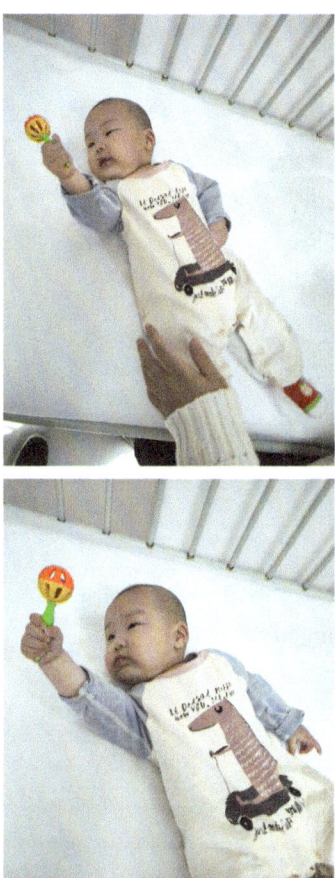

Item #35: Watch and shake the bell stick

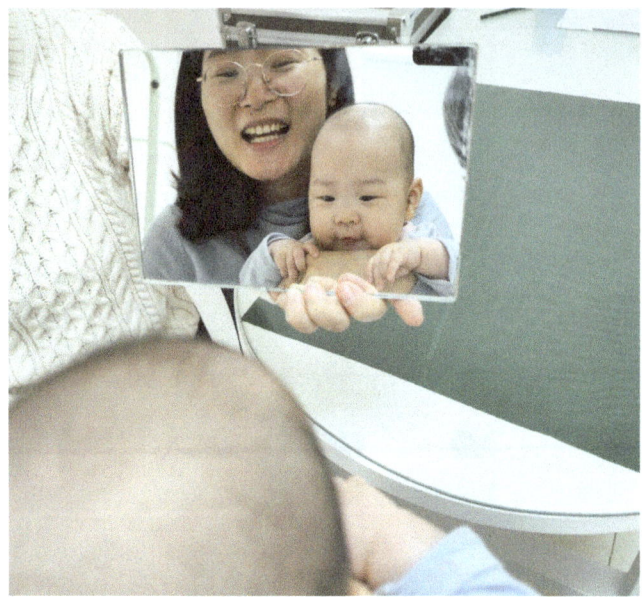

Item #41: Watch the figure in the mirror

Pictures of a child at 1 year and 16 days undergoing assessment

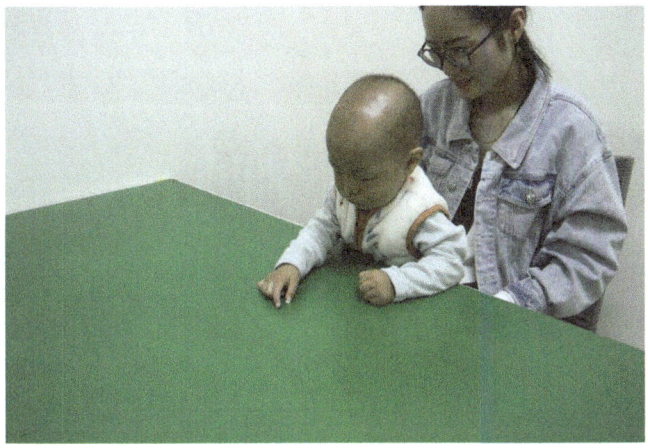

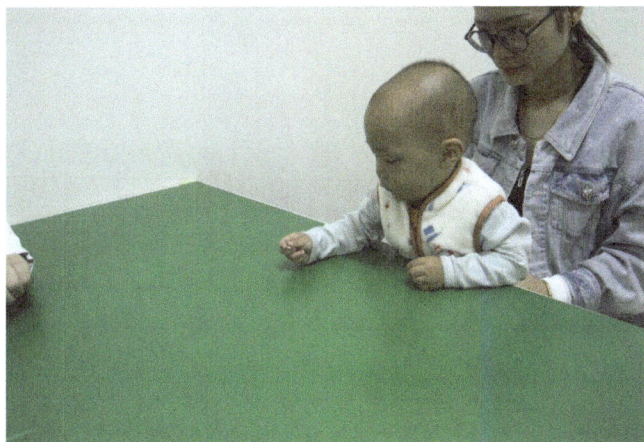

Item #87: Pinch a pellet with thumb and index finger

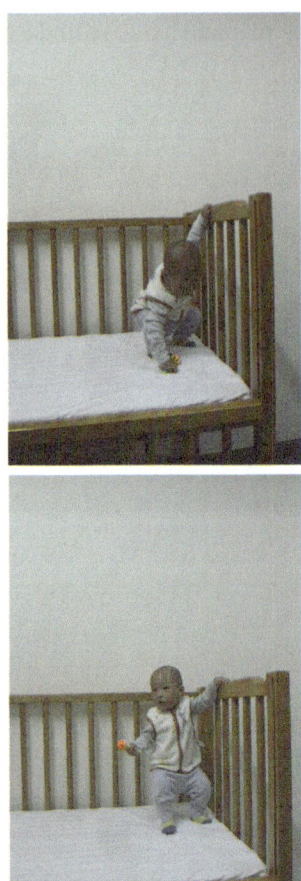

Item #105: Hold onto the railing to squat down and pick something up

10 APPENDICES A, B, AND C 313

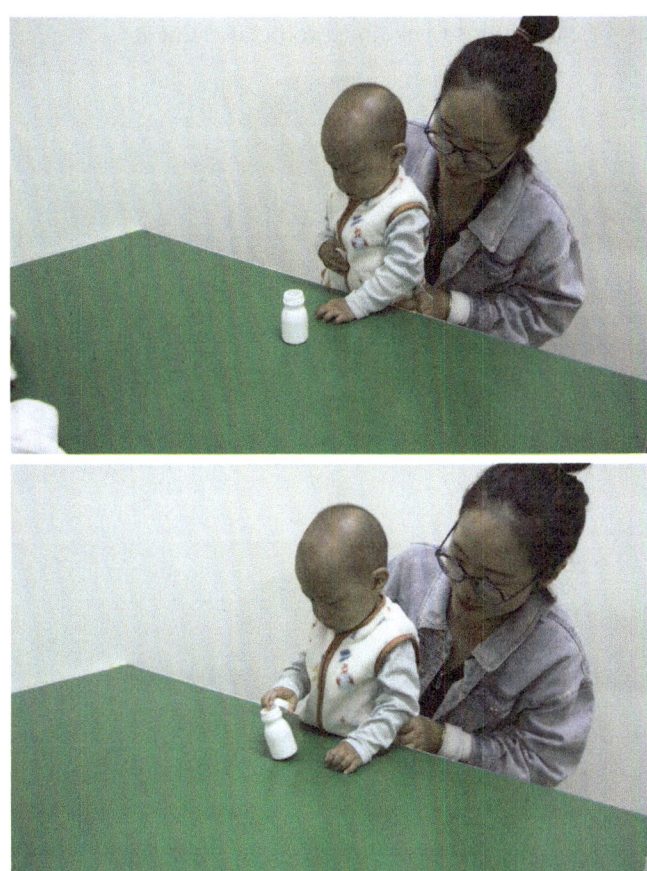

Item #118: Cap the bottle

Pictures of a child at 3 years undergoing assessment

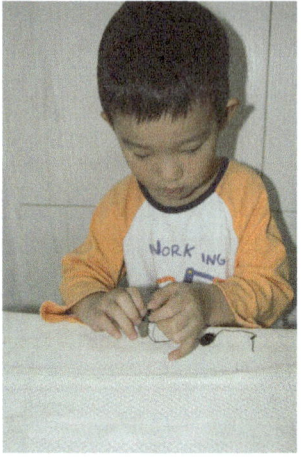

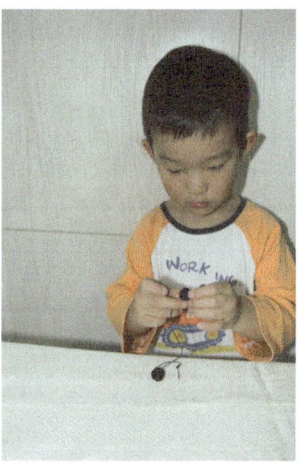

Item #176: Thread through 3–5 buttons

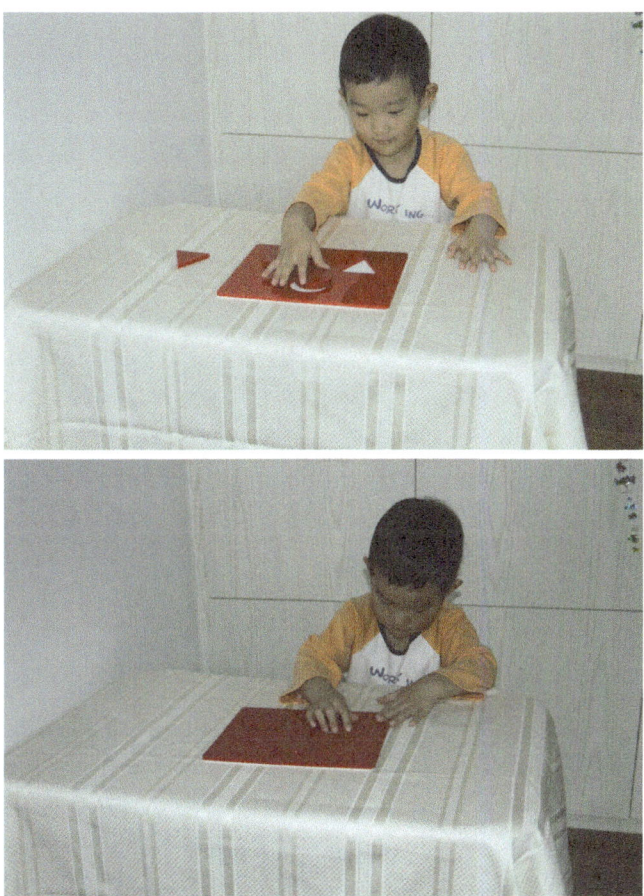

Item #179: Correctly put the building blocks of different shapes into the inverted template

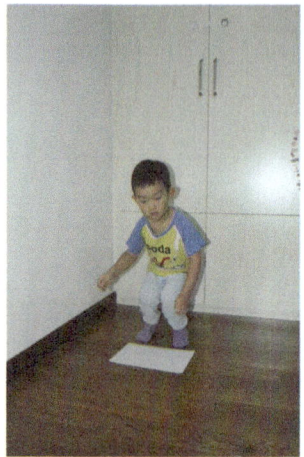

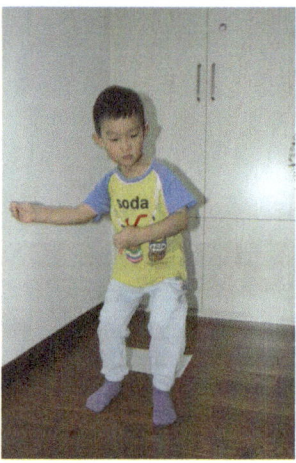

Item #186: Perform standing long jump

10 APPENDICES A, B, AND C 317

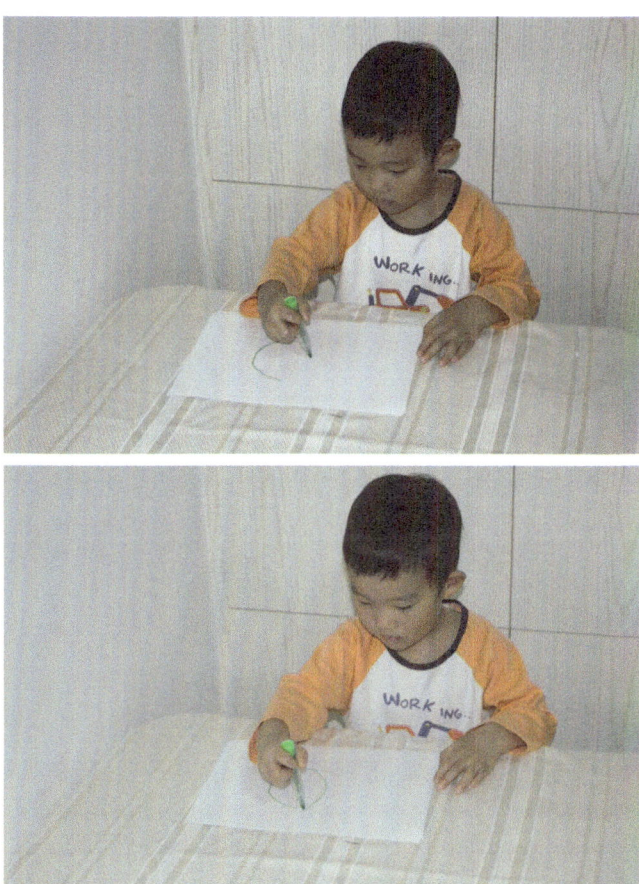

Item #187: Imitate drawing a circle

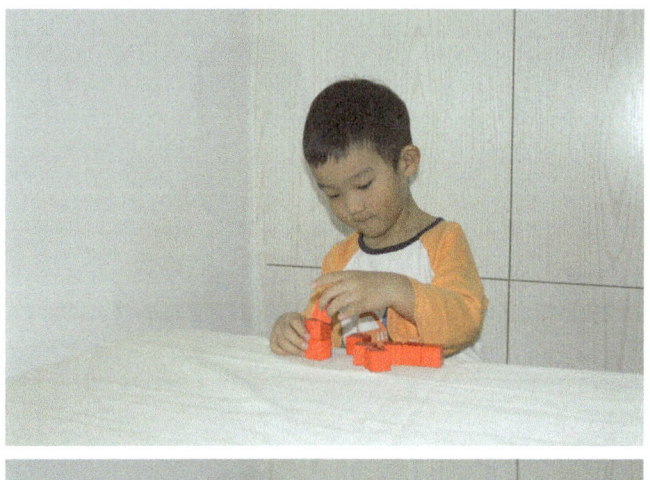

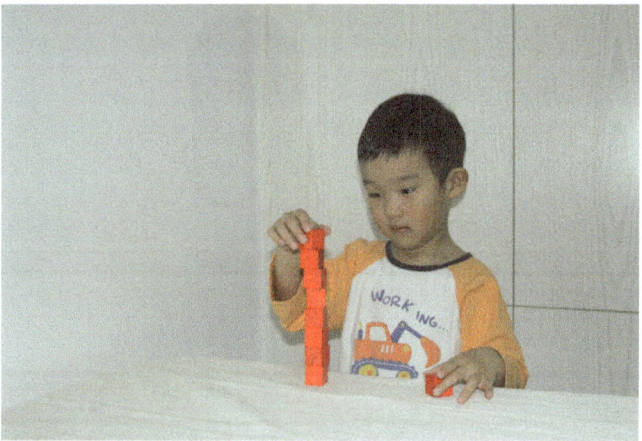

Item #189: Stack 10 building blocks

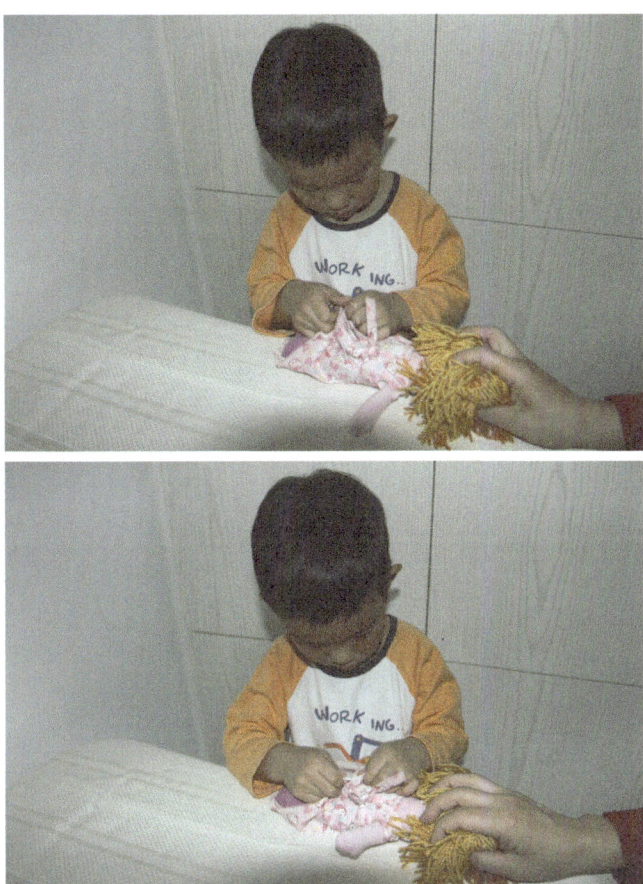

Item #194: Can unbutton

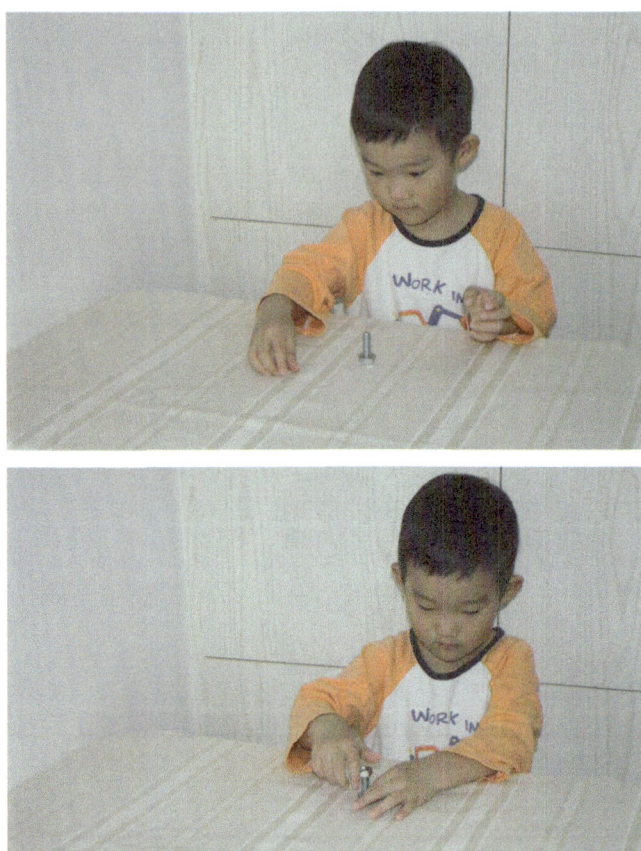

Item #199: Tighten the screw

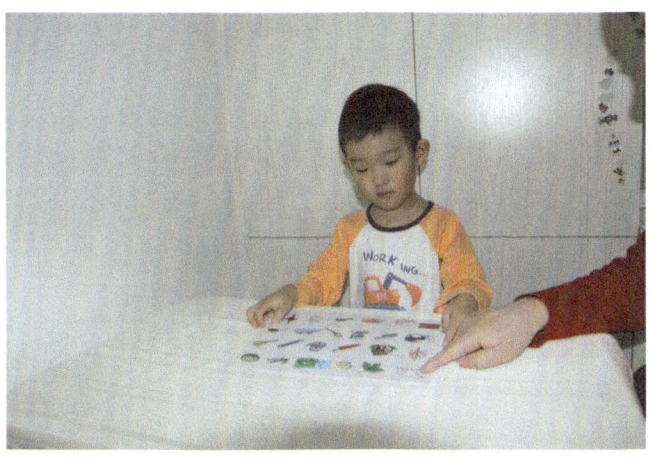

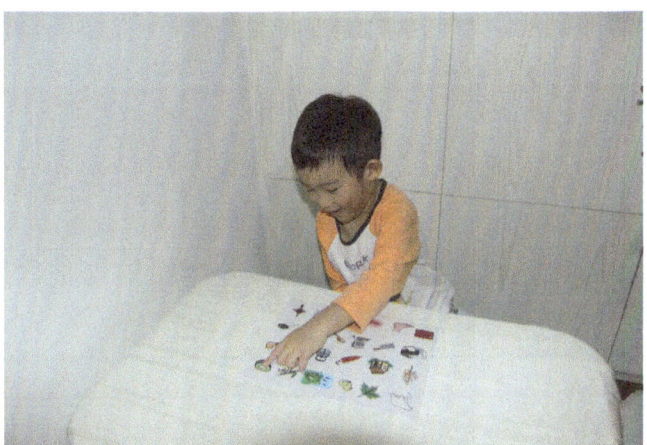

Item #202: Tell the names of 14 pictures

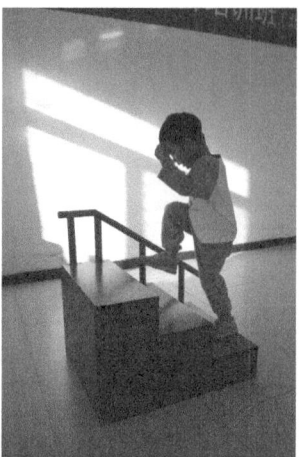

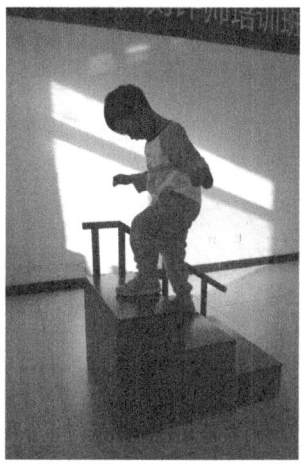

Item #208: Go upstairs with alternating feet

10 APPENDICES A, B, AND C   323

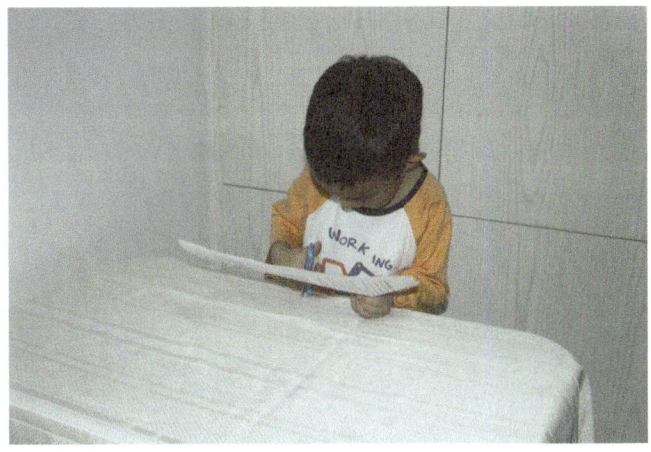

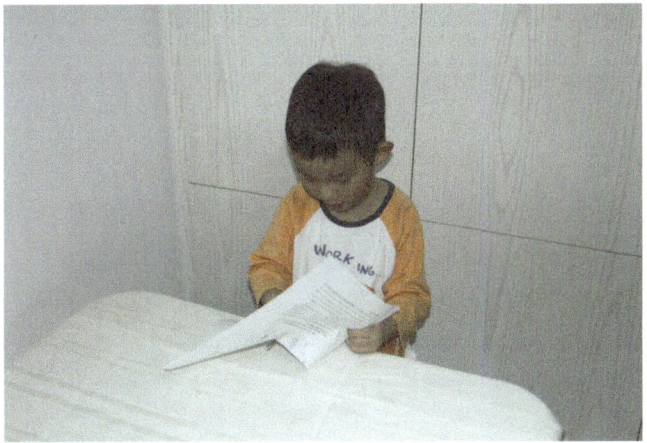

Item #211: Can use scissors

Pictures of a child at 5 years undergoing assessment

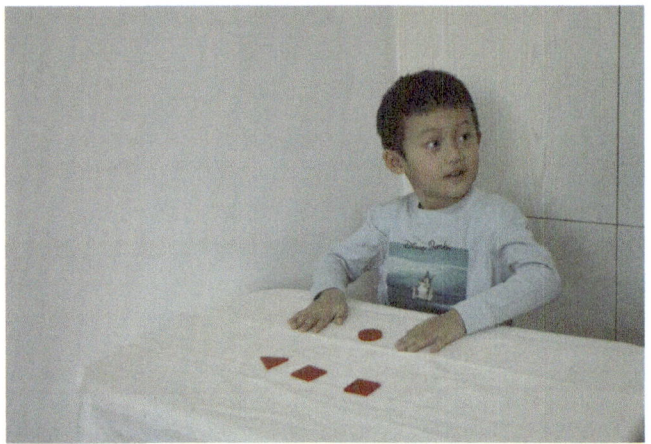

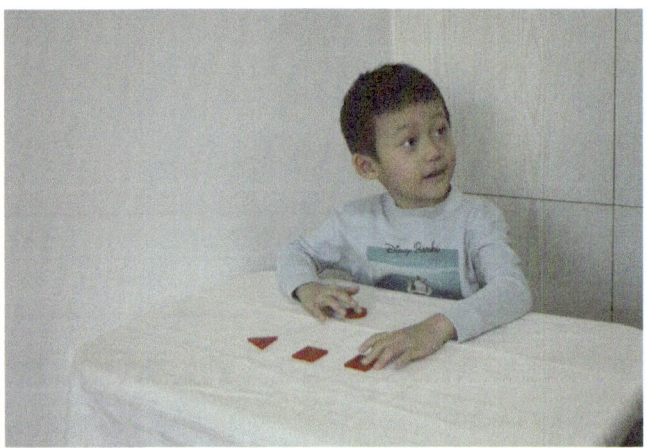

Item #234: Categorization

10 APPENDICES A, B, AND C 325

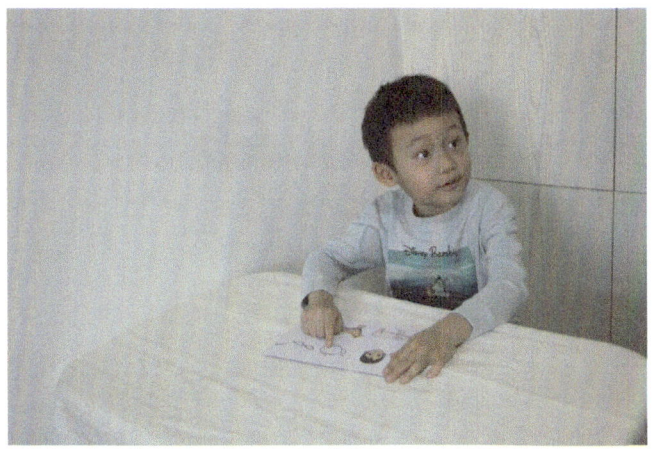

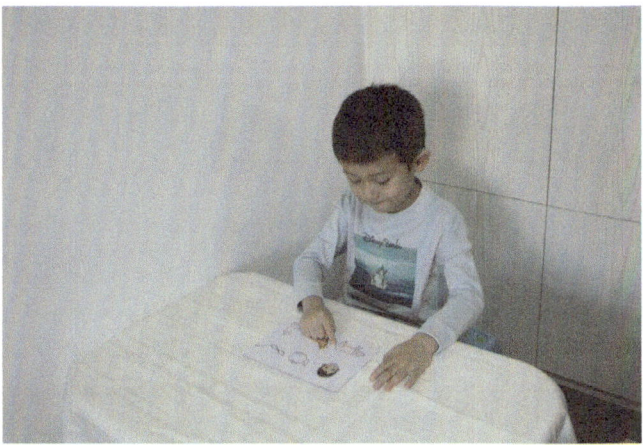

Item #235: Identify the missing parts in pictures (4/6)

Pictures of a child at 6 years and 4 months undergoing assessment

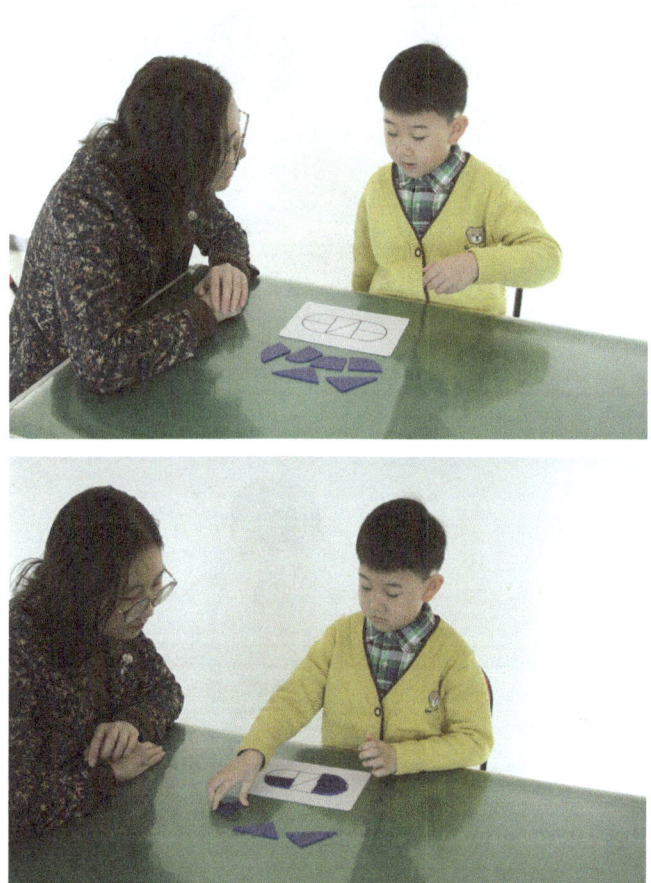

Item #243: Assemble an oval according to the picture

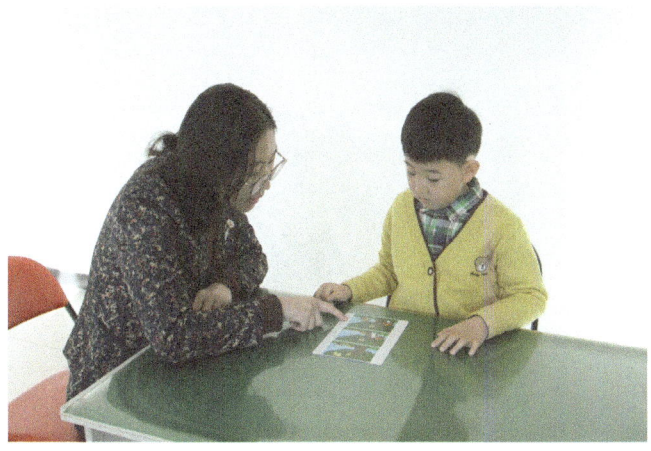

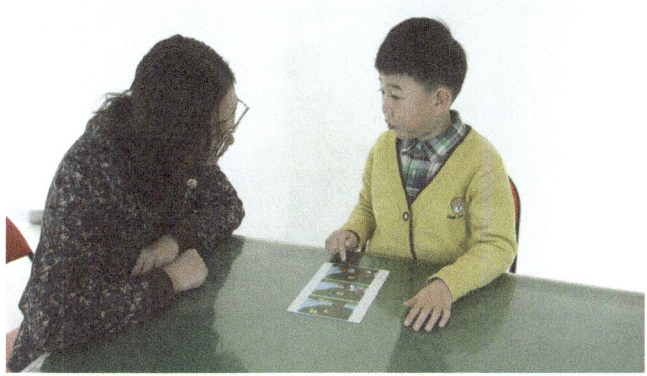

Item #268: Describe the picture contents

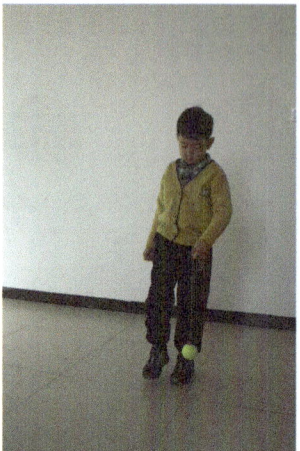

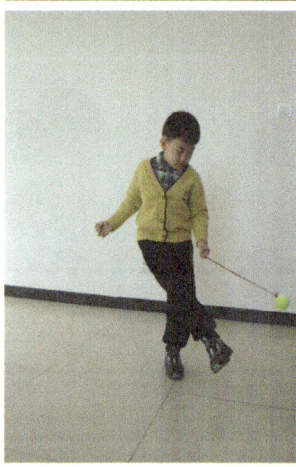

Item #273: Kick a ball with string

10 APPENDICES A, B, AND C   329

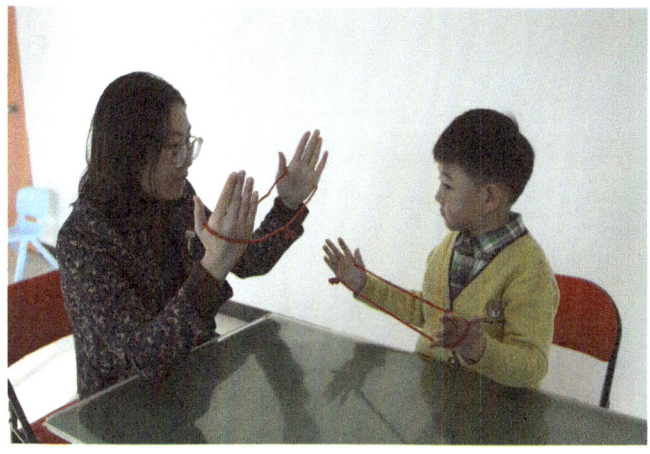

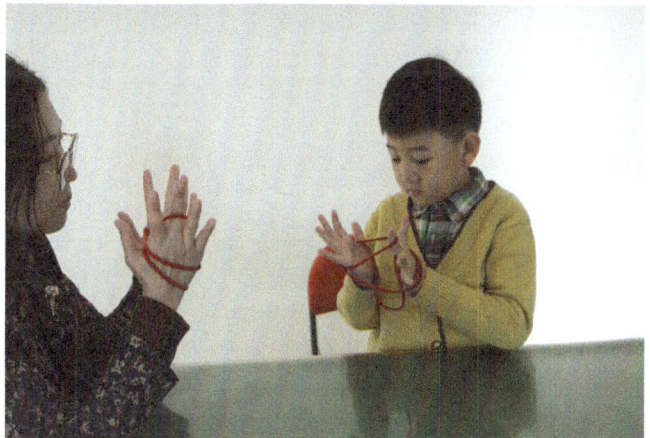

Item #286: Learn to play the Cat's Cradle game

Correction to: Erxin Scales: Child Developmental Scale of China

Correction to:
C. Jin et al., *Erxin Scales: Child Developmental Scale of China*,
https://doi.org/10.1007/978-981-99-9997-2

The original version of this book has been revised since some figures and tables have been replaced in Chapters 7 and 9. The book and the chapters have been updated with the changes.

The updated versions of these chapters can be found at
https://doi.org/10.1007/978-981-99-9997-2_7
https://doi.org/10.1007/978-981-99-9997-2_9

© The Author(s), under exclusive license to Springer Nature
Singapore Pte Ltd. 2025
C. Jin et al., *Erxin Scales: Child Developmental Scale of China*,
https://doi.org/10.1007/978-981-99-9997-2_11

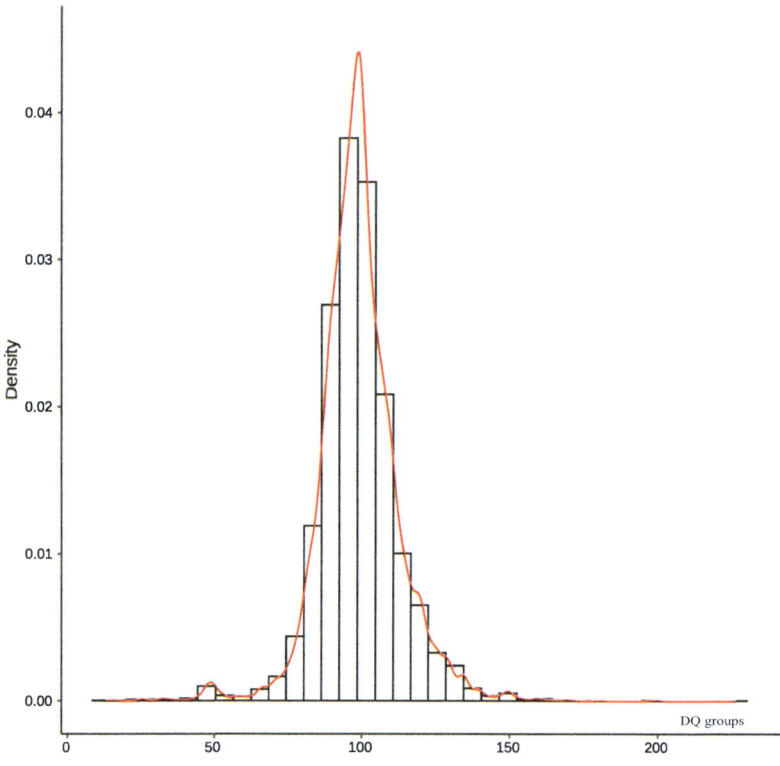

Fig. 11.1 Histogram and probability density curve of overall DQs grouped with an interval of 6 for the sample of 8,914 children

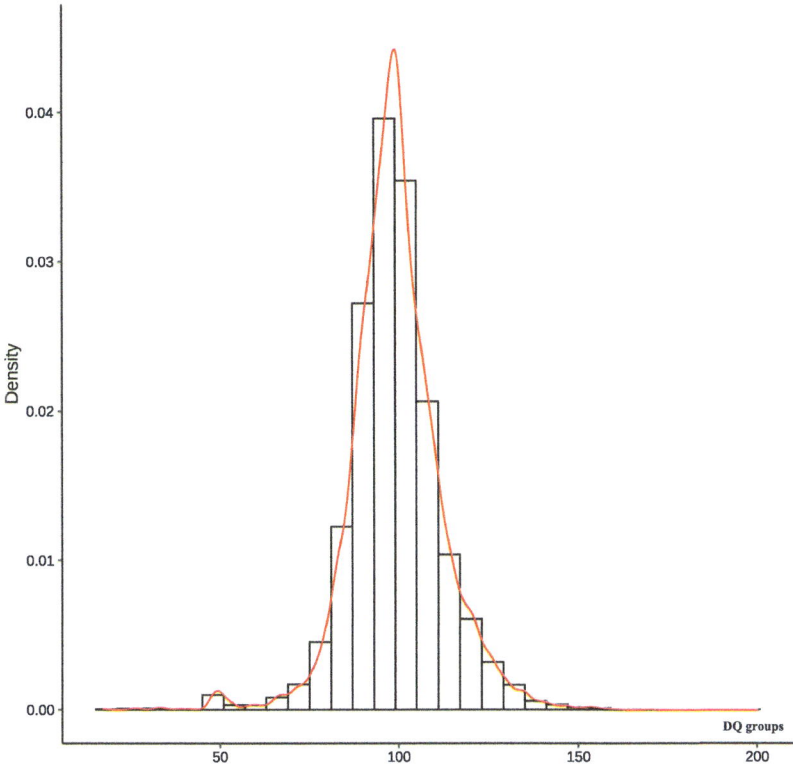

Fig. 11.2 Histogram and probability density curve of overall DQs grouped with an interval of 6 for the 8,612 children aged 2–84 months

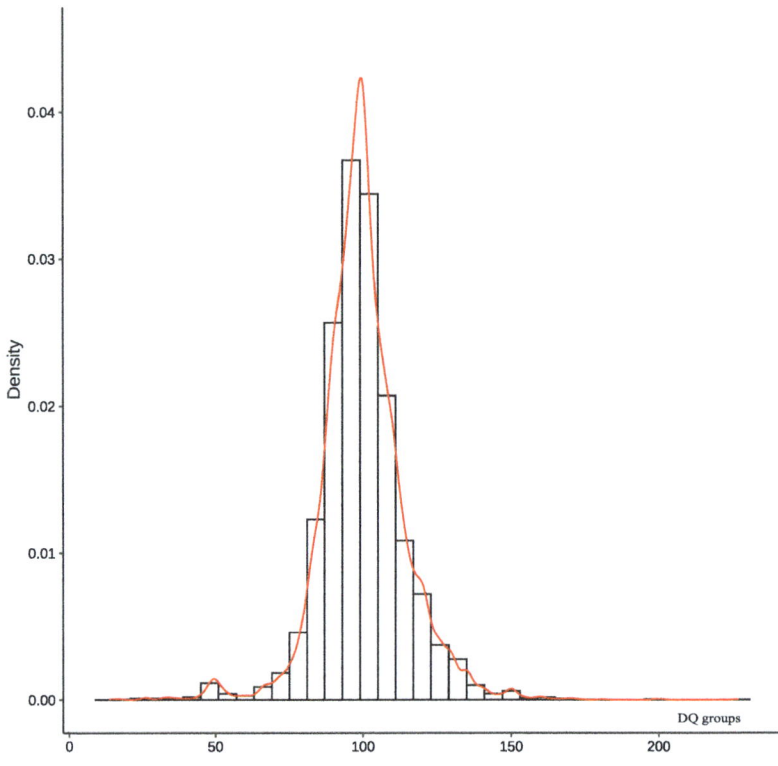

Fig. 11.3 Histogram and probability density curve of DQs grouped with an interval of 6 for the 7,658 children aged 1–60 months

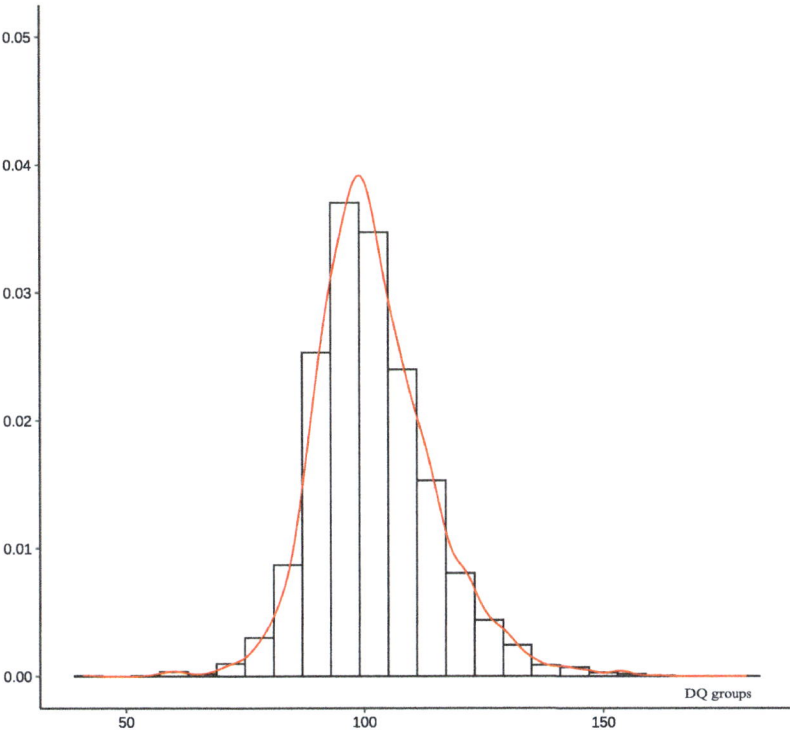

Fig. 11.4 Histogram and probability density curve of overall DQs grouped with an interval of 6 for the 2,872 children aged 4–6 years (36–84 months)

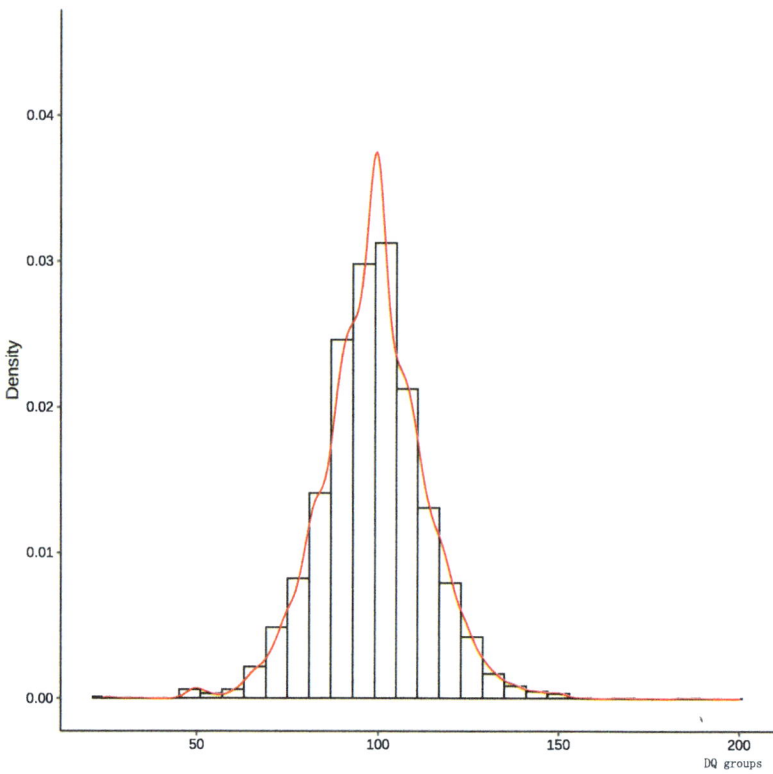

Fig. 11.5 Histogram and probability density curve of gross motor DQs grouped with an interval of 6 for the 8,612 children aged 2–84 months

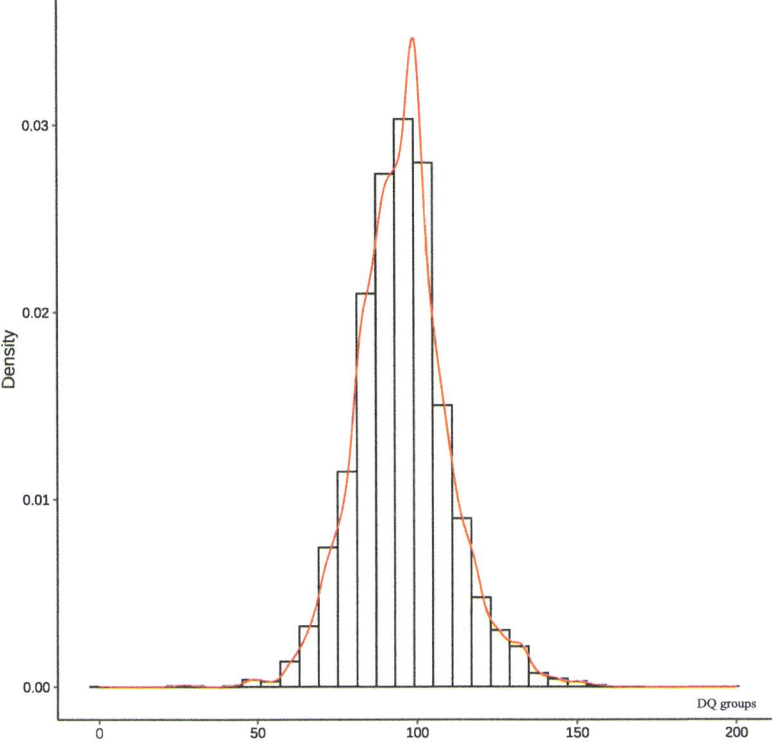

Fig. 11.6 Histogram and probability density curve of fine motor DQs grouped with an interval of 6 for the 8,612 children aged 2–84 months

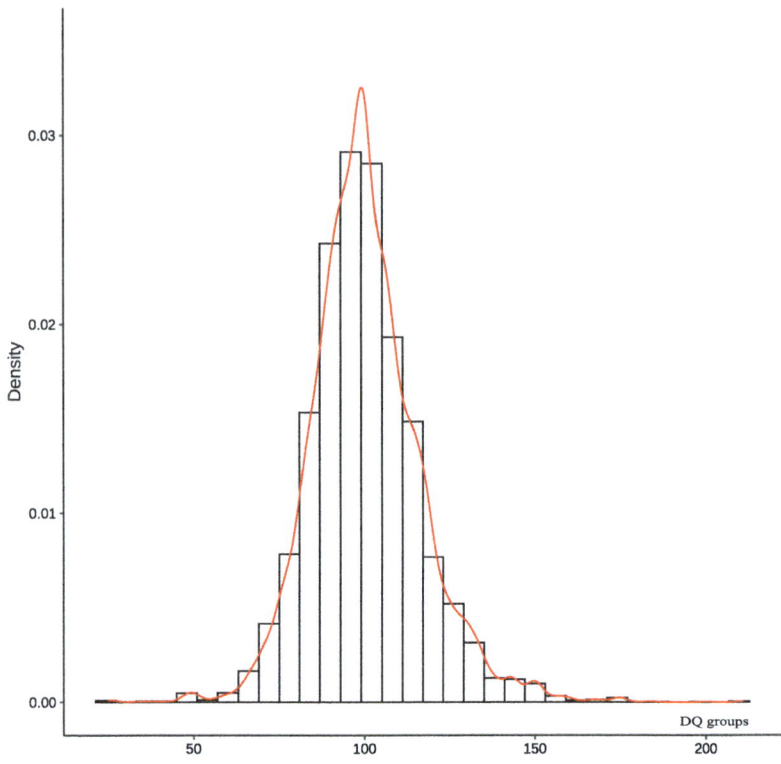

Fig. 11.7 Histogram and probability density curve of adaptability DQs grouped with an interval of 6 for the 8,612 children aged 2–84 months

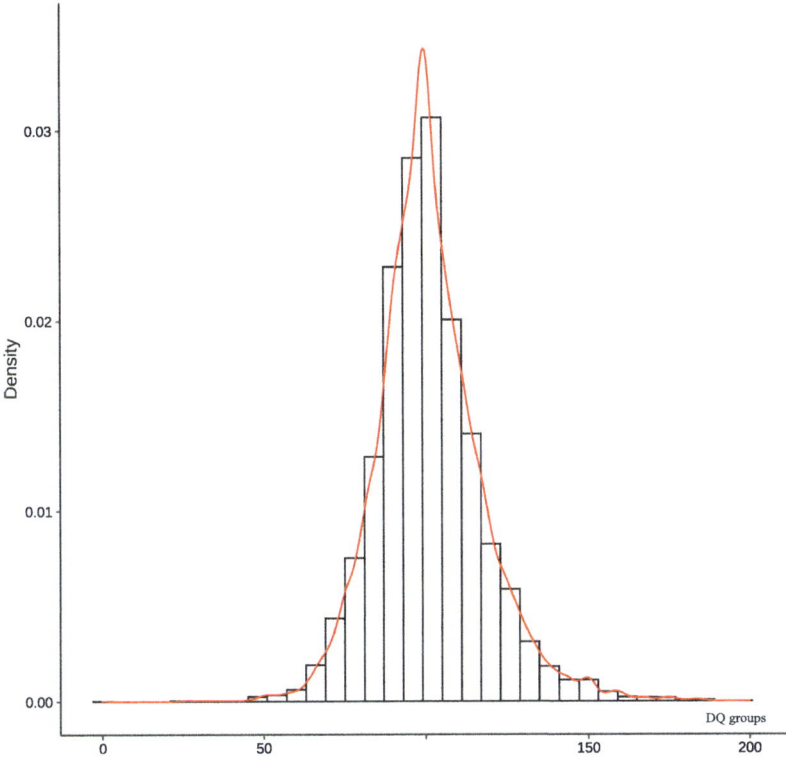

Fig. 11.8 Histogram and probability density curve of language DQs grouped with an interval of 6 for the 8,612 children aged 2–84 months

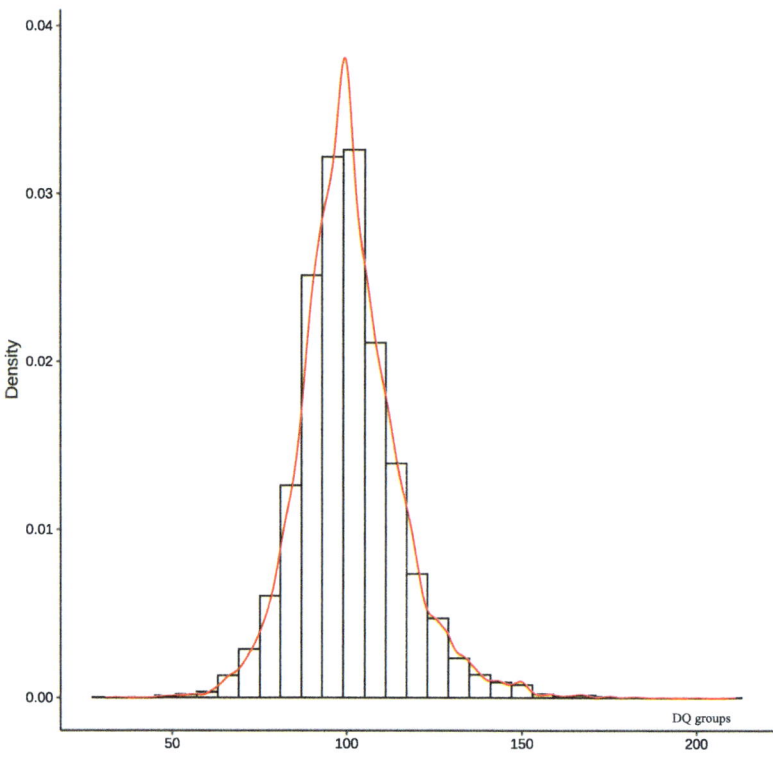

Fig. 11.9 Histogram and probability density curve of social behavior DQs grouped with an interval of 6 for the 8,612 children aged 2–84 months

Index

A

Adaptive Behavior Assessment System-Second Edition (ABAS-II), 31, 36, 52

Adaptive behavior scales, 29

Age correction, 175–178

Application, vi, vii, 2, 25, 26, 29, 34, 35, 48, 49, 52, 53, 61, 63, 68, 69, 128

Assessment, v, vi, ix, x, 2, 3, 8, 29, 30, 32, 35, 37, 46–49, 54, 61, 64, 72, 90, 91, 102, 117, 119–121, 126, 127, 129, 133, 139, 141, 145, 146, 172, 175, 177, 179, 181, 182, 184

Assessor(s), 3, 32, 35–37, 69, 72, 73, 75, 86, 175, 177, 179, 181–183, 306

Autism spectrum disorder (ASD), vi, 3, 4, 47–49, 64, 70, 72, 117, 131–136, 138, 142, 145, 146, 175, 183

B

Bayley Scales of Infant and toddler Development-Third Edition (BSID-III), 31, 35, 36, 51, 124

Bayley Scales of Infant Development (BSID), v, 7–9, 30, 31, 35, 37, 45, 51, 52, 54, 61, 166, 172

Behavior, 15, 19, 20, 22, 26, 131

Behavioral patterns, 17, 91, 132, 134

Brain development, 9, 12, 29, 38, 42, 172

Brain plasticity, 12

C

Case-control study, 93, 135, 136

Cognition
  memory, 7, 11, 13–17, 30, 70, 153
  perception, 7, 12, 13, 15–17, 63, 70, 128, 145, 153
  thinking, 13–17, 19, 22–26, 68, 70, 127

Cognitive assessment scales, 29

Cognitive development, 12, 13, 18–20, 26, 49, 68, 124, 127

© The Editor(s) (if applicable) and The Author(s), under exclusive license to Springer Nature Singapore Pte Ltd. 2024
C. Jin et al., *Erxin Scales: Child Developmental Scale of China*,
https://doi.org/10.1007/978-981-99-9997-2

Cognitive development theory, 3, 9, 16, 20, 26, 27, 45, 53, 120
  accommodation, 16, 20, 24
  assimilation, 16, 20
  equilibration, 17, 19, 26
  schemas, 13, 15–17, 20–22, 24
  symbols, 13, 15–17, 19, 23, 24, 183
Communication, vi, vii, 1, 3, 28, 30, 43, 45, 48, 71, 145, 177, 182
Comparative Fit Index (CFI), 104, 110
Conditioned reflex, 10, 20
Confirmatory factor analysis, 4, 28, 71, 104, 110, 121, 125
Construct validity, 27, 46, 103, 113, 121, 123, 135, 141
Content validity, 46, 119, 120, 123
Criteria, 28, 46, 50, 66, 71, 86, 90, 92, 131, 132, 150, 166
Criterion scales, 102, 126
Cross-sectional validation, 2, 27, 62, 119

D

Database on neuropsychological development of infants and toddlers, 2
Delayed development, 166, 167
Denver Developmental Screening Test (DDST), 33, 34, 36–38, 48, 51, 54
Developmental degree (mental age), 5
Developmental delays, 8, 29, 30, 32, 33, 35, 38, 43, 45, 47, 48, 51, 53, 64, 68, 117, 132, 138, 146, 151, 173, 181
Developmental evaluation, 141
Developmental quotient (DQ), 5, 32, 47–49, 53, 96, 102, 126, 140, 146, 149–151, 154–156, 161, 162, 172, 173, 175, 176, 183
  at main test ages, 5, 175
Developmental scale
Erxin Scale
  appropriate age, 165
  extensibility, 53, 54
  industry standard, 4, 5
  scale application, 27, 46
  scale management, 49
  universality, 53, 54
  instruction manual for the Erxin Scale, x, 69, 180, 184, 185
  instructions, 5, 63, 72, 92, 179, 184
  operational methods, 28, 36, 71, 92
  predictive validity, 38
  scoring criteria, 36, 46, 180, 185
  subscales
    adaptability, 4, 47, 50, 62, 68, 70, 72, 81, 96, 97, 102–104, 122–124, 146, 156, 164, 175, 181, 185
    communication warning behavior, vi, 4, 44, 47, 64, 67, 70–72, 78, 89, 90, 93, 120, 133, 135, 136, 138–142, 145, 146, 165, 175, 181, 183–185
    fine motor, 4, 11, 30–33, 37, 39, 47, 50, 62, 68, 70, 72–74, 96, 97, 104, 122, 124, 128, 146, 150, 155, 156, 160–164, 175, 177, 181, 185
    gross motor, 4, 23, 30–33, 37–39, 47, 48, 50, 62, 68, 70, 72, 96, 97, 103, 122–124, 156, 164, 175, 177, 181, 183, 185
    language, 4, 11, 32, 33, 37, 39, 44, 47, 50, 62, 68–70, 72, 96, 97, 103, 104,

122–124, 146, 156, 164, 172, 175, 181, 185
 social behavior, 4, 32, 47, 62, 68, 70, 72, 96, 97, 104, 122, 124, 133, 146, 156, 164, 175, 181, 185
Diagnostic scales, 2, 49, 62, 120, 173
Difficulty coefficient, 4, 95, 96, 119, 120
Discrimination index, 4, 110, 135

E
Early screen exposure, 43, 44
Environment, v, ix, x, 2, 8, 12, 21, 29, 31, 38, 40, 42, 44, 45, 51, 63, 78, 91, 152, 179
Evaluation, vii, x, 15, 47, 48, 50, 51, 63, 117, 126, 136, 146, 149, 151, 166, 173
Examiner(s), 179, 180

F
Factor analysis, 4, 103, 110, 121, 123–125, 134, 135, 141, 142
Features, 13–15, 24, 134, 173

G
Gesell Developmental Observation-Revised (GDO-R), 32, 52
Gesell Development Schedules (GDS), v, 3, 8, 9, 31, 32, 35–38, 45, 46, 50, 54, 61, 102, 118, 126
Greenspan Social-Emotional Growth Chart: A Screening Questionnaire for Infants and Young Children, 31
Griffiths Mental Development Scales (GMDS), 8, 33, 37, 54

H
Homogeneity reliability (internal consistency), 97–99

I
Instruction manual, x, 69, 180, 184, 185
Intelligence quotient (IQ), 29, 40, 149, 172
 deviation, 166
Inter-rater reliability, 97, 122
Intervention, vi, 12, 32, 43, 47, 49, 53, 68, 117, 128, 132, 133, 177
Interviews, 27, 134, 146
Inventory, 302
Item weights, 27, 72

K
Key ages, 32, 36, 51
Kurtosis, 150, 152, 154, 155

L
Living environment, x, 35, 69, 121, 128
Longitudinal follow-up, 5, 39, 40, 120, 175, 177

M
Main test ages, 28, 48, 51, 64, 66, 67, 71, 72, 75–78, 80–82, 84, 87, 88, 90, 96–98, 102, 122, 136, 155, 162, 175, 181, 185, 296–301
Management, 66, 67, 179
Maturity, 17, 19, 22, 45, 50, 120, 150, 153
Mental Development Index (MDI), 31, 34
Mental representations, 15, 16, 23
Mind, 9, 14, 16

Model fit, 28, 104, 110, 113, 114, 125
Multicenter research team, x, 2, 27, 28, 53, 62, 67
Myelination, 9, 10

N
Nervous system, 9, 10, 12, 13, 17, 29, 32, 41, 77
Non-Normed Fit Index (NNFI), 104, 110
Norm(s), x, 3, 4, 38, 126, 167
classification, 173
evaluation of, 28, 173, 174

O
Original items, 63, 120
Original revised scale, 3, 4, 28, 67, 88–90, 96

P
Piaget's stages of cognitive development
concrete operational stage, 19
deferred imitation, 23
formal operational stage, 19
preoperational stage, 18, 20, 23, 25, 26
sensorimotor stage, 18, 20, 26
Preterm infants, 86, 175, 177
Probability density function, 149–150
Psychological measurement, 8, 27
Psychological tests, v, 27, 64, 180
Psychometric properties, 4, 27, 28, 98, 160
Psychometrics, 6, 27, 33, 53, 64, 135, 167, 180
Psychomotor Development Index (PDI), 31, 34

Q
Qualification certification, 179
Quality control, 3, 27, 28, 33, 53, 54, 66, 67, 86

R
Reliability, x, xiv, 2, 4, 27, 28, 34, 46, 53, 54, 64, 122, 126, 134, 146, 167
Representative sample, x, 3, 27, 33, 34, 46, 53, 63, 88, 119, 150, 152, 160, 173, 180
Research and development, 45
Responsive caregiving, 42
Revision, vi, xiv, 1, 3, 6, 9, 20, 26–28, 33, 47, 49, 54, 63, 64, 92, 93, 95, 119, 120, 133, 146, 163, 179, 180
Revision principles, 68
Risk index, 4, 44, 47, 136, 175, 176
Risk(s), vi, x, 44, 48, 64, 67, 70, 86, 128, 133, 136, 146, 175, 183
ROC curve
sensitivity, 136, 138–140
specificity, 136, 138, 140

S
Sampling, x, 3, 53, 67, 92, 93
Scale dimensions, 72
Scale validity, 127
Sensitive periods, 12
Sensory perception, 24, 50, 104, 134, 151
Skewness, 150, 152, 154, 155
Social-Emotional Scale, 31, 36, 52
Social environment, 17, 26, 42, 45, 47
Split-half reliability, 98, 100, 101, 122, 123

Standardization, x, 3, 4, 8, 34, 37, 46, 53, 61, 62, 66, 69, 88, 90, 92, 126, 128, 167, 180
Standardization of measurement tools, 3, 63, 90
Stanford-Binet Intelligence Scale: Fifth Edition (SB5), 51
Subscale DQ
- distribution, 150, 152
- frequency distribution, 156, 160, 162, 164, 166, 168
- histogram, 6–10, 159, 161, 163, 165, 167
- percentile, 175
- probability density curve, 6–10, 159, 161, 163, 165, 167
- quartile, 160, 168

T
Technical roadmap, 54, 66, 134
  for scale revision, 64, 65
Test-retest reliability, 99, 101, 102, 122, 135
Tracking, 1, 7, 8, 27, 45, 62, 133

V
Validity, x, xiv, 2, 4, 27, 28, 34, 53, 54, 61, 64, 123, 126, 134, 167

W
Wechsler Preschool and Primary Scale of Intelligence-Revised (WPPSI-R), 29, 102, 126

The manufacturer's authorised representative in the EU is Springer Nature Customer Service Centre GmbH, Europaplatz 3, 69115 Heidelberg, Germany. If you have any concerns regarding our products, please contact ProductSafety@springernature.com

Printed and bound by CPI Group (UK) Ltd, Croydon, CR0 4YY

25/03/2026

02078175-0007